Multiple Organ Failure

Multiple Organ Failure

Pathophysiology and Basic Concepts of Therapy

Edwin A. Deitch, M.D.
Department of Surgery
Louisiana State University
School of Medicine
Shreveport, Louisiana

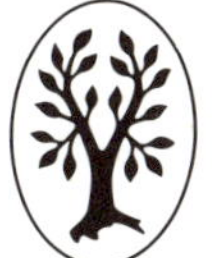
1990
Thieme Medical Publishers, Inc.   New York
Georg Thieme Verlag   Stuttgart • New York

Thieme Medical Publishers, Inc.
381 Park Avenue South
New York, New York 10016

MULTIPLE ORGAN FAILURE: PATHOPHYSIOLOGY
AND BASIC CONCEPTS OF THERAPY
Edwin A. Deitch

Library of Congress Cataloging-in-Publication Data

Multiple organ failure: pathophysiology and basic concepts of therapy
    / [edited by] Edwin A. Deitch
        p.   cm.
    Includes bibliographical references.
    ISBN 0-86577-282-7
    1. Multiple organ failure.   I. Deitch, Edwin A.
    [DNLM: 1. Multiple Organ Failure—physiopathology.   2. Multiple
Organ Failure—therapy.   QZ 140 M961]
    RB150.M84M853   1990
    617'.01—dc20
    DLC   90-10723
    for Library of Congress   CIP

Multiple organ failure: Pathophysiology
    and basic concepts of therapy/[edited by]
    Edwin A. Deitch

Important note: Medicine is an ever-changing science. Research and clinical experience are continually
broadening our knowledge, in particular our knowledge of proper treatment and drug therapy.
Insofar as this book mentions any dosage or applications, readers may rest assured that the authors,
editors, and publishers have made every effort to ensure that such references are strictly in accor-
dance with the state of knowledge at the time of production of the book. Nevertheless, every user
is requested to carefully examine the manufacturers' leaflets accompanying each drug to check on
his own responsibility whether the dosage schedules recommended therein or the contraindications
stated by the manufacturers differ from the statements made in the present book. Such examination
is particularly important with drugs that are either rarely used or have been newly released on the
market.

Some of the product names, patents, and registered designs referred to in this book are in fact
registered trademarks or proprietary names even though specific reference to this fact is not always
made in the text. Therefore, the appearance of a name without designation as proprietary is not to
be construed as a representation by the publisher that it is in the public domain.

Printed in the United States of America.

5   4   3   2   1

TMP ISBN 0-86577-282-7
GTV ISBN 3-13-747301-2

*This book is dedicated
to my wife, Jean, and
my two sons, David and Joseph.*

Contents

Contributors

George Babikian, M.D.
Resident in Orthopaedics
State University of New York at Buffalo
Erie County Medical Center
Buffalo, New York

Christopher C. Baker, M.D.
Professor
Head Trauma Section
Department of Surgery
University of North Carolina
Chapel Hill, North Carolina

Arthur E. Baue, M.D.
Vice-President for the Medical Center
St. Louis University
St. Louis, Missouri

Palmer Q. Bessey, M.D.
Associate Professor of Surgery
Director of Trauma, Burn, and Critical Care
Washington University School of Medicine
St. Louis, Missouri

Lawrence Bone, M.D.
Assistant Professor of Surgery and Orthopaedics
State University of New York at Buffalo
Erie County Medical Center
Buffalo, New York

John R. Border, M.D.
Professor of Surgery and Orthopaedics
State University of New York at Buffalo
Erie County Medical Center
Buffalo, New York

Jill Burk, Ph.D, R.N.
Research Nurse Coordinator, Burn Center
New York Hospital-Cornell Medical Center
New York, New York

Michael D. Caldwell, M.D., Ph.D.
Professor of Surgery
Brown University
Rhode Island Hospital
Providence, Rhode Island

Frank B. Cerra, M.D.
Professor
Department of Surgery
University Of Minnesota
Minneapolis, Minnesota

Irshad H. Chaudry, Ph.D.
Professor
Departments of Surgery and Physiology
Michigan State University
East Lansing, Michigan

Nicolas V. Christou, M.D., Ph.D., F.R.C.S.C., F.A.C.S
Associate Professor of Surgery
McGill University
Montreal, Canada

Steven A. Conrad, M.D., Ph.D.
Assistant Professor
Departments of Medicine, Physiology and
Biophysics, and Director, Medical/Cardiac ICU
LSU Medical Center-Shreveport
Shreveport, Louisiana

Edwin A. Deitch, M.D.
Professor
Department of Surgery
LSU Medical Center-Shreveport
Shreveport, Louisiana

David L. Dunn, M.D., Ph.D.
Assistant Professor
Division of Surgical Infectious Diseases
Department of Surgery
The University of Minnesota
Minneapolis, Minnesota

Jerome L. Finkelstein, M.D.
Clinical Assistant Professor
Department of Surgery
Cornell University Medical College
Associate Director, Burn Center
New York Hospital-Cornell Medical Center
New York, New York

Donald E. Fry, M.D.
Professor and Chairman
Department of Surgery
University of New Mexico School of Medicine
Albuquerque, New Mexico

Richard L. Gamelli, M.D.
Professor
Department of Surgery
University of Vermont College of Medicine
and Associate Chief of Surgery
Medical Center Hospital of Vermont
Burlington, Vermont

Cleon W. Goodwin, M.D.
Associate Professor
Department of Surgery
Cornell University Medical College and
Director, Burn Center
New York Hospital-Cornell Medical Center
New York, New York

James M. Harkema, M.D.
Professor
Department of Surgery
Michigan State University
East Lansing, Michigan

David N. Herndon, M.D.
Annie Laurie Howard Professor of Surgery
The University of Texas Medical Branch and
Chief of Staff
Shriners Burns Institute
Galveston, Texas

Paul Kispert, M.D.
Assistant Professor of Surgery
University of Pittsburgh
VA Medical Center
Pittsburgh, Pennsylvania

Marc Eric Lanser, M.D.
Assistant Professor of Surgery
Harvard Medical School and
Associate in Surgery
Beth Israel Hospital
Boston, Massachusetts

Stephen F. Lowry, M.D.
Associate Professor of Surgery
Cornell University Medical College
The New York Hospital-Cornell Medical Center
New York, New York

Michael R. Madden, M.D.
Professor
Department of Surgery
Cornell University Medical College
New York, New York

Hiram C. Polk Jr., M.D.
Professor
Department of Surgery
The Price Institute of Surgical Research
University of Louisville
School of Medicine
Louisville, Kentucky

Jorge Rodriguez, M.D.
Assistant Professor of Surgery
State University of New York at Buffalo
Erie County Medical Center
Buffalo, New York

Geoffrey M. Silver, M.D.
Surgical Resident
Department of Surgery
University of Vermont College of Medicine
Burlington, Vermont

Daniel L. Traber, Ph.D.
Professor of Anesthesiology, Physiology, and
Biophysics
The University of Texas Medical Branch and
Coordinator of Research
Shriners Burns Institute
Galveston, Texas

Craig Walvatne, M.D.
Fellow in Surgery
University of Minnesota
Department of Surgery
Minneapolis, Minnesota

Roger W. Yurt, M.D.
Associate Professor and Vice-Chairman
Department of Surgery
Cornell University Medical College and
Director, Trauma Center
The New York Hospital-Cornell Medical Center
New York, New York

Foreword

The appearance of a major monograph on the subject of multiple system organ failure, in this case authored by many of the major players in the field, is an important recognition of an area of research, concern, and interest that has dominated surgical care and investigation for more than two decades.[1,2] The illness is defined elegantly within the book to follow but clearly represents the functional failure of a variety of organs, which, to one degree or another, are essential to bodily function. Gastric mucosal failure is just as surely fatal as oliguric renal failure and just as dangerous as so-called adult respiratory distress syndrome. In some measure, organ failure is a disease of progress; patients who have developed this illness typically would have died in the late resuscitative period in decades past. It has been the surgeon's ability, with precise and effective resuscitation and a full range of support, including the vigorous use of safe systemic antibiotics, to bring some patients through their most acute illness only to be challenged after the first or second week of hospitalization by the emergence of organ failure. Organ failure is unequivocally related to our ability to accomplish the initial save and then provide, to a significant degree, temporary support for many of the organs involved.

On the contrary, multiple system organ failure has represented the Achilles' heel in the practice of surgery since the Vietnam War, and certainly pervades the units and services of all tertiary care hospitals in America, particularly institutions that truly care for badly hurt individuals. Indeed, one can argue that it is an unfortunate, depressing, and all too common final pathway for the surgical patient who does not die of a closed head injury, exsanguination, or neoplasm.

The near simultaneous discovery that infection is the most common underlying cause of organ dysfunction is now 15 years old.[3-5] Even today the majority of patients who develop organ failure have infection as its underlying cause, whether in the failing organ itself, such as pneumonia in the lung, or in a remote location such as oliguric renal failure associated with a subphrenic abscess. It is the effective and definitive treatment of the underlying cause that seems to matter most in recovery. Effective treatment of the infection is almost never by antibiotics alone—with the exception of pneumonia—but requires some significant mechanical intervention to achieve a successful outcome.[6]

Curiously, the idea that pelvic abscess might produce alveolar membrane dysfunction was slow to be realized. The lonely, pioneering work of Blaisdell, who likened this to the pulmonary injuries seen after washout of long ischemic, revascularized extremities, has been particularly impressive to me.[7,8] Again several groups simultaneously identified infection as triggering a series of events which aggregated a variety of organs, such as leukocytes, platelets, and other material, and may well have microembolized the lung.[9-11] The mechanics do not hold together quite so well for other organs, but clearly there is a redistribution of nutritive blood flow under these conditions which deserves continued investigation. The infection-induced aggregation of vital particles and embolic occlusion of small vessels is a most comfortable hypothesis. The mechanisms of organ failure of other sites and origin are obviously less well understood.

Supportive measures have been refined and patients are living longer, some are truly coming to the correction of their illness and being discharged from the hospital, when the underlying cause of their organ failure is recognized and corrected. It clearly has been a most exciting time in the history of medicine; the mainstream of modern surgery during the last 25 years flows through the story of multiple system organ failure as told by the authors of this well-organized monograph.

Hiram C. Polk, Jr.

References

1. Fry DE, Pearlstein L, Fulton RL, et al. Multiple system organ failure. Arch Surg 1980;115:136–140.
2. Eiseman B, Beart R, Norton L. Multiple organ failure. Surg Gynecol Obstet 1977;144:323–326.
3. Fulton RL, Jones CE. The cause of post-traumatic pulmonary insufficiency in man. Surg Gynecol Obstet 1975;40:179–186.
4. Horovitz JH, Carrico CJ, Shires GT. Pulmonary response to major injury. Arch Surg 1974;108:349–355.
5. Norton L, Moore G, Eiseman B. Liver failure in the postoperative patient: the role of sepsis and immunologic deficiency. Surgery 1975;78:6–13.
6. Polk HC Jr, Shields CL. Remote organ failure: a valid sign of occult intraabdominal infection. Surgery 1977;81:310–313.
7. Blaisdell FW, Lim RC, Stallone RJ. The mechanism of pulmonary damage following traumatic shock. Surg Gynecol Obstet 1970;130:15–22.
8. Blaisdell FW. Pathophysiology of the respiratory distress syndrome. Arch Surg 1974;108:44–49.
9. Hohn DC, Meyers AJ, Gherini ST, Beckmann A, Markison RE, Churg AM. Production of acute pulmonary injury by leukocytes and activated complement. Surgery 1980;88:48–58.
10. Thörne LJ, Kuenzig M, McDonald HM, Schwartz SI. Effect of denervation of a lung on pulmonary platelet trapping associated with traumatic shock. Surgery 1980;88:208–214.
11. Manwaring D, Curreri PW. Platelet mediation of fragment D-induced respiratory distress syndrome. Surg Forum 1980;31:242–243.

Preface

Multiple organ failure has reached epidemic proportions in most intensive care units and is fast replacing single organ failure as a cause of death in these patients. Multiple organ failure is not limited to any one group of patients or the provence of any one medical specialty. It occurs in patients of all ages, in patients with medical as well as surgical diseases, and in all parts of the world. Once the syndrome of multiple organ failure is fully manifest, even the best attempts at therapy are generally fruitless. Although specific therapeutic interventions are not yet clinically available to consistently halt the progression of organ dysfunction, there are some bright spots. The aim of this book is to examine and evaluate these new areas of knowledge as well as to explore objectively the limits of our current knowledge with the ultimate goal of improving the clinical outcome of our patients.

In structuring this book, an attempt was made to include not only what is known clinically, but also to explore potential pathophysiologic mechanisms responsible for the development and/or perpetuation of multiple organ failure. This approach mandates that the reader develop an understanding of systemic homeostatic mechanisms as well as the specifics of normal organ function. Since only by understanding these dynamic interrelationships in health, will it be possible to apply and develop effective therapeutic interventions in these critically ill patients. I am grateful to the outstanding clinician-scientists who have accepted this difficult task. To accomplish this goal, topics were divided into general chapters dealing with the history, epidemiology, and staging of organ failure, as well as specific chapters on individual organs and physiologic systems. Since current and future therapy is multimodal, the final chapter of this book provides an overview of the information presented in the previous chapters.

Edwin A. Deitch

Multiple Organ Failure

1

Historical Perspective

Arthur E. Baue

A chain is only as strong as its weakest link. When links are strengthened where the chain is broken previously, new weak spots appear simply because the chain holds to test them. The obvious weak link in the severely wounded in this war (WW II) is the kidney.

—Edward D. Churchill[1]

Describing a Syndrome

Throughout the short history of modern surgery—whether one begins with Ambrose Paré, John Hunter, or Theodor Bilroth—there have been limits to surgical capability. Whether these limits were imposed by pain requiring the development of anesthesia or hemorrhage and fluid loss requiring hemostasis and intravenous fluids or infection requiring antisepsis and then asepsis, there have always been challenges to develop technical resources and biologic understanding beyond existing capability. This striving by the surgical practitioner, academician, or investigator to extend the limits of surgery is part not only of our heritage but of our responsibility to our patients and the profession. Certainly, there are limits in the treatment of certain types of disease, with extirpation of cancer and bypass grafts for atherosclerotic occlusions serving as prime examples. There are limits or weak links also in our overall capability to care for patients after severe injury, major life-threatening operations, or catastrophic

1

illnesses requiring operations for treatment and in patients with significant chronic illness who face any of these problems.

Multiple organ failure is a syndrome of surgical progress. As the care of injured patients has evolved and improved, various organ systems have, in turn, been the limiting factor affecting recovery after a severe injury or major operation. Although patients after operation or injury may die from a number of specific or general injuries and complications, there has usually been—in any one time in surgical history—a particular organ system that has been the most common and difficult problem. The major wars have provided larger experiences and more concentrated documentation of what was occurring simultaneously in civilian hospitals to patients traumatized by injury or operation.

Thus, Dr. Churchill, our chief at the Massachusetts General Hospital, wrote about his experiences during World War II in *Surgeon to Soldiers*. Although this book was published in 1972, it recounted clearly some of the many lessons learned during World War II about war wounds, injury, and the care of injured and operated patients. When I read Professor Churchill's book in 1972, the concept of "weak links in the chain" fascinated me. At that time, we were developing a cardiac surgical program in St. Louis at the Jewish Hospital of St. Louis and the Washington University School of Medicine. The support of failed organs had come into being, but the concept of remote organ failure had not yet developed fully. Low cardiac output was a frequent postoperative problem.

I decided to review the autopsy reports on our patients who died after a prolonged period of resuscitation and support in our intensive care units. Review of these reports and of the problems detailed within them began to suggest a pattern of problems in various organs remote from the primary site of injury or pathologic condition. For example, in a patient who, following a colon resection, had anastomotic breakdown with peritonitis and died after 6 weeks of progressive difficulty, the following were among the findings at autopsy: pulmonary congestion and edema; focal organizing pneumonia; thrombi in the renal glomerular capillaries with acute tubular necrosis in a stage of early healing; icterus; massive acute, noninflammatory hepatic necrosis; multiple infarcts of the spleen; and autolysis of the adrenal glands. Thus, this patient, although dying essentially of peritonitis, had the findings of multiple organ failure including evidence of failure of the lungs, liver, kidneys, and adrenal glands.

In a patient who died after a prolonged period of support for hemorrhagic pancreatitis, the autopsy findings indicated generalized jaundice, pleural fluid, aspiration pneumonia, acute tubular necrosis, extensive necrosis of the liver, and ulcerations of the gut. A third example was a patient with necrotizing bacterial arteritis, interstitial pulmonary edema with hyaline membranes, acute renal failure in a stage of healing, massive acute centrilobular necrosis of the liver, and passive congestion of the spleen. This patient died about a month and a half after an aortic and mitral valve replacement for valvular heart disease, with a continuous low cardiac output after operation. Again, however, the final pathologic manifestations were those of multiple organ failure. Thus, these three patients had very different initial diseases, but the final problem and syndrome were very similar.

This, in combination with Professor Churchill's weak links, led me to contemplate and try to define the problem in my editorial in the *Archives of Surgery* in July 1975 entitled "Multiple, Progressive, or Sequential Systems Failure: A Syndrome of the 1970's."[2] As I searched for an appropriate name for this syndrome, I came across the article by Tilney et al.[3] in 1973 entitled "Sequential Systems Failure After Rupture of Abdominal Aortic Aneurysms: An Unsolved Problem in Postoperative Care."[3] The term "sequential systems failure" was unique. I wish that I had thought of it, and I cited their observations about patients with abdominal aortic aneurysms in my original editorial.

Tilney et al. described 18 patients who required hemodialysis after surgical treatment of ruptured abdominal aortic aneurysms. After reviewing the clinical events and autopsy findings, they found a similar progression of organ system failure that began with pancreatic or pulmonary disease and progressed to upper gastrointestinal bleeding. They said that the lethality of renal failure after a ruptured aneurysm is explained as superimposition of preexisting chronic cardiovascular disease on the mechanical and metabolic consequences of the operation. The mortality in this group of patients was more than 90%.

Many other persons have contributed to the development of these concepts and to our knowledge of organ failure. It is often as difficult to determine the origin of ideas and concepts as it is to recognize all who have contributed. Claude Welch, one of the senior attending surgeons at the Massachusetts General Hospital when I was a resident, taught us the concept of refunctionalization of the gastrointestinal tract.[4] Welch had observed that, in an otherwise normal patient with peritonitis, if bowel function that allowed oral intake did not return in approximately 2 weeks, it was necessary to operate immediately to refunctionalize the gastrointestinal tract so that the patient could begin to eat again. If there was further delay, then by 3 weeks the patient began to deteriorate and would eventually die. This, of course, was well before the time of total parenteral nutrition and the capability to prevent or delay metabolic failure by parenteral means.

This led to a report in 1963 by Burke et al.[5] in which they described high-output respiratory failure in patients with peritonitis. Most of these patients eventually died of renal failure, but in the process they had overbreathing (hypoxic hyperventilation) and respiratory failure. Skillman et al.[6] found a high mortality rate in patients with peritonitis who developed respiratory failure, as did Clowes and his group[7] and Border et al.[8] Siegel et al.[9] described myocardial failure with sepsis. Skillman et al.[10] found that a syndrome of respiratory failure, hypotension, sepsis, and jaundice was associated with lethal hemorrhage from acute gastric stress ulcerations. Thus, the beginning concepts of remote organ problems developing, particularly with sepsis, came into the literature and to surgical recognition.

Following my report in 1975, Eiseman and colleagues[11] described a number of patients with multiple organ failure, emphasizing hepatic failure, and they coined the expression "multiple organ failure," which has continued today. Polk and Shields[12] reported on remote organ failure as a sign of occult intra-abdominal infection. They pointed out at that time that if a patient developed remote organ failure, the chances were at least 50% that the cause of the problem would be found in the peritoneal cavity and require surgical therapy by drainage or extirpation.[12] Thus, the recommendation was made at that time that a patient with remote organ failure should have an exploratory laparotomy to try to get at the problem and resolve it. The concept of a blind laparotomy for sepsis and remote organ failure was developed. Patients without abdominal infection or a necrotic organ such as acalculous cholecystitis (a frequent finding) would likely die anyway, so the blind laparotomy seemed justified. Now, we recognize that this blind approach is no longer necessary for the following reasons: (1) better means of identifying an intra-abdominal problem are available, such as ultrasound and computed tomography scanning; (2) inflammation or the nonbacteremic septic state defined by Meakins and Marshall[13] is the cause about half the time, and a laparotomy is not helpful. The emphasis on the role of uncontrolled infection in organ failure came from Fry et al.,[14] along with Polk and colleagues. Shortly thereafter, Border et al.[15] provided extensive observations and measurements of metabolic alterations in patients with multiple systems organ failure, as they now called it. Subsequently, they provided a series of very worthwhile articles in the *Journal of Trauma*, too numerous to cite here.

Many others have written about and contributed to our knowledge of multiple organ failure, including Trunkey and Miller,[16] Marshall and Dimick[17] and Cassone.[18] Extensive metabolic studies have been contributed by a number of groups, including those of John Seigel, John Border, Frank Cerra, and the late George Clowes and their groups. These immense contributions will, I am sure, be referred to elsewhere in this book.

Limiting Organ Systems

At any particular time in recent surgical history, there has been a single limiting organ system that was the primary factor resulting in morbidity and mortality after injury. I use the generic meaning of "injury," which includes both types of trauma—accidental trauma and an operation or planned trauma in the operating room.

The development of the concept of multiple organ failure also required a knowledge of the pathophysiologic aspects of surgical problems and of organ failure, and also the development of means to support various organ systems when they have failed, which then allowed the appearance of multiple organ difficulties.

Shock

> *Now tell us all about the war, and what they killed each other for.*
> —Robert Southey (1774–1843). The Battle of Blenheim[1]

In his book, Churchill provides an excellent description of wound shock and blood transfusion. In World War I, wound shock was believed to be a complex, mysterious problem. Various hypotheses had been proposed, including vasomotor exhaustion, acapnia, adrenal exhaustion, and traumatic toxemia. Wound shock was thought to be different and not accounted for by hemorrhage, infection, brain injury, blast injury, fat embolism, or other recognized problems in injured patients. It remained for Parsons and Phemister[19] and for Alfred Blalock[20] to demonstrate in the 1930s that shock after injury in experimental animals was due to blood loss and a deficiency in circulating vascular volume.

Despite this, a concept of irreversible shock developed and was still prevalent in World War II. This began with another concept in which plasma was to be used to restore the bulk of the blood lost from the intravascular space and sodium chloride solution would be used for dehydration and electrolyte depletion. No plans were made for the use of whole blood. In fact, it was the position of the United States Army that blood would not be made available. It became apparent through Churchill's work and the contributions of the British in the North African campaign that blood was necessary and that wound shock is blood volume loss identical to hemorrhage. The thing that seemed to convince the Army was a conversation by Churchill with a correspondent, reported in the *New York Times* on August 26, 1943: "Plasma Alone Is Not Sufficient—Colonel Edward D. Churchill of Boston, Professor of Surgery at Harvard and now consulting surgeon for troops here, has pioneered in setting up blood banks similar to the Red Cross blood deposits in the United States. In a report to the Surgeon General's Office, Colonel Churchill declared, 'There is need for whole blood transfusions in the treatment of a significant proportion of wounded. Plasma is not an adequate substitute in these cases.' "

This broke the bottleneck in North Africa. Refrigerators were made available for mobile hospitals. The opportunity to draw blood and use it became available from then on through the war. Thus, the concept of support of the circulation and the prevention and treatment of shock after injury evolved during World War II, despite extensive experimental knowledge in animal studies in the 1930s preceding the war. Churchill states: "In view of the present liberal use of whole blood adequate to reestablish equilibrium in a wounded man, it is amazing to recall that World War II was started with the concept of plasma for the intravascular space and sodium chloride for the interstitial space with therapeutic measures. In World War II, replacement of lost blood reached an extraordinary high level of effectiveness. It is certain that hundreds of injured men survived the immediate effects of wounds that under slightly less favorable circumstances would have proved fatal. Irreversible shock as such was not encountered. An appreciable number of the wounded survived, however, only to die about the tenth day with complete anuria."[1] This led to Churchill's realization that the obvious link in the severely wounded in this war was the kidney.

Renal Failure

> *I would remind you again how large and various was the experience of the battlefield, and how fertile the blood of warriors in rearing good surgeons.*
>
> —Edward D. Churchill[21]

Churchill, in an address to the medical services of the French, British, and American armed forces and the physicians and surgeons of the Department of Oran, Algeria, said, "War offers to the military surgeon an opportunity and responsibility for the development of this science that is non-existent during time of peace."[1] The teaching shortly after World War II was that the response to injury indicated that there was sodium retention due to aldosterone secretion. Potassium was lost from the urine. Therefore the injured or operated patient needed blood, plasma, or both, but not a great deal of saline, since salt was being conserved. Injured and operated patients were kept on the dry side. Thus, during the Korean conflict, a major cause of death in otherwise normal young persons after injury was acute renal failure.

The United States Army Surgical Research Unit in Korea first used the phrase "post-traumatic renal insufficiency," which occurred 20 to 30 times more commonly in Korea than it would later in the Vietnam conflict.[22] The studies in Korea demonstrated the most common cause of delayed death in those patients who had been successfully resuscitated from severe injury was the development of acute renal failure. At that time, 1 in 200 seriously injured soldiers developed acute renal failure with a mortality close to 90%. Benjamin Rush,[23] who was part of the research team in Korea, indicated that this was a time when sodium retention with injury had been recognized and sodium solutions were not given to any particular extent to these injured and operated patients. It was thought that the sodium retention would perhaps lead to edema. Recognition of this problem of post-traumatic renal insufficiency led to development of the concept by Shires and others of a decrease or loss of extravascular water and a decrease in the size of the extracellular fluid space after injury.[24] The need then for larger volumes of intravenous water and sodium, such as with Ringer's lactate solution, was recognized, leading to better support of this organ system. As the factors that produce renal insufficiency were better understood, this problem was often prevented by rapid fluid resuscitation of the patient and the support of the kidneys by improving renal blood flow and promoting adequate urine output.

Renal failure thus decreased in frequency. When it did occur, it was treated much more satisfactorily. Failure of the circulatory system could be prevented or treated adequately by rapid volume resuscitation. This would simultaneously produce a diuresis and decrease the likelihood of acute renal failure. It is interesting that in the four-volume set of reports from Korea by the Army Surgical Research Unit, there was no mention of pulmonary problems.[25] These were not recognized as a difficulty at that time.

Ventilatory Failure

As the circulation and renal function were better supported after injury, a new problem came into focus: pulmonary failure. By better support of the kidneys and the circulation, the lungs then emerged as the next organ system to be in jeopardy. Rapid resuscitation also tended to overwhelm the lungs, and this produced other difficulties. Patients with more severe injuries, who were now able to survive for longer periods of time, were therefore subjected to the possibility of the development of pulmonary problems. At the time of the Vietnamese conflict, this was called "post-traumatic pulmonary insufficiency." The lungs became the limiting organ system after injury, both in civilian and in military practice.[26]

This raised several questions. Did pulmonary failure develop because better resuscitation and support of the cardiovascular and renal systems exposed the lungs as the next limiting organ system? Or did aggressive and, perhaps on occasion, excessive fluid resuscitation jeopardize the lungs? It seems likely that both of these problems occurred, along with direct pulmonary injury from blunt injury as well.

Adequate, but not excessive, fluid resuscitation after injury and recognition of the lungs as a limiting organ system after injury have since both contributed to more frequent prevention of respiratory failure. When not prevented, respiratory failure can now be treated much more satisfactorily. In order to make this possible, however, adequate means of support of ventilation became necessary. The first ventilators, the Engstrom units, were developed in Sweden in the late 1950s. Our group at the Massachusetts General Hospital—led by Hennings Pontoppidan and others in anesthesia and surgery—developed in 1960 and 1961 the first intensive care unit in the United States for respiratory failure. Initially there was considerable morbidity, even mortality, associated with the mechanics of ventilatory support. The problems included the need for constant supervision, technical failures, barotrauma, tracheal injury, vascular injury, and sepsis. Many of these problems have now been solved, and short-term ventilatory support should be quite safe. At the present time, the mortality from ventilatory failure alone should be fairly low. Thus, post-traumatic pulmonary insufficiency no longer was the single most-limiting organ system after injury.

Multiple Organ Failure

The next limiting organ system that appeared was not a single organ but the complex or syndrome that we now call multiple organ failure. Morbidity and death after operation or injury still occur from various complications such as thromboembolism, acute vascular occlusions or infarctions, shock, post-traumatic renal failure, post-traumatic pulmonary failure, sepsis, and peritonitis. However, each of these problems occurring by itself can often be treated successfully. Certain combinations of such complications, however, were recognized some years ago as being particularly lethal.[27,28] For example, renal failure associated with sepsis and respiratory and hepatic failure still had a very grave prognosis, even though renal failure itself was no longer the critical event. The incidence of renal failure in the injured in Vietnam was only 0.1 to 0.2%, but the mortality of those who developed it was still quite high (63 to 77%), owing to associated injuries and sepsis rather than to renal failure per se.[29] Liver problems with hepatomegaly and jaundice with trauma or sepsis were recognized more frequently, and the term "post-traumatic hepatic insufficiency" came into use.[30] The gastrointestinal tract, which heretofore seemed to wait quietly during starvation and sepsis, is now recognized as causing problems by such difficulties as bleeding or perforation, translocation of organisms,[31] and altered immune function.[32] Metabolic failure with alterations of peripheral metabolism and the

Table 1–1   Listing of the Systems That Can Fail

Post-traumatic
    Circulatory failure—shock
    Renal failure
    Pulmonary insufficiency
    Hepatic failure
    Coagulation problems
    Immunosuppression—immune failure
    Gastrointestinal failure
    Metabolic failure
    Neuroendocrine failure
    Musculoskeletal failure
    Central nervous system failure

autocannibalism of skeletal muscle[33] and subsequent hepatic failure were recognized.

Thus, all systems can fail (Table 1–1). Whether this occurs in a simultaneous or a sequential (domino) fashion is determined more by the state and severity of the injury and the complications that develop.

As clinical reports of patients who developed multiple organ failure mounted, a clear definition of organ failure and the factors contributing to it emerged. The setting was clearly identified as follows: (1) a severe metabolic insult secondary to trauma, operation, or both; (2) often the occurrence of a clinical or technical error that was not initially recognized; (3) frequent development of sepsis, often accompanied by peritonitis or a severe inflammatory process; (4) low cardiac output and circulatory problems; (5) limitations in organ function from prior disease.

Soon it became apparent that severe inflammation, in itself, associated with tissue necrosis or other problems could produce or activate mediators that depressed the circulation and altered organ function. These descriptions of clinical factors by Goris et al[34] indicated clearly that infection was not necessary. It was also apparent that persons with limitations of functions of one or more organ systems before operation or injury were much more susceptible to this problem than were otherwise normal persons. This was especially true in patients with vascular occlusive disease, chronic obstructive lung disease, hepatic damage, immunosuppression from various disease processes or organ transplantation, and cardiac disease. The common thread underlying all of these problems seemed to be an altered circulation, reduced blood flow, inadequate tissue perfusion, and ischemia. The recognition that patients developing multiple organ failure often developed what appeared to be a septic state—but without bacterial infection—led to the description of the nonbacterial septic clinical state by Meakins and Marshall.[13]

ORGAN ASSOCIATIVE OR SYSTEMS RELATIONSHIP PERIOD

As further documentation of problems of multiple organ failure occurred, the relationships between systems and the occurrence of sequential or domino effects were studied. The frequency and possible causes of an organ failing in association with a disease process remote to that organ led to a number of relationships. For example, pancreatitis is frequently associated with ventilatory failure and a form of pulmonary edema. There has been speculation that this may be due to pulmonary alveolar-capillary membrane damage produced by some factor from the necrotic pancreas, such as pancreatic enzymes, phospholipase A, vasoactive substances, or circulating free fatty acids. Many other factors, however, may contribute to this problem in pancreatitis because the patient, who is catabolic, may have sepsis, a distended abdomen, elevated hemidiaphragms, pleural effusions, and a depressed circulation. Patients with pancreatitis may also have myocardial depression due to a toxin, such as has been described as the myocardial depressant factor.

The association of abdominal sepsis and peritonitis with pulmonary failure has led to extensive studies of complement activation, neutrophil aggregation, superoxide production, and many other events that could potentially damage the pulmonary capillary endothelium. Thus, an extensive series of studies was carried out on these organ-associative relationships, such as the hepatorenal syndrome. There have been studies concerning how a septic process remote from the kidneys could result in renal damage and whether this could be due to immune complex deposition and other such difficulties involved in a septic process. One of the hazards in the study of such system relationships is the possibility of post hoc ergo propter hoc reasoning. This means that two events occurring simultaneously or sequentially may or may not have a cause and effect relationship. Thus, things may occur simultaneously or sequentially but may not be related to one another.

Acute renal failure and multiple organ failure have also been described in the Peoples Republic of China. Shen and Zhang[35] report that 23 patients with acute renal failure developed multiple organ system failure, with an overall mortality of approximately 50%, and that this was associated with ventilatory failure and sepsis. Thus, the problems of single and multiple organ failure are similar in China to those problems occurring in other countries. Similar documentation of difficulties in patients with multiple organ failure and postoperative acute gastrointestinal bleeding also come from Buenos Aires, Argentina.[36] There have been a number of major reviews and symposia on multiple organ failure, all better defining the syndrome and its complications and problems.[37,38]

Central Nervous System Failure

A major limitation after accidental injury remains, of course, the central nervous system (CNS). It has been well documented by Baker et al.,[39] at the San Francisco General Hospital, as well as by Faist et al.[40,41] at the University of Munich and by Baker and our group[42] at Yale that 50% of patients who died after accidental injury did so from primary CNS causes. This is true whether the trauma was due to gunshot or knife wounds or to high-speed accidents on the autobahn and is consistent with all experiences. This provides a major challenge in the prevention of injury and the care of the injured. Patients with primary CNS injury may die from that injury alone or may develop multiple organ problems.

However, the CNS remains the major single limiting organ system after injury and is a challenge for those who would like to decrease the impact of accidental injury.

System Management—Problem Orientation

Another avenue of thought that helped to promote the concept of an organ or systems basis for consideration of disease and injury was the organization of clinical thinking and patient care on this basis. Just as the systems review in the history of a patient helps to assure completeness of evaluation, so can such methods assist in overall patient care. Weed[43] proposed the use of a problem orientation for medical records, particularly when, as with most patients, there are multiple problems. Even better for surgical patients is a system or organ structure method of record-keeping and management. As the problems of patients after injury and operation become increasingly complex and abnormalities occur, in a number of body systems, it is necessary to develop different methods for recording information about the patient's course in the hospital record. Katz and Ottinger[44] developed an approach that requires consideration of each system and documents the patient's course by writing follow-up notes and orders. The function of each system is analyzed, and a plan for each is defined. Data display can be arranged by systems rather than by problems, and this becomes compatible with modern computer technology. It also provides a constant frame of reference applicable to all acutely ill patients. Thus, this approach allows one to define the extent and nature of multiple organ failure and its progress or regression.

Summary

It is apparent now that many different disease processes and injuries can result in multiple organ difficulties. An unsuspected pheochromocytoma can produce a multiple system crisis, as can other acute processes. What began as a surgical problem—the leading edge of our capabilities—has now become a general intensive care unit syndrome. The term and concept are now used by emergency physicians and by our colleagues in anesthesia and critical care medicine.

The term "multiple organ failure" is currently used in the lay press as well. An Associated Press report from Pittsburgh a short time ago offered this description: "The patient Rolandria Dodge, three, was with her parents, Brandon and Cindy Dodge of Fruitland, New Mexico, when she died of multiple organ failure at 4:45 p.m. at Children's Hospital, Pittsburgh. The child had earlier received an abdominal transplant of multiple organs including the liver, pancreas, stomach, small intestine and part of her large intestine."

As we learn more about acute illness, life-threatening injury, and the interrelatedness of our biologic responses to injury, we will better be able to prevent multiple organ failure.[45–48] What then will be the next "weak link in the chain"?

References

1. Churchill ED. Surgeon to soldiers. Philadelphia: JB Lippincott, 1972.
2. Baue AE. Multiple, progressive, or sequential systems failure: a syndrome of the 1970s. Arch Surg 1975;110:779–781.
3. Tilney NL, Bailey GL, Morgan AP. Sequential system failure after rupture of abdominal aortic aneurysms: an unsolved problem in postoperative care. Ann Surg 1973;178:117–122.
4. Welch CE. Treatment of combined intestinal obstruction and peritonitis by refunctionalization of the intestine. Ann Surg 1955;142:739.
5. Burke JF, Pontoppidan H, Welch CE. High output respiratory failure: an important cause of death ascribed to peritonitis or ileus. Ann Surg 1963;158:581–595.
6. Skillman JJ, Bushnell LS, Hedley-Whyte J. Peritonitis and respiratory failure after abdominal operations. Ann Surg 1969; 170:122–127.
7. Clowes GHA Jr, Zuschneid W, Turner M, Blackburn G, Rubin J, Toala P, Green G. Observations on the pathogenesis of the pneumonitis associated with severe infections in other parts of the body. Ann Surg 1968;167:630.
8. Border JR, Tibbets JC, Schenk WG. Hypoxic hyperventilation and acute respiratory failure in the severely stressed patient: massive pulmonary arteriovenous shunts? Surgery 1968;64:710.
9. Siegel JH, Greenspan M, DelGuercio LRM: Abnormal vascular tone, defective oxygen transport and myocardial failure in human septic shock. Ann Surg 1967;165:504.
10. Skillman JJ, Bushnell LS, Goldman H, Silen W. Respiratory failure, hypotension, sepsis and jaundice. Am J Surg 1969;117:523–530.
11. Eiseman B, Beart R, Norton L. Multiple organ failure. Surg Gynecol Obstet 1977;144:323–326.
12. Polk HC Jr, Shields CL. Remote organ failure: a valid sign of occult intra-abdominal infection. Surgery 1977;81:310–313.
13. Meakins JL, Marshall JC. The gastrointestinal tract: the 'motor' of MOF (part of SIS panel discussion). Arch Surg 1986;121:197–201.
14. Fry DE, Pearlstein L, Fulton RL, Polk HC Jr. Multiple system organ failure. Arch Surg 1980;115:136–140.
15. Border JR, Chenier R, McMenamy RH, LaDuca J, Seibel R, Birkhahn R, Yu L. Multiple systems organ failure: muscle fuel deficit with visceral protein malnutrition. Surg Clin North Am 1976;56:1147–1167.
16. Trunkey DD, Miller CL. Multiple organ failure and sepsis. In Najarian JS, Delaney JP (eds): Emergency surgery. Year Book Medical Publishers, 1982, pp. 273–285.
17. Marshall WG Jr, Dimick AR. The natural history of major burns with multiple subsystem failure. J Trauma 1983;23:102–105.
18. Cassone E. Clinical and laboratory signs of multiple organ failure. Infecti Surg, 1983;2:857–862.
19. Parsons E, Phemister DB. Hemorrhage and "shock" in traumatized limbs: an experimental study. Surg Gynecol Obstet 1930;51:196–207.
20. Blalock A. Acute circulatory failure as exemplified by shock and hemorrhage. Surg Gynecol Obstet 1934;58:551.
21. Allbutts TC. The historical relations of medicine in surgery to the end of the sixteenth century. London: Macmillan, 1905.
22. U.S. Army. Battle casualties in Korea—studies of the Surgical Research Team, volume IV: "Post-traumatic renal insufficiency." Army Medical Service Graduate School, Walter Reed Army Medical Center, Washington, DC, 1955.
23. Rush B. Personal communication.
24. Shires GT, et al. Alterations in cellular membrane function during hemorrhagic shock in primates. Ann Surg 1972;176:288.
25. U.S. Army. Battle casualties in Korea—studies of the Surgical Research Team, volumes I–IV. Brooke Army Medical Center and Army Medical Service Graduate School, Walter Reed Army Medical Center, Washington, DC, 1955.
26. Moore FD, Lyons JH, Pierce EF Jr, Morgan AP, Drinker PA, MacArthur JD, Mannin GJ. Post-traumatic respiratory insufficiency. Philadelphia: WB Saunders, 1969.
27. Baue AE. Sequential or multiple systems failure. In Najarian J, Delaney J (eds): Critical surgical care. Miami: Symposia Specialists, 1977, pp 293–300.
28. Baue AE, Chaudry IH. Prevention of multiple systems failure. Surg Clin North Am 1980;60:1167–1178.
29. Fischer RP. High mortality of post-traumatic renal insufficiency in Vietnam: a review of 96 cases. Am Surg 1974;40:172–177.
30. Baue AE. Multiple organ or systems failure. In Haimovici H (ed): Vascular emergencies. New York: Appleton-Century-Crofts, 1981, chapter 7.

31. Deitch EA, Winterton J, Berg R. Effect of starvation, malnutrition, and trauma on the gastrointestinal tract flora and bacterial translocation. Arch Surg 1987;122:1019–1024.
32. Border JR, Hassett J, LaDuca J, et al. The gut origin septic states in blunt multiple trauma (ISS = 40) in the ICU. Ann Surg 1987;206:41–59.
33. Cerra FB, Siegel JH, Colman B, Border J, McMenamy RH. Autocannibalism, a failure of exogenous nutritional support. Ann Surg 1980;192:570.
34. Goris RJA, te Boekhorst TPA, Nuytinck JKS: Multiple organ failure: generalized autodestructive inflammation? Arch Surg 1985;120:1109–1115.
35. Shen P-F, Zhang S-C. Acute renal failure and multiple-organ-system failure. Arch Surg 1987;122:1131–1133.
36. Bumaschny E, Doglio G, Pusajo J, et al. Postoperative acute gastrointestinal tract hemorrhage and multiple-organ failure. Arch Surg 1988;123:722–726.
37. Carrico CJ, Meakins JL, Marshall JC, et al. Multiple-organ-failure syndrome. Arch Surg 1986;121:196–208.
38. Polk HC, Baue AE, Trunkey DD, Frye DE. Multiple system organ failure, symposium. Contemp Surg 1981;19:107–139.
39. Baker CC, Oppenheimer L, Stephens B, et al. Epidemiology of trauma deaths. Am J Surg 1980;140:144–150.
40. Faist E, Baue AE, Dittmer H, Heberer G. Multiple organ failure in polytrauma patients. J Trauma 1983;23:775–787.
41. Faist E, Heberer G, Baue AE. Das mehrorganversagen beim polytraumatisierten patienten. Krankenhausarzt 1983;56:1–14.
42. Baker CC, Degutis LC, DeSantis J, Baue AE. Impact of a trauma service on trauma care in a university hospital. Am J Surg 1985;149:453–458.
43. Weed LL. Medical records that guide and teach. N Engl J Med 1968;278:593–600.
44. Katz NM, Ottinger LW. System-structured management of acutely ill surgical patients. Arch Surg 1976;111:239–242.
45. Baue AE. Multiple systems failure and circulatory support. Jpn J Surg 1983;13:69–85.
46. Baue AE. Recovery from multiple organ failure. Am J Surg 1985;149:120–121.
47. Baue AE, Guthrie D. Modern aspects of multiple organ failure. In Eigler FW, Peiper H-J, Schildberg FW, Witte J, Zumtobel V, (eds): Stand und Gegenstand Chirurgischer Forschung. Berlin: Springer-Verlag, 1986.
48. Baue AE. Multiple organ or systems failure. In Delaney JP, Najarian JS (eds): Trauma and critical care surgery. Year Book Medical Publishers, 1987, pp 363–371.

2

Diagnosis and Epidemiology of Multiple Organ Failure

Donald E. Fry

Organ failure complexes have been identified in severely injured and critically ill patients for many decades. Early on, prior to general recognition in civilian practice, military casualties were generally acknowledged to be at risk for the development of various organ failure syndromes.[1] Traditionally, organ failure complexes were identified by a single-organ system. Thus, cardiovascular failure, renal failure, and pulmonary failure were each considered as isolated entities.

During the 1970s and 1980s, advances in health care ushered into medical practice an unprecedented support technology. Aggressive volume support, monitoring with Swan-Ganz catheters, and a spectacular array of pharmacologic agents have permitted effective support of circulatory function. Dialysis, ventilators, and nutritional support have each added to the patient's physiologic reserve during stress and critical illness. The total of these support measures has resulted in solitary organ failure being a rather uncommon observation in the critically ill surgical patient. Rather, multiple organ system failure has become a well-recognized final pathway to death in intensive care unit patients.

This chapter will discuss the development of criteria used to define a failed organ system. Since these definitions are arbitrary, I shall illustrate how those criteria and definitions were used in previous studies. Finally, these definitions will be used to characterize the epidemiology of the multiple organ failure syndrome.

Diagnosis of Organ Failure

Those organ systems that have been studied most completely are those that can be monitored clinically. For example, cardiac, pulmonary, renal, and hepatic failure each can be clinically defined using commonly identified clinical criteria. Stress bleeding is similarly identified as an expression of gastrointestinal failure.

Other organ systems can also be identified as failing or having disordered function in the critically ill patient, but definition of organ failure is more difficult in these systems. Disseminated intravascular coagulation represents a functional failure of the coagulation system. However, objective information confirming disseminated intravascular coagulation requires the presence of elevated levels of fibrin split products. This test is not specific, since in critically ill patients some elevation of fibrin split products can be identified without clinical bleeding and in many patient care scenarios clinical bleeding may occur without elevation of fibrin split products. Regulation of substrate metabolism is clearly disordered in the critically ill patient but, depending on the sophistication of the monitoring system used, every patient with a major stress response can be viewed as having failure of this "system." Elevated serum amylase concentration has been reported to reflect potential pancreatic dysfunction but may in reality represent perturbed excretion of amylase by the kidney.[2] Finally, neurologic dysfunction clearly occurs in many of these patients but is extraordinarily difficult to quantitate.

In our early studies of multiple organ failure[3–6] we chose to study those organ functions that could be readily identified using standard clinical and laboratory information. The selection of which organ systems to study was also affected by certain prejudices. For example, the emergence of visceral organ dysfunction did not appear to be the consequence of a failed central circulation. Arterial pressure and measurements of cardiac output in patients with sepsis have appeared to be adequate until the immediate preagonal period.[7,8] Thus, pulmonary hepatic, renal, and gastrointestinal (stress bleeding) failure were considered as organ systems that could be evaluated by readily available clinical information.

Definitions

The diagnosis of a specific organ dysfunction required definitions that could readily be applied to large populations of patients. Definitions for diagnostic purposes were developed that were arbitrary but had some supporting rationale.

PULMONARY FAILURE

The definition of pulmonary failure was adopted from the studies of Fulton and Jones.[9] A patient was not considered to have pulmonary failure unless five or more days of continuous ventilator support at an FiO_2 equal to, or greater than, 0.4 was required to combat hypoxia. Many patients require transient ventilator support after major operations, trauma, or massive resuscitation. These patients commonly show a nadir of pulmonary gas exchange immediately following their primary physiologic insult, but progressively improve and by 2 to 3 days into the convalescent period they can be successfully weaned from ventilatory support. Thus, we chose the 5-day interval of ventilatory support to eliminate this favorable group of patients and to include principally only those patients with progressive pulmonary dysfunction.

HEPATIC FAILURE

A clinical diagnosis of hepatic failure proved difficult, particularly when reviewing a large number of trauma patients with associated direct hepatic trauma. We chose two criteria for the diagnosis of liver failure: (1) a total serum bilirubin level greater than 2 mg/dl; and (2) doubling of accepted normal serum concentrations of liver enzymes (serum glutamic oxaloacetic and lactate dehydrogenase). Both criteria had to be met, since even isolated and relatively uncomplicated liver trauma caused "liver enzyme" concentrations to increase, whereas elevations in bilirubin levels can be due to multiple transfusions or the presence of a retroperitoneal, or pelvic hematoma. By requiring both criteria to be met, we hoped to avoid the spurious diagnosis of liver dysfunction that might be secondary to nonhepatic variables.

RENAL FAILURE

A diagnosis of renal failure is clearly recognized when the patient develops severe oliguria or anuria. However, patients with trauma and sepsis will commonly develop a high output or normal output renal dysfunction. Creatinine concentrations will increase to very high levels (5 to 8 mg/dl) in many of these patients before oliguria appears. Thus, our group believes that oliguria and anuria were too rigorous for making the diagnosis of renal failure. We chose an elevation of serum creatinine above 2 mg/dl as the threshold for the diagnosis of renal failure, regardless of urine output volume. Blood urea nitrogen concentrations invariably doubled in concert with the creatinine.

STRESS GASTROINTESTINAL BLEEDING

Stress gastrointestinal bleeding has been identified as a common complication in critically ill and multiply transfused patients and has been viewed as a clinical manifestation of failure of the gastrointestinal tract. During our initial studies of multiple organ failure, routine upper gastrointestinal endoscopy had not yet received consistent application in all patients with upper gastrointestinal bleeding. Thus, the diagnosis of stress gastrointestinal bleeding was considered when patients had upper gastrointestinal bleeding of two units or more without an otherwise documented source of blood loss. Modern endoscopic technology allows stress bleeding to be diagnosed more accurately, and currently it is the standard technique for making this diagnosis.

Frequency of Multiple Organ Failure

In 1976, Eiseman and associates[10] reported on a group of patients with multiple organ failure that they had identified at the Denver General Hospital. In that

Table 2–1   Frequency and Mortality Rate of Individual Organ Failure Complexes Among 553 Patients Undergoing Emergency Surgical Procedures

Organ System	No. Patients	Frequency of Occurrence (%)	No. Deaths	Mortality Rate (%)
Lung	42	7.6	28	67
Liver	47	8.5	25	53
Stress bleeding	17	3.1	10	59
Kidney	39	7.1	28	72

series, they used diagnostic criteria that were similar to our own. The mortality rate of their patients with the multiple organ failure syndrome was 70%. Since the patients were identified from an unknown total population of patients, the frequency of the development of this syndrome could not be defined.

To determine the incidence of the multiple organ failure syndrome, Fry et al.[3] reviewed a consecutive series of 553 emergency surgical procedures from all surgical disciplines at the Louisville General Hospital. All patients who died within 24 hours of admission were excluded from evaluation, since these patients were considered to have died from their primary disease process and were not considered to be at risk for developing subsequent multiple organ failure. In the group of patients studied, two thirds were trauma patients and one third required emergency surgery.

As defined in Table 2–1, pulmonary, hepatic, and renal failure each occurred in approximately 7 to 9% of the patients, whereas gastrointestinal bleeding occurred less frequently. Although in this series stress gastrointestinal bleeding appeared to occur infrequently, with the greater utilization of upper gastrointestinal endoscopy the rate of identification of stress-induced gastritis has increased. Thus, our initial observations may have underestimated the frequency of stress gastritis by virture of having critieria that were not sensitive enough. As is noted in Table 2–1, the identified mortality rate by organ system was formidable. Since the mortality rate for the entire series of patients was 10%, the greater than 50% mortality rate by organ system clearly documented the significance of compromised organ function on patient outcome.

When the mortality rate of these patients was correlated with the number of organ systems that failed, a virtual linear relationship was found between the number of organ systems that failed and death (Table 2–2). Although failure of each organ system contributed to an increased mortality, renal failure appeared to be associated with the greatest adverse impact on patient survival. In fact, all patients with two organ systems in addition to kidney failure died. Thus, if patients were defined as having multiple organ failure when two or more organ systems fail, more than 50% of the deaths in this series of patients were associated with multiple organ failure.

The failure of organ systems that are functionally and anatomically separate from one another has led to considerable speculation that a common pathophysiologic mechanism may be responsible for multiple organ system failure. Because military casualties have traditionally been the prototype patient to de-

Table 2–2   Frequency and Mortality Rate Related to the Number of Organ Systems Involved, and Not Related to a Specific Organ, in 553 Patients Undergoing Emergency Surgical Procedures

No. Organ Systems	No. Patients	Frequency of Occurrence (%)	No. Deaths	Mortality Rate (%)
One	46	8.3	14	30
Two	20	3.6	12	60
Three	13	2.4	11	85
Four	5	0.9	5	100
Two or more	38	6.9	28	74

velop organ failure complexes, clinical variables commonly identified among the war-injured patient have received the greatest scrutiny.

Shock, hypotension, and inadequate tissue perfusion have been commonly implicated as etiologic agents of the multiple organ failure syndrome. "Shock lung," "shock kidney," and "shock liver" are terms that were commonly heard in military hospitals that managed severe military injuries that survived the acute insult, operation, and immediate resuscitation. Presumably, the hypoperfusion state resulted in cellular injury, which in turn led to clinically definable impairment of organ function. The experience of Tilney et al.[2] with civilian patients with ruptured aortic aneurysms reflects a similar experience in which hypovolemic and hypoperfused patients developed distant organ failure.

Hypoxemia represents another clinical variable that has been implicated in end-organ failure. While hypoxemia and shock represent different clinical insults, they are physiologically similar, since in both clinical conditions tissue oxygenation is inadequate. Those who believe in the importance of adensoine triphosphate supply as a requirement for cellular homeostasis will readily accept that sustained suboptimal tissue oxygenation may be manifested by end-organ failure. The patient with chronic obstructive pulmonary disease has been associated with having stress gastritis, especially during periods of acute decompensation, and provides some credibility to this concept.

Blood transfusion has been implicated as an important clinical variable in end-organ failure, since histopathologic assessment of tissues from multiple organ failure patients has identified microaggregates of blood cellular elements within the capillaries and microcirculation of tissues known to fail. This finding has led some investigators to suggest that microaggregates from the transfusion of bank blood may be a contributory variable to the development of this syndrome. Obviously, making the distinction between the impact of transfusion-associated particulate matter and the roles of blood loss and shock on the development of organ failure is very difficult.

Uncontrolled infection has been viewed by many workers to be of primary etiologic significance in the evolution of multiple organ failure. However, the mechanism of end-organ failure secondary to infection must clearly be different from that of simple hypoperfusion or hypoxia, since, unlike shock and hypoxemia, the hemodynamic response to infection is a hyperdynamic one.[11,12] Likewise, unlike hypovolemic shock, infection is associated with peripheral vasodilation and reduced systemic vascular resistance. The interest in infection as a cause of disordered cellular homeostasis has precipitated an avalanche of research that has focused on red cell oxyhemoglobin dissociation,[13] mitochondrial metabolism,[14–16] microarteriovenous shunts,[7] systemic redistribution of blood flow,[17] and the microaggregation hypothesis of the septic microcirculatory arrest.[18,19]

Other variables have been proposed as potential factors in the pathogenesis of organ failure. Long bone fractures have been associated with remote organ failure, presumably due to the fat embolism syndrome. Head injury has been implicated in organ failure potentially because of autonomic nervous system influences in the periphery. Many treatment regimens and pharmaceutical agents have end-organ toxicity and may have additive effects to other insults in the pathogenesis of this syndrome.

In our review of 553 surgical patients at risk for organ failure, we identified 38 patients with multiple organ failure.[3] These 38 patients had a mortality rate of 74%. We then proceeded to study all the previously mentioned clinical variables in these patients to establish associations.

To establish clinical relationships, we had to establish definitions of the clinical variables that we wanted to study. As with the definitions for organ failure syndromes, definitions for clinical variables may suffer from being too lenient or too strict. The clinical definitions used were the following.

HYPOVOLEMIC SHOCK

Patients were defined as having hypovolemic shock if admission systolic blood pressure was 80 mmHg or less or if an intraoperative systolic blood pressure of 60 mmHg or less was observed. The more severe criterion for intraoperative hypotension was chosen to compensate for the vasodilatory effects of general anesthesia. Any patient requiring greater than 10 L of resuscitation in the first 6 hours of hospitalization also was considered as having hypovolemic shock, regardless of blood pressure measurement.

MASSIVE BLOOD TRANSFUSION

Patients who received 6 units or more of blood during the initial 6 hours of management were defined as having this clinical variable.

MASSIVE CRYSTALLOID RESUSCITATION

Patients were defined as having massive crystalloid resuscitation in this clinical group if they received 6 L or more of crystalloid resuscitation in the initial 6 hours of management.

MASSIVE VOLUME RESUSCITATION

By adding all crystalloid, colloid, blood, and blood products together, a total volume of resuscitation was established., The threshold for massive fluid resuscitation was 6 L total volume in a 6 hour period or 14 L in 24 hours.

Table 2–3   Statistically Significant Clinical Variables in Patients Who Developed Multiple Organ Failure (MOF) from the 553 Emergency Surgical Patients Studied

Variable	No. Patients	No. MOF	Statistical Significance (p)
Hypovolemic shock	67	16	<0.01
Massive blood therapy	32	9	<0.01
Massive crystalloid therapy	35	10	<0.01
Chest injury	113	14	<0.01
Septicemia	123	34	<0.01

INFECTION

A patient was considered as having major infection, or sepsis, based on fulfillment of any one of the following criteria: (1) a maximum core body temperature of 39°C for 5 consecutive days; (2) visceral suppuration (such as abscess or empyema) that required operative intervention for drainage; (3) reoperation, for debridement of an infected site; (4) positive blood culture; or (5) septic shock (systolic pressure less than 80 mmHg) in the postoperative period. Lesser infections, such as wound, urinary tract, or pulmonary infection that did not meet at least one of the previously described criteria were not considered as a septic event for purposes of this study.

Using these criteria and definitions, the frequency of these clinical variables was identified in the whole population of surgical patients that was reviewed. Table 2–3 identifies those clinical variables that were present among patients with multiple organ failure more often than in the population as a whole. Neither head injury nor long bone fractures were found to have statistical significance.

From this preliminary assessment, several observations could be made. Shock, blood resuscitation, crystalloid resuscitation, total volume resuscitation, and sepsis had a similar relationship to multiple organ failure as outcome; that is, 24 to 29% of patients who had each variable identified subsequently developed multiple organ failure. Furthermore, 34 of the 38 patients (89%) who developed multiple organ failure had sepsis as an associated clinical variable. The high frequency of sepsis among the patients with multiple organ failure suggested that uncontrolled infection may be an important process.

Accordingly, uncontrolled infection was then examined as a single variable that may have the greatest significance for the emergence of multiple organ failure. When the entire population of 123 patients with sepsis was eliminated from the study population, none of the previously significant variables remained statistically valid. However, the elimination of 67 patients with shock from the study population left sepsis as a highly significant variable in association with the emergence of multiple organ failure. Similarly, the deletion of the other significant clinical variables from the whole population also identified sepsis as a highly significant variable.

Because shock and large volume resuscitation were significant variables until sepsis was removed, this suggested that there was a relationship between hypovolemia or shock and the subsequent development of invasive infection. We then examined the 67 patients who were identified as having oligemic shock. Twenty-seven of these patients developed sepsis. This relationship between shock and sepsis was statistically significant (p < 0.001). These data led to the conclusion at that time (1980) that shock had immunosuppressive sequelae that may render the host more vulnerable to invasive infection and, hence, to multiple organ failure.

However, recent evidence has focused on the immunosuppressive effects of blood transfusion.[20,21] Although not specifically emphasized in our original publication, massive blood transfusion was as statistically valid a predictor of sepsis as oligemic shock. Indeed, all 67 patients with shock received blood transfusions even though not all met the criteria of massive transfusion. The only valid conclusions that can be implied from these data are that shock and its treatment appear to be associated with the development of severe infection, and that uncontrolled infection has the strongest association with the development of multiple organ failure.

Site-Organism Specificity in Multiple Organ Failure

In initial publications, Eiseman et al.[10] and Polk and Shields[22] emphasized the necessity for aggressive surgical management of the patient with multiple organ failure. Organ failure became an indication for laparotomy, and infection-associated organ failure became identified with intra-abdominal sepsis. However, in reviewing our 123 patients with sepsis from the initial population of 553 postoperative subjects, it was interesting to note that pleuropulmonary sepsis and intra-abdominal sepsis occurred with equal frequency.[3] Furthermore, when patients were categorized by their site of most severe infection, many of the patients with intra-abdominal infection subsequently developed secondary pulmonary infection during their hospital course. Among the 32 deaths from sepsis in the total population of patients in this series, pulmonary infection was the principal septic focus in 14 patients, whereas lethal intra-abdominal infections occurred in 14 patients. Thus, pleuropulmonary sepsis appears to be at least as significant as intra-abdominal infection in multiple organ failure. In subsequent studies, we have shown that intra-abdominal infection is statistically associated with intercurrent pulmonary sepsis and that intra-abdominal infection impairs pulmonary bacterial clearance.[23,24] My recent experience has been consistent with the studies of Hunt[25] in that patients with intra-abdominal infection are as likely to die of intercurrent pulmonary sepsis as they are from the inciting intra-abdominal process. As has been emphasized by Siegel et al.[12] and Cerra et al.,[26] multiple organ failure is a response of the host to infection and is not site specific.

The role of specific organisms as mediators of the organ failure cascade has been the subject of considerable speculation. The lipopolysaccharide-bearing bacterial organisms have been most commonly associated with sepsis and septic shock. For that reason, endotoxemia has been considered by many researchers to be important in the pathogenesis of organ failure. However, we have identified enterococcemia,[27] *Bacteroides fragilis* bacteremia,[5] and candidemia[28] as being

Table 2–4   Temporal Sequence of Organ Failure in Those Patients with Sepsis

Clinical Event	No. Days After Operation ($\pm$ SD)
Clinical sepsis	2.6 $\pm$ 5.6
Pulmonary failure	2.3 $\pm$ 3.8
Hepatic failure	5.7 $\pm$ 7.6
Stress gastrointestinal bleeding	9.9 $\pm$ 8.9
Renal failure	11.6 $\pm$ 19.1

equally important in the development of organ failure complexes. Deutschman et al.[29] have shown that the septic response of patients with viral infection is similar to that seen in patients with bacterial infection. Vary et al.[30] have even suggested that the severity of the septic response may be greater with anaerobic pathogens than the commonly identified endotoxin-laden enteric gram-negative bacteria. At present, the septic response and subsequent organ dysfunction must be viewed as a sustained and exaggerated nonspecific response of the host, and no organism-specific relationship has yet been identified.

Sequence of Organ Failure

In our initial studies, we were interested in whether a definable sequence of organ failure could be characterized.[3] Important questions to be addressed included whether systems failure occurred in nearly a simultaneous fashion or whether a prototype model of sequential organ failure could be defined. Furthermore, if infection is the clinical variable that is causally related to multiple organ failure, then it would be important to identify the onset of infection prior to the subsequent cascade of events.

All patients who had one or more failed organ systems that were associated with infection were reviewed. The day of onset of clinical sepsis was determined from clinical criteria in the patient's record. The day of the initial emergency operation was used as day 0 for reference. The date of onset of infection and the initial day of onset of organ failure were then identified relative to the day of operation.

The day of onset of infection and of failure of each organ system is illustrated in Table 2–4. For the entire group, sepsis began 2.6 $\pm$ 5.6 days after operation. Pulmonary failure characteristically occurred first and tended to occur on the same day that clinical infection was recognized. The sequence was completed with hepatic failure occurring second and then stress gastrointestinal bleeding. Renal failure occurred last and generally was the harbinger of a fatal outcome.

Although this prototype sequence could be identified by averaging all patients together, individual patients commonly followed a totally independent se-

Table 2–5   **Frequency and Mortality Rates of Multiple Organ Failure Identified in Patients with Abdominal Abscess (n = 143), Bacteroides Bacteremia (n = 98), and Splenic Trauma (n = 337)**

Organ System: No. Organs	ABDOMINAL ABSCESS[4]		BACTEROIDES BACTEREMIA[5]		SPLENIC TRAUMA[6]	
	No.	% Mortality	No.	% Mortality	No.	% Mortality
Lung	46	74	23	87	61	48
Liver	66	50	42	62	61	39
Stress bleeding	17	65	11	55	17	53
Kidney	38	82	37	73	24	75
One	31	23	26	42	40	10
Two	15	53	15	67	22	41
Three	29	79	15	80	17	59
Four	4	100	3	100	7	100

quence. The reason for variation potentially relates to the physiologic reserve of each organ system. For example, patients with occult or overt underlying liver disease may demonstrate hepatic failure first. Patients with a creatinine clearance of 30% of normal frequently manifested renal failure at a much earlier point in the natural history of the process than would ordinarily be the case. Because the subjects in this series were relatively young and healthy trauma patients, we believe that the sequence of organ failure identified in this study group should most closely approximate the sequence of organ failure in patients with no or minimal underlying major organ dysfunction.

Validation of Patterns in Multiple Organ Failure

In an effort to validate the observations made in our initial study, three additional groups of patients were studied. Individual series of 143 patients with intra-abdominal abscess,[4] 98 patients with Bacteroides bacteremia,[5] and 337 patients undergoing spenectomy for trauma[6] were studied. Identical criteria were used to define organ failure as were used in the original study. The overall frequency of multiple organ failure was increased in the patients with intra-abdominal abscess or Bacteroides bacteremia, but was less frequent in the patients undergoing splenectomy for trauma.

The mortality rate by organ system for each of these three patient groups is illustrated in Table 2–5. Mortality rates were similar in the intra-abdominal abscess series as were noted in the original group of patients requiring emergency operations. In the Bacteroides bacteremia series, pulmonary failure had an apparent increase in mortality rate for undefined reasons. In the splenic trauma series, both pulmonary and liver dysfunction had relatively high frequencies of occurrence but very low mortality rates. These latter observations in the patients with splenic trauma are probably secondary to associated blunt chest and liver trauma.

In these series of patients, an effort was made to define those clinical variables that were associated with a fatal outcome. Numerous variables were identified as having statistical significance, including organ failure, presence of bacteremia, and age greater than 50 years.[4] The largest chi-quare value was identified for those patients in whom multiple organ failure occurred. These observations further support the association of uncontrolled infection with multiple organ failure.

Epidemiologic Considerations

The results of our studies, as well as observations by others, have led to the conclusion that the septic response is clearly associated with the evolution of multiple organ failure. Although numerous investigators are vigorously pursuing the mechanism that will explain the pathophysiologic events that translate infection into organ failure, no clear explanation is presently available.

Because uncontrolled infection appeared as the preeminent variable, we and others have advocated an aggressive approach to infection management in the hope that better control of established infections will reverse the cascade of events.[4,22,31] Aggressive antibiotic use and liberal application of reoperation have had their advocates. However, some workers have suggested that empirical reoperation is a futile effort, regardless of whether or not suppurative collections are identified.[32,33]

Indeed, patients whom we have studied with enterococcal bacteremia[27] and candidemia[28] seem to have entered a futile phase of organ failure that defies conventional methods of antimicrobial chemotherapy or surgical drainage. In these groups of patients, the role of the gastrointestinal tract serving as a reservoir to fuel the process of the systemic septic response, and hence multiple organ failure, appears to be a reality.[34] The translocation of bacteria or bacterial cell products, or both, from the gastrointestinal tract may even have significance in the hypovolemic shock state.[35,36]

Thus, for many patients, infection, severe trauma, shock, and even soft tissue trauma appear to mediate the onset of multiple organ failure. It is of interest that multiple organ failure and the catabolism of the septic process may then in turn provoke the loss of gut host defenses, which in turn permits a polymicrobial sepsis that fuels the organ failure complex. A self-energizing cycle of sepsis that begets multiple organ failure, which begets more sepsis, creates a futile cycle that is unresponsive to conventional management. Clearly, the challenge of the future is to unravel this complex process and pave the way for new and innovative treatment modalities.

References

1. Baue AE. Multiple, progressive, or sequential systems failure. Arch Surg 1975;110:779–781.
2. Tilney NL, Bailey GL, Morgan AP. Sequential system failure after rupture of abdominal aortic aneurysms: an unsolved problem in postoperative care. Ann Surg 1973;178:117–122.

3. Fry DE, Pearlstein L, Fulton RL, Polk HC Jr. Multiple system organ failure: the role of uncontrolled infection. Arch Surg 1980;115:136–140.

4. Fry DE, Garrison RN, Heitch RC, et al. Determinants of death in patients with intraabdominal abscess. Surgery 1980;89:517–523.

5. Fry DE, Garrison RN, Polk HC Jr. Clinical implications in Bacteroides bacteremia. Surg Gynecol Obstet 1979;149:189–192.

6. Fry DE, Garrison RN, Williams HC. Patterns of morbidity and mortality in splenectomy for trauma. Am Surg 1980;46:28–32.

7. MacLean LD, Mulligan WG, McLean AP, et al. Patterns of septic shock in man—a detailed study of 56 patients. Ann Surg 1967;166:543–548.

8. Siegel JH, Greenspan M, Del Guercio LR. Abnormal vascular tone, defective oxygen transport and myocardial failure in human septic shock. Ann Surg 1967;165:504–511.

9. Fulton RL, Jones CE. The cause of post-traumatic pulmonary insufficiency in man. Surg Gynecol Obstet 1975;140:179–186.

10. Eiseman B, Beart R, Norton L. Multiple organ failure. Surg Gynecol Obstet 1977;144:323–326.

11. Clowes GHA Jr, O'Donnell TF Jr, Ryan NT, et al. Energy metabolism in sepsis; treatment based on different patterns in shock and high output stage. Ann Surg 1974;179:684–693.

12. Siegel JH, Cerra FB, Coleman B, et al. Physiologic and metabolic correlations in human sepsis. Surgery 1979;86:63–93.

13. Miller LD, Oski FA, Diaco JF, et al. The affinity of hemoglobin for oxygen: its control and in vivo significance. Surgery 1970;68:187–192.

14. Schumer W, Das Gupta TK, Moss GS, et al. Effect of endotoxemia on liver cell mitochondria in man. Ann Surg 1970;171:875–882.

15. Mela L, Bacalzo, LV Jr, Miller LD. Defective oxidative metabolism of rat liver mitochondria in hemorrhage and endotoxin shock. Am J Physiol 1971;220:571–577.

16. Fry DE, Silver BB, Rink RD, et al. Hepatic cellular hypoxia in murine peritonitis. Surgery 1979;85:652–661.

17. Rutherford RB, Balis JV, Trow RS, et al. Comparison of hemodynamic and regional blood flow changes at equivalent stages of endotoxin and hemorrhagic shock. J Trauma 1976;16:886–897.

18. Scovill WA, Saba TM, Kaplan JE, et al. Deficits in reticuloendothelial humoral control mechanisms in patients after trauma. J Trauma 1976;16:898–904.

19. Fry DE. Multiple system organ failure. Surg Clin North Am 1988;68:107–122.

20. Waymack JP, Warden GD, Alexander JW, et al. Effect of blood transfusion and anesthesia on resistance to bacterial peritonitis. J Surg Res 1987;42:528–535.

21. Waymack JP, Robb E, Alexander JW. Effect of transfusion on immune function in a traumatized animal model. II. Effect on mortality rate following septic challenge. Arch Surg 1987;122:935–939.

22. Polk HC Jr, Shields CL. Remote organ failure: a valid sign of occult intra-abdominal infection. Surgery 1977;81:310–313.

23. Richardson JD, Fry DE, Van Arsdall LR, et al. Pulmonary bacterial clearance in peritonitis. J Surg Res 1979;26:499–503.

24. Richardson JD, DeCamp MM, Garrison RN, et al. Pulmonary infection complicating intra-abdominal sepsis: clinical and experimental observations. Ann Surg 1982;195:732–738.

25. Hunt JL. Generalized peritonitis: to irrigate or not to irrigate the abdominal cavity. Arch Surg 1982;117:209–212.

26. Cerra FB, Siegel JH, Coleman B. Septic autocannibalism: a failure of exogenous nutritional support. Ann Surg 1980; 192:570–578.

27. Garrison RN, Fry DE, Berberich S, et al. Enterococcal bacteremia: clinical implications and determinants of death. Ann Surg 1982;196:43–48.

28. Dyess DL, Garrison RN, Fry DE. Candida sepsis: implications of polymicrobial blood-borne infection. Arch Surg 1985;120:345–349.

29. Deutschman CS, Konstantinides FN, Tsai M, et al. Physiology and metabolism in isolated viral septicemia: further evidence of an organism-independent, host-dependent response. Arch Surg 1987;122:21–25.

30. Vary TC, Siegel JH, Tall B, Morris JG. Role of anaerobic bacteria in intra-abdominal septic abscesses in mediating septic control of skeletal muscle glucose oxidation and lactic acidemia. Presented at the annual meeting of the American Association for the Surgery of Trauma, Newport Beach, CA, October 6, 1988.

31. Hinsdale JG, Jaffe BM. Reoperation for intra-abdominal sepsis: indications and results in modern critical care setting. Ann Surg 1984;199:31–36.

32. Norton LW. Does drainage of intra-abdominal pus reverse multiple organ failure? Am J Surg 1985;149:347–351.

33. Bunt TJ. Non-direct relaparotomy for intra-abdominal sepsis: a futile procedure. Am Surg 1986;52:294–298.

34. Carrico CJ, Meakins JL, Marshall JC, et al. Multiple organ failure syndrome. Arch Surg 1986;121:196–203.
35. Fine J, Moore FD. Irreversible shock. N Engl J Med 1963;268:107–108.
36. Deitch LA, Bridges W, Baker J, et al. Hemorrhagic shock-induced bacterial translocation is reduced by xanthine oxidase inhibition or inactivation. Surgery 1988;104:191–198.

3

Role of Scoring Systems in Multiple Organ Failure

Christopher C. Baker

Life can be understood backwards, but it must be lived forwards.
—Kierkegaard

The syndrome of multiple organ failure (MOF) has emerged in the 1980s as one of the major clinical problems vexing clinicians caring for critically ill and injured patients. Although MOF can certainly affect pediatric and medical patients, the comments here will be directed toward surgical patients. Part of the problem in evaluating the MOF syndrome has been in defining MOF. The reader is directed elsewhere for a complete discussion of this issue.[1] Suffice it to say that the definition of MOF has centered around a characterization of the MOF syndrome. It is clear that sepsis is a concomitant problem and may even be a causal factor in 50 to 75% of patients with MOF.[2-4] Part of the problem in defining MOF from a clinical standpoint has been that the patient populations in reported series tend to be diverse (such as trauma or general surgical patients) rather than homogeneous (such as burn patients). In addition, until recently, there have not been any reproducible sublethal animal models of MOF.

Since our clinical efforts to treat established MOF so often fail, a major clinical challenge in MOF has been to identify patients at risk for developing the MOF syndrome in order to concentrate intensive efforts toward preventing MOF. To aid in prognostication and to allow comparison of different groups of patients from different institutions, a number of scoring systems have been advanced in recent years. Although the predictive accuracy of the current scoring systems for the individual patients is limited, they are very accurate when applied to large patient populations. Thus, these scoring systems are potentially powerful tools for comparing outcome between different patient populations. In fact, only by using these scoring systems to stratify patients according to severity of injury or physiologic dysfunction, will it be possible to evaluate critically the modalities directed toward the prevention or treatment of MOF. Therefore it is important for the practicing clinician to be familiar with the various scoring systems. To that end, this chapter will address three issues. First, the major scoring systems will be summarized and analyzed. Second, data from the surgical intensive care unit (SICU) at Yale-New Haven Hospital (YNHH) will be presented to illustrate the clinical utility of scoring systems. Finally, an attempt will be made to put the role of scoring systems into a useful clinical perspective.

Background

In 1973 Tilney et al.[5] identified the pattern of MOF in patients undergoing surgery for ruptured abdominal aortic aneurysms. In 1975, Baue[6] was one of the first investigators to analyze and stress the sequential nature of organ failure that occurs in MOF. Eiseman et al.[3] made a major contribution in 1977 by identifying risk factors for MOF in a carefully analyzed but diverse group of 42 patients. In this study, Eiseman et al. characterized risk factors as follows: (1) premorbid factors such as diabetes, cancer, cirrhosis, and cardiopulmonary disease; (2) pathophysiologic factors, such as prolonged hypotension, hypothermia, or acidosis; (3) injury factors, such as drug overdose, major trauma or thermal injury, major surgery; (4) treatment factors, including massive transfusions, prolonged immobilization, antibiotic abuse, steroids, and malnutrition; and (5) complications, such as untreated sepsis, coagulopathies, necrotic tissue, and nosocomial infections.[3] One of the most important clinical lessons of Eiseman et al.'s study was that patients with MOF often have been subject to a clinical error of omission (for example, missed esophageal injury) or commission (24 of 42 cases).[3] Intra-abdominal sepsis was present in 22 of the 29 patients with sepsis and MOF,[3] a point that has been emphasized more recently by Fry et al.[7]

Given this plethora of information, how does the clinician identify the patient at risk for MOF and avoid making errors that might lead to MOF? The former question can be answered with a crystal ball and intuition, but some of the scoring systems discussed later may help in identifying the high-risk patient. The latter goal can only be approached asymptotically with a high index of suspicion, expert care from medical and nursing staff, and superb clinical judgment. Remember the old adage about judgment: "Good judgement comes from experience, and experience comes from bad judgement."

Scoring Systems

A number of authors have written on the subject of scoring systems for critically ill and injured patients.[8–12] Some of these systems have been designed specifically for trauma patients, such as the trauma score (TS) developed by Sacco and Champion[8] and the Injury Severity Score (ISS) originated by Susan Baker.[9] The TS is a physiologic system that can be used prospectively, whereas the ISS rates injury on an anatomic basis after all injuries have been assessed. Other scoring systems than the TS and ISS are more applicable to intensive care unit (ICU) patients, since they combine physiologic and anatomic information with demographic and risk factor data. Examples of these systems are the Acute Physiology and Chronic Health Evaluation (APACHE) score first described by Knaus et al.[10] in 1981 or a sepsis severity scoring system, such as those proposed by Elebute and Stoner[11] or Stevens.[12] Although a number of these systems are complex, they share two common features. First, they allow comparison of patients with comparable levels of severity of injury or illness (comparing apples to apples rather than apples to oranges). Second, they attempt to identify prospectively those patients who are at increased risk for morbidity or mortality in the SICU. A summary of these scoring systems follows.

Trauma Scoring Systems

Patients with thermal injury constitute a relatively homogeneous population, and their risk factors for morbidity and mortality have been well characterized. The major factors predicting outcome after thermal injury are age, percent body surface area burned, percent full-thickness burn, the presence or absence of inhalation injury, and premorbid diseases. In fact, these data are so reproducible that they have been incorporated into a formula allowing prediction of likelihood of survival following thermal injury by Zawacki et al.[13] On the other hand, trauma patients—with their multiple fractures, contusions, torso and head injuries—represent a much more heterogeneous group of patients that makes analysis and prediction of outcome more difficult.

The first major advance in the scoring of trauma patients occurred in 1974 when Teasdale and Jennet[14] introduced a simple system for assessing neurologic status after head injury. This system has been popularized as the Glasgow Coma Scale (GCS) and is outlined in Table 3–1. Although GCS is a powerful tool in the acute prognostic assessment of trauma patients, when the GCS is combined with anatomic information on the nature of the head injury, the ability to predict outcome is substantially improved.[15] Obviously, a number of factors unrelated to head injury (such as shock, alcohol, drugs, hypothermia, acidosis, intubation) can confound the GCS. In addition, a number of us have seen patients with severe isolated head injury with a GCS of 3 who have survived and made a substantial recovery to a productive existence. Nonetheless, the GCS remains a remarkably simple and reliable physiologic tool in assessing the neurologic status of acutely injured patients.

Utilizing the GCS with other physiologic variables of respiratory and cardiovascular function, Sacco and Champion devised the TS and reported on its use in trauma patients in 1981.[8] This scoring system has been validated in more than 50,000 multiple trauma patients throughout the country and been found to be a powerful means of predicting outcome in diverse populations of trauma patients (Table 3–1). Because of some difficulties in the use of the original TS in

Table 3–1   Trauma Score*

Component	Clinical Evaluation	Score	Total GCS Points
Respiratory rate	10–24/min	4	
	24–35/min	3	
	≥ 36/min	2	
	1–9/min	1	
	None	0	
Respiratory expansion	Normal	1	
	Retractive	0	
Systolic blood pressure	≥ 90 mmHg	4	
	70–89 mmHg	3	
	50–69 mmHg	2	
	0–49 mmHg	1	
	No pulse	0	
Glasgow Coma Scale			
Eye opening	Spontaneous	4	
	To voice	3	
	To pain	2	
	None	1	
Verbal response	Oriented	5	14 – 15 = 5
	Confused	4	11 – 13 = 4
	Inappropriate words	3	8 – 10 = 3
	Incomprehensible words	2	5 – 7 = 2
	None	1	3 – 4 = 1
Motor response	Obeys commands	6	
	Localizes pain	5	
	Withdraws (pain)	4	
	Flexion (pain)	3	
	Extension (pain)	2	
	None	1	
Total trauma score			1–16

*From Champion, et al.[37] Reprinted with permission.

the field, two items—respiratory expansion and capillary refill—were dropped in 1986, leading to the revised TS.[16] Predicted mortality rates for various levels of TS are shown in Table 3–2.

In addition to the physiologic TS, an anatomic assessment of severity of injury was introduced by Susan Baker in 1974 and updated in 1976.[9] The ISS, because of its complexity, will not be outlined in detail here. Basically, the ISS depends on coding of injuries using the Abbreviated Injury Scale (AIS) promulgated in 1971.[17] After the AIS scores for various areas of the body (such as central nervous system, respiratory, cardiovascular, abdomen, skin, and musculoskeletal) are determined, the ISS is obtained by adding the squares of the AIS scores for the three most seriously injured anatomic regions. The maximum score is 75, which correlates with a fatal injury. In general, mortality is proportional to ISS,[18] although patients with advanced age (older than 70 years) and those with penetrating abdominal trauma may have higher mortality rates than predicted for a given ISS. More recently, the TS and ISS have been utilized in the so-called TRISS methodology,[19] which graphs mortality as a function of ISS and TS for

Table 3–2 Survival Rates Indicated by Trauma Score*

Trauma Score	Survival (%)
16	99
15	98
14	96
13	93
12	87
11	76
10	60
9	42
8	26
7	15
6	8
5	4
4	2
3	1
2	0
1	0

*From Champion, et al.[37]
Reprinted with permission.

individual patients. This technique has been incorporated into the Major Trauma Outcome Study of the American College of Surgeons and has allowed hospitals to compare their results to a national standard and to compare results between hospitals. In addition, quality assurance programs within hospitals can evaluate patients who were predicted to live by TRISS but actually died, or vice versa.

Despite these major advances in trauma scoring systems, most trauma surgeons would agree on several points: (1) the ideal scoring system has not been developed (witness the plethora of other systems in the literature not discussed); (2) a number of other factors that are difficult to quantify (such as mechanism of injury, transport time, level of prehospital care, quality of hospital care, premorbid state) may affect an individual patient's response to injury; and (3) current systems aid in categorizing trauma patients but are not yet sophisticated enough as prognostic indices to aid in clinical decision-making for an individual patient (that is, to treat or not to treat, as per Zawacki et al.[13] in burns).

Scoring Systems in the Intensive Care Unit

If trauma patients represent a heterogeneous group, the critically ill patients residing in an SICU bring new meaning to the term "mixed bag." Nonetheless, there are certain physiologic and pathophysiologic derangements that these patients share. Sepsis, single-organ failure, and MOF are often multifactorial in nature; unfortunately, the resultant effects of organ dysfunction are the same, and death is the final common pathway. The challenge in evaluating MOF in the SICU has been as follows: (1) to categorize heterogeneous patients so that they can be compared within and between institutions; (2) to identify prospectively those patients at high risk for sepsis and MOF; and (3) to understand better the basic mechanisms leading to sepsis and MOF so that prophylactic and therapeutic measures can be devised to attack these dreaded complications in high-risk patients.

There have been a plethora of scoring systems advanced for scoring severity of illness and for categorizing patients in the ICU setting. Dellinger[20] recently collated an excellent review on this subject with detailed tabular and graphic summaries. The interested reader is referred to this valuable resource for further information.

In the early 1980s, the first major attempt to score severity of illness in the ICU was advanced by Knaus et al.[10] The original APACHE scoring system combined the patient's chronic health status with 34 physiologic data points collected on admission to the ICU. The patient was placed in one of four chronic health categories (A–D):

- A: no functional limitations
- B: mild to moderate limitation of activity due to chronic disease
- C: serious, but not incapacitating, restriction of activity due to chronic disease
- D: severe restriction of activity, including bedridden and institutionalized patients

The 34 physiologic data points included cardiovascular, respiratory, renal, gastrointestinal, hematologic, neurologic, septic, and metabolic measurements. The data are scored from 0 to 4. Thus, depending on the degree of disruption of physiologic homeostasis (4 being the farthest from normal), the final APACHE score can range from 0 to 124. The APACHE system has been validated as a reliable predictor of mortality in the ICU in both the United States and France.[21] More recently, Knaus and coworkers[22] have streamlined their system by decreasing the number of measured physiologic variables from 34 to 12 and by modifying the weight of certain variables. In this new system, APACHE II, the maximum possible score is 71.[22] APACHE II is simpler than the original system and yet is slightly better than the original in predicting mortality.

In a study of 5677 ICU patients, of whom 2719 (48%) developed acute failure of one or more organs, Knaus et al.[23] documented that mortality was related to the patient's age, the number of organs failing, and the duration of organ failure. For example, the mortality rate for patients with organ failure of a single organ that lasted longer than 1 day was 40%, which increased to 60% when two organs failed. In 99 patients with MOF (more than three organs) lasting more than 3 days, mortality was 98%.[23] Unfortunately, this important article did not include data on APACHE scores. They did mention data on the Therapeutic Intervention Scoring System (TISS) of Cullen et al.,[24] but since this system seems to measure epiphenomena rather than physiologic indices, it is less widely used.

Clearly, none of us wish to prolong the inevitable in the ICU patient in whom survival is unprecedented. Nonetheless, as pointed out by Feinstein,[25] our technologic and therapeutic abilities have outstripped our scientific understanding of prediction and risk stratification. Regarding these powerful but complex systems of scoring ICU patients, the following quotation by Dellinger[20] remains relevant:

> All of the systems are more accurate in predicting death than in predicting survival. All do well for populations of patients, but are inappropriate for use in therapeutic decisions concerning an individual patient.

Sepsis Scoring Systems

Several investigators have utilized the acute physiology score (APS) from the APACHE system to evaluate patients with sepsis, particularly intra-abdominal infections.[26-28] Pine et al.[26] confirmed the validity of the APS in intra-abdominal sepsis and added the following predictive factors: age, shock, malnutrition, and alcoholism. In 1984, Meakins and Solomkin[27] proposed a stratification scheme that combined the APS with a general and specific anatomic classification. In 1985, Dellinger et al.[28] evaluated the APS in 187 patients with intra-abdominal sepsis and found striking correlation between APS and mortality rate. Although age and malnutrition again emerged as risk factors, many other clinical factors (such as shock, site and degree of infection, peritonitis, diabetes) did not emerge as independent predictors of mortality when the data were controlled for APS.

Somewhat earlier in 1983, Stevens[12] in the United States and Elebute and Stoner[11] in England attempted to devise actual scoring systems for sepsis. The system developed by Stevens, dubbed the sepsis severity score (SSS), was based on scoring organ dysfunction (1, least; 5–6, most) for seven organ systems: lung, kidney, coagulation, cardiovascular, liver, gastrointestinal tract and neurologic.[12] Because of his recognition of the cumulative effect of MOF in sepsis, Stevens adopted the geometric model that had been utilized for the ISS by Susan Baker.[9] Therefore the overall SSS was determined by adding the squares of the scores for the three organ systems with the most severe dysfunction. Steven's original report, pithy, as are so many seminal papers, described the SSS and tested it prospectively in 30 patients with "surgical" sepsis. The mean SSS in survivors was 29 versus 49 in nonsurvivors ($p < 0.001$), and the SSS appeared to be effective in tracking the progress of individual patients.[12] The SSS was later compared with the APS by Skau et al.[29] from Sweden, who modified the SSS slightly to decrease subjectivity. They studied 58 patients, 16 or whom died (28%). There was good correlation between the two scoring systems; the mortality rate was 83% when the APS or SSS was greater than 30, whereas no patient with a score of less than 10 died. Both methods show a significant correlation with mortality, although the value for SSS ($r = 0.68$) was slightly higher than for APS ($r = 0.56$). Analysis of other factors showed that there was an added predictive value for the combination of age over 60 years and chronic disease with APS but only age over 60 years was a factor with the SSS. The points that come out in the discussion of this and the previously mentioned articles are as follows: (1) it is important to have an objective, reproducible system (or systems) that can be used to describe patients and to compare patients for multicenter trials; (2) the physiologic response of the host to the disruption of homeostasis following sepsis is probably far more critical to predicting outcome than traditional clinical factors; and (3) future studies need to incorporate immunologic and metabolic data and to define their role better in predicting outcome after sepsis and MOF.

Another approach to the problem of scoring in sepsis was advanced by Elebute and Stoner.[11] They divided the response to sepsis into four classes: local effects, temperature response, systemic effects, and laboratory data. Subjective degrees of severity were scored on an analogue scale. The values for the sepsis score (SS) ranged from 0 to 45, and the breaking point for survival or nonsurvival in the initial report of 15 patients was an SS of 20.[11] The SS was later tested in a larger group of 135 critically ill ICU patients (56% mortality) by Dominioni and associates[30] from Italy. The initial SS was a strong predictor of outcome; the mortality rates were 100% for a SS above 30 (n = 8), 89% for a SS above 20 (n = 71), and 20% for a SS of 20 or less (n = 64). Clearly, this was a severely ill group of patients, since only 12% had an initial SS less than 16. If an SS of 20 is chosen as the point above which death is predicted, the overall accuracy in this study was 84% (114 of 135).

The Dominioni study, in addition to supporting the SS, added the important dimension of measuring acute-phase proteins (APP). In 85 of their 135 patients they monitored the following APP on a serial basis: α_1-acid glycoprotein; α_1-antitrypsin, complement factor B, and complement products C3 and C3a.[30] Thirty-five of these patients survived (41%), and the survivors had significantly higher levels of all the APP than nonsurvivors (p <0.001). Interestingly, C3a levels, elevated in all patients, were slightly higher in nonsurvivors. These data suggested that excessive complement activation appears to be associated with increased mortality. Based on these studies, Dominioni and coauthors proposed yet another scoring system to assess probability of survival from severe surgical sepsis, the Sepsis Index of Survival (SIS). It is ironic, if not touching, that this acronymic designation is the same as that for the Surgical Infection Society, where this study was first presented (Chicago, April, 1986). At any rate, the SIS derives from the following formula:

$$\text{SIS\%} = 121 + 0.26 \times (\text{factor B}) + 0.36 \times (\alpha_1\text{-acid glycoprotein}) - 6 \times (\text{SS})$$

The SIS correctly predicted outcome in 74 patients (87%) in Dominioni's study of 85 patients. The SIS score uses a cutoff of 50% in predicting survival versus death. Survival is predicted when the SIS score is 50% or greater, death is predicted in patients who score less than 50%. The sensitivity and specificity of the SIS in predicting outcome in this study were 88% and 86%, respectively.[30] Presumably, modifications in decision analysis[25] or further variables may be able to improve the predictive accuracy of the SIS. Nonetheless, the added laboratory data for the SIS are somewhat cumbersome to obtain and did not substantially improve on the predictive value of the SS alone (84%).

Before closing this section, I should mention that recent studies in the area of scoring of sepsis have added some new ideas and fueled some old controversies. In a small study of 45 patients with sepsis (14 deaths), Dudley and coworkers tested their hypothesis that the local effects portion of the sepsis score was less important than the physiologic response to sepsis by comparing the SS of Elebute and Stoner to the APACHE II.[31] Although the SS for nonsurvivors (21.5) was higher than for survivors (14, p <0.05), there was overlap between the two groups and there was no difference between the two groups in the local component of the SS. Both the APACHE II and the systemic component of SS were significantly increased in the nonsurvivors; the Apache II correctly identified 13 of the 14 nonsurvivors and appeared to be better at predicting survival than the SS. The investigators suggest that SS "is more relevant to the grading of the metabolic effects of sepsis than to prediction of survival,"[31] but clearly larger multicenter trials are needed to address this question.

Yale SICU Experience

While the scoring systems just discussed were being developed and published, we were reorganizing the care of trauma and SICU patients at YNHH. The results of this reorganization will be summarized briefly.[32] Prior to the institution of a dedicated trauma service, the mortality rate for trauma patients in our ICU setting was 16.1% (31 of 193), and one third of these patients died with sepsis or MOF, or both. Following the creation of a dedicated trauma service in July 1983, mortality for ICU trauma patients decreased to 11% in the first year and was 4 to 5% thereafter. Much of this improvement appeared to be due to a decrease in the incidence and mortality of sepsis and MOF.

In 1982 and 1983, data were accumulated on outcome of all SICU patients by Joseph DeSantis as part of the M.D. thesis requirement for the Yale University School of Medicine.[33] Initially retrospective data on 216 patients admitted to the SICU (June 1 to September 30, 1982) were analyzed in a detailed fashion in order to determine the relationship between putative predictive parameters and subsequent morbidity and mortality. Prospective data collection was then undertaken in a second group of 150 patients (January 1 to August 31, 1983), and the prognostically important variables identified in the retrospective study were tested to verify their ability to predict morbidity and mortality.

Data accumulated in this study include demographic information, surgical service, APACHE score, certain multiple additional laboratory tests (such as lipase), cardiovascular hemodynamic data (when available). Data were compared for survivors and nonsurvivors and for retrospective and prospective patients by appropriate use of the two-tailed *t* test or chi-square analysis. An attempt was made to stratify the risk of subsequent complications using a categorical response program (FUNCAT) as described by Landis et al.[34] Complications were divided into four classes according to their relative threat to life:[33]

1. Class 1: remotely life-threatening (such as fever, anemia, chest pain without electrocardiac (ECG) changes)
2. Class 2: mildly life-threatening (such as ECG changes, ileus, mild congestive heart failure)
3. Class 3: moderately life-threatening (such as myocardial infarction, pneumonia, intra-abdominal abscess, fistula)
4. Class 4: immediately life-threatening (such as septic shock, respiratory failure, renal failure, hypotension requiring pressor agents, cardiac arrest)

Table 3–3 SICU Length of Stay Versus Mortality

Total Days in SICU	Total No. Patients	Mortality (%)
1	152	6.0
2	78	10.8
3	58	7.4
4	18	11.1
5	16	18.8
6	10	30.0
7–14	24	26.1
15–21	4	25.0
>21	6	83.3
Total	366	11.2

Table 3–4 Complications by Class

Group	CLASS 1		CLASS 2		CLASS 3		CLASS 4	
	No.	%	No.	%	No.	%	No.	%
Retrospective Population	44	20	59	27	109	50	74	34
Prospective Population	37	25	34	23	59	39	30	19*
Total Population	81	22	93	25	168	46	104	28

*Significantly lower than retrospective population (chi-square, p <0.01).

The mortality for the entire study population was 11.2% (41 of 366). As in previous studies,[35,36] length of stay (LOS) was inversely related to the chance of survival, as shown in Table 3–3.[33] The survivors had a mean LOS in the ICU of 2.6 days compared with 7.9 days in nonsurvivors (p = 0.007). A total of 444 complications developed in 176 patients (48%). The data on development of complications outlined in Table 3–4 are particularly interesting, since the incidence of class 4 complications was significantly lower in the later prospective group,[33] paralleling the results seen after implementation of a dedicated trauma service.[32] The most common of the severe class 4 complications was sepsis, which occurred in 26 patients (7.1%), followed by profound hypotension (17 patients, 4.6%), respiratory failure requiring intubation (16 patients, 4.4%), renal failure (10 patients, 2.7%), neurologic failure (5 patients, 1.4%) hepatic failure (2 patients, 0.5%), and adult respiratory distress syndrome (2 patients, 0.5%). Not surprisingly, all but 2 of the 244 patients without complications or with complication scores of 1 or 2 (defined as the class of the most severe complication the patient sustained) survived. The 55 patients with class 3 complications also

Table 3–5   Health Status Versus Outcome

Group	A No.	A %	B No.	B %	C No.	C %	D No.	D %
Survivors	62	97	111	93	125	83	15	88
Nonsurvivors	2	3	8	7	25	17	2	12*
Total[†]	64	18.6	119	34	150	42.6	17	4.9

*Significantly higher mortality in C and D versus A and B (chi-square, p <0.001).

[†]Total number of patients is 345 because complete data were not available on 21 patients.

had a low mortality rate (3.7%), whereas the 67 patients with class 4 complications had a significantly increased mortality rate of 55.2% (p <0.001).

Analysis of the predictive power of admission parameters in the study were somewhat disappointing. Admission parameters that were significantly different between survivors and nonsurvivors include the following: age, lowest level of systolic blood pressure (first 24 hours), peak and low diastolic blood pressure, peak level of pulmonary artery diastolic pressure, peak temperature, peak potassium, blood urea nitrogen, white blood cell count, and albumin. Risk of mortality was particularly high in patients who were intubated, had sepsis, had a temperature less than 36°C, were comatose (mortality of 47%), or who sustained respiratory (78%) or cardiac (83%) arrests. The numbers of patients in the latter three groups were not sufficient to perform a valid statistical analysis. Analysis of APACHE data revealed a significantly higher mortality in patients with C or D status than in those with A or B status, as shown in Table 3–5.

After exhaustive analysis of the retrospective data, four variables were chosen as most valuable in predicting a complication score of 4 based on the FUNCAT procedure:[32] low systolic blood pressure, peak blood urea nitrogen, peak total bilirubin, and intubation. The following equation was devised:

$$X = 0.3873 \times A + 0.5180 \times B + 0.2315 \times C + 0.08451 \times D - 0.8568$$

where A = 1 if systolic blood pressure is less than 90 mmHg, B = 1 if patient is intubated, C = 1 if blood urea nitrogen is more than 20 mg/dl, and D = 1 if total bilirubin is more than 1.5 mg/dl.

The variable X in this equation is indicative of the relative risk of having a complication score of 4. Individual patients were categorized as being low risk ($X \leq -0.1$), intermediate risk ($-0.1 < X \leq 0.05$), and high risk ($X \geq 0.05$). When this equation and these risk categories were applied to the prospective data, it was found that 78% of patients predicted to be in the high-risk group went on to develop complication scores of 4, whereas 93% of patients at low risk had complication scores of less than 4. Remember that a complication score of 4 in this study was also highly predictive of a fatal outcome (55% mortality). Unfortunately, the sensitivity of the formula was poor, since only one third of the patients who actually had a complication score of 4 were predicted to be high risk by the formula. Although it has some intriguing elements, the complication scoring system developed in this study is limited in its ability to factor the number and severity of a patient's complications. Despite its limitations and (like other formulas) its inability to assist in clinical decision-making, this formula and data analysis does have a role in the SICU. Perhaps the role is to assist in allocation of critical care resources, by targeting those patients who are at low risk for complications (and therefore might benefit from early discharge) as well as those high-risk patients with long ICU stays (in whom ICU care has diminishing returns and may no longer be warranted).

Conclusion

This chapter has outlined the background and nature of various scoring systems for injury and sepsis as they relate to multiple organ failure. In addition, our experience in the Yale SICU and our efforts to predict morbidity and mortality from admission parameters have been outlined. Several lessons can be learned and suggestions tendered from the analysis.

First of all, MOF and sepsis are complex and profound disorders of homeostasis that can be well characterized as clinical syndromes in the SICU despite our incomplete understanding of the basic pathophysiology of these entities. Secondly, objective and reproducible systems are needed to allow us to categorize and compare patients who are at risk for developing or who have developed MOF. The trauma score (and the revised TS) is a valid, prospective tool that is a good, simple measure of the physiologic status of injured patients.[8] It can help in quality assurance of prehospital care and should be used in centers caring for multiple trauma patients. Susan Baker's ISS, and anatomic scaling of injury,[9] takes longer to assess but can be particularly powerful as a predictor and as a quality assurance tool.[19]

The scoring of physiologic status and the prediction of outcome (particularly survival) in the ICU is a more difficult issue. The APACHE[10] and APACHE II[22] scores, particularly the APS portion, seem to have the best results in quantitating the magnitude of disruptions in homeostasis of ICU patients. Of the various scoring systems for sepsis, the best appear to be the SSS of Stevens[12,29] or the SS of Elebute and Stoner.[11] The addition of APP data, as recommended by Dominioni,[30] seems to me to be a "long run for a short slide" in terms of added predictive power.

From the just-mentioned systems and our data analysis attempts at Yale, several concepts emerge. First, the ideal scoring system for MOF has not yet been defined. Second, even the perfect scoring system cannot replace clinical decision-making for individual patients. Third, future efforts in this area should concentrate on including simple and reproducible measures of other critical determinants of risk for developing MOF or sepsis, such as the patient's nutritional status, the metabolic aspects of energy production, and the immune host defense status. Finally, clinicians and investigators should study their own patient populations to see what lessons can be learned regarding ICU care and utilization of ICU resources.

What is the role of scoring systems in MOF? First, such systems can be used to compare patients in different institutions and to compare different forms of treatment. Second, they can predict the relative risk of death for SICU patients (with or without MOF) and can aid in following the response to treatment. Third, they allow one to test the role of various other factors as risks for sepsis and MOF, such as the recently demonstrated role of steroids as a risk factor independent of APACHE II scoring.[34] Finally, they can play a major role in quality assurance and resource utilization by helping us to evaluate objectively the care of critically ill and injured patients in our own institutions.

Acknowledgments.   The author thanks Joseph DeSantis, M.D., for permission to refer to his M.D. Thesis, Linda Degutis, M.S.N., for her editorial assistance, and Sandra Oronzo for preparing the manuscript.

References

1. Baker CC: Trauma in the 1980's: The "Success Story" of Multiple Organ Failure. In Maull KI, Cleveland HC, Strauch GO, Wolferth CC (eds): Advances in trauma, vol. III. Chicago: Year Book Medical Publishers, 1988:37–51.
2. Baker CC, Oppenheimer L, Stephens. B, et al. Epidemiology of trauma deaths. Am J Surg 1980;140:144–150.
3. Eiseman B, Beart R, Norton L. Multiple organ failure. Surg Gynecol Obstet 1977;144:323–326.
4. Faist E, Baue AE, Dittmer H, et al. Multiple organ failure in polytrauma patients. J Trauma 1983;23:775–787.
5. Tilney NL, Bailey GL, Morgan AP: Sequential systems failure after rupture of abdominal aortic aneurysms: an unsolved problem in postoperative care. Ann Surg 1973;178:117–122.
6. Baue AE: Multiple, progressive, or sequential systems failure: a syndrome of the 1970's. Arch Surg 1975;110:779–781.
7. Fry DE, Pearlstein L, Fulton RL, et al. Multiple system organ failure. Arch Surg 1980;115:1316–1400.
8. Sacco WJ, Carnazzo AJ, et al. Trauma score. Crit Care Med 1981;9:672–676.
9. Baker SP, O'Neill B: The injury severity score: an update. J. Trauma 1976;16:882–885.
10. Knaus WA, Zimmerman JE, Wagner DP, et al. APACHE—acute physiology and chronic health evaluation: A physiologically based classification system. Crit Care Med 1981;9:591–597.
11. Elebute EA, Stoner HB: The grading of sepsis. Br J Surg 1983;70:29–31.
12. Stevens LE: Gauging the severity of surgical sepsis. Arch Surg 1983;118:1190–1192.
13. Zawacki BE, Azon SP, Imbus SA, Chang YT. Multifactorial profit analysis of mortality in burned patients. Ann Surg 1979;189:1–5.
14. Teasdale G, Jennett B: Assessment of coma and impaired consciousness: a practical scale. Lancet 1974;2:81–83.
15. Levati A, Farina M, Vecchi G, et al. Prognosis of severe head injuries. Neurosurgery 1982;57:779–783.
16. Champion HR, Copes WW, Sacco WJ: Trauma registries. In Maull KI, Cleveland HC, Strauch GO, Wolferth CC (eds): Advances in trauma, vol. III. Chicago: Year Book Medical Publishers, 1988:241–261.
17. Committee on Medical Aspects of Automotive Safety. Rating the severity of tissue damage: I The Abbreviated Injury Scale. JAMA. 1971;215:277–280.
18. Gerritsen SM, van Loenhort T, Gimbrere JSF. Prognostic signs and mortality in multiply injured patients. Injury 1982;14:82–92.
19. Boyd CR, Tolson MA, Copes WS. Evaluating trauma care: the TRISS method. Trauma score and injury severity score. J Trauma 1987;217:370–378.
20. Dellinger EP: Use of scoring systems to assess patients with surgical sepsis. Surg Clin North Am 1988;68:123–145.

21. Knaus WA, LeGall Jr, Wagner DP, et al. A comparison of intensive care in the USA and France. Lancet 1982;2:642–646.
22. Knaus WA, Draper EA, Wagner DP, Zimmerman JE: APACHE II: a severity of disease classification system. Crit Care Med 1985;13:818–829.
23. Knaus WA, Draper EA, Wagner DP, Zimmerman JE: Prognosis in acute organ-system failure. Ann Surg 1985;202:685–693.
24. Cullen DJ, Civetta J, Briggs BA, Ferrara LC: Therapeutic intervention scoring system: a method for quantitative comparison of patient care. Crit Care Med 1974;2:57–60.
25. Feinstein AR. An additional basic science for clinical medicine: I. The constraining fundamental paradigms. Ann Intern Med 1983;99:393–397.
26. Pine RW, Wertz MJ, Leonard ES, et al. Determinants of organ malfunction or death in patients with intra-abdominal sepsis. Arch Surg 1983;118:242–249.
27. Meakins JL, Solomkin JS, Allo MD, et al. A proposed classification of intra-abdominal infections. Arch Surg 1984;119:1372–1378.
28. Dellinger EP, Wertz, MJ, Meakins JL, et al. Surgical infection stratification system for intra-abdominal infection. Arch Surg 1985;120:21–29.
29. Skau T, Nystrom P-O, Carlsson C: Severity of illness in intra-abdominal infection: a comparison of two indices. Arch Surg 1985;120:152–158.
30. Dominioni L, Dionigi R, Zanello M, et al. Sepsis score and acute-phase protein response as predictors of outcome in septic surgical patients. Arch Surg 1987;122:141–146.
31. Ponting GA, Sim AJW, Dudley HAF. Comparison of the local and systemic effects of sepsis in predicting survival. Br J Surg 1987;74:750–752.
32. Baker CC, Degutis LC, SeDantis JG, Baue AF. The impact of a trauma service on trauma care in a university hospital. Am J Surg 1985;149:453–458.
33. DeSantis JG. The value of admission parameters in predicting mortality and complications in surgical intensive care unit patients. M.D. Thesis. New Haven: Yale University School of Medicine, 1984.
34. Landis J, Stonish W, Freeman J, Koch G. A computer program for generalized chi-square analysis of categorical data using weighted least squares (Gen cat). Comp Prog Biomed 1976;6:196–231.
35. Scheffler RM, Knaus WA, Wagner DP, Zimmerman JE: Severity of illness and the relationship between intensive care and survival. Am J Public Health 1982;72:449–454.
36. Bohnen JMA, Mustard RA, Oxholm SE, Schouten D. APACHE II score and abdominal sepsis: a prospective study. Arch Surg 1988;123:225–229.
37. Champion HR, Sacco WJ, Carnazzo AJ, et al. Trauma score. Crit Care Med 1981;9:672–676.

4

Gut Failure: Its Role in the Multiple Organ Failure Syndrome

EDWIN A. DEITCH

The development of progressive sequential organ failure has emerged as a leading cause of death in the critically ill patient over the last two decades. Although this syndrome has been the focus of extensive clinical and laboratory study, the exact mechanisms responsible for its development and perpetuation are just beginning to be unraveled. One hypothesis that has received increasing attention is that gut failure plays an important role in the initiation or perpetuation of the multiple organ failure syndrome (MOFS). The clinical recognition that the gut may be the reservoir for bacteria-causing systemic infections in critically ill intensive care unit (ICU) patients has led Border and coworkers[1] to coin the term "gut septic states" to describe this phenomenon. The recognition that gut failure and distant organ failure may be causally related has prompted Meakins and others to consider the gut as the "motor" of multiple organ failure (MOF).[2,3]

In evaluating the hypothesis that gut failure is causally related to the development or perpetuation of MOF, several clinical facts must be considered. First, in most patients who develop the MOFS, many of the organs that fail are not directly injured or involved in the primary disease process. Additionally, there is a lag period of days and in some patients weeks between the initial insult and the development of distant organ failure. These two clinical facts indicate that MOFS is a systemic process mediated by endogenous or exogenous cir-

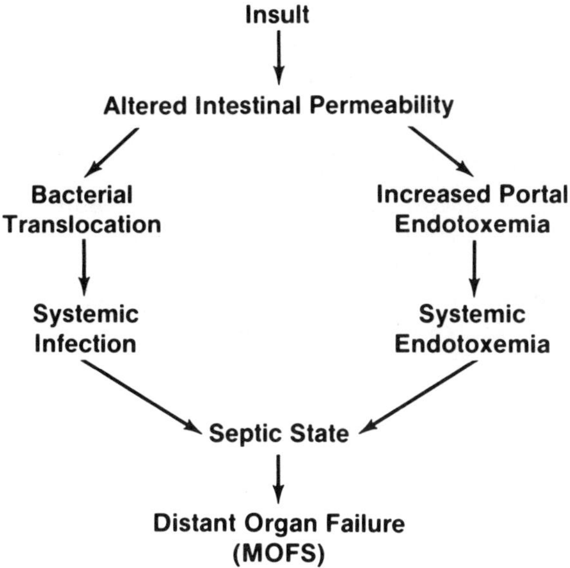

Figure 4–1. Schematic illustration of potential relationship between injury or stress-induced alterations in intestinal permeability and the development of MOFS.

culating factor or factors whose effects are not immediately apparent after the initiating event or events. These findings prompted Fry et al.,[4] Baue,[5] and others[6] to propose that MOF was the external expression of a septic syndrome due to an occult septic focus. This concept was widely accepted by the medical and surgical communities and MOF in the absence of a clinically identifiable source of infection was considered an indication for an exploratory laparotomy.[6,7] However, as more patients with MOF were empirically explored looking for occult intra-abdominal abscesses, it became clear that MOFS could exist in the absence of an identifiable focus of infection.[8,9] This was true of bacteremic patients with MOFS as well as nonbacteremic patients, since no septic focus could be identified clinically or at autopsy in more than 30% of bacteremic patients dying of clinical sepsis and MOF.[10]

Thus, many patients with MOFS appear to have infections originating in the gut, yet they do not have an identifiable septic focus. The reason for this paradox appears to lie in the fact that under certain circumstances bacteria can cross the intestinal mucosal barrier and cause systemic infections, a process termed "bacterial translocation."[11,12] In patients with MOFS who die a clinically septic death in the absence of positive blood cultures or septic foci[8,10] gut barrier failure also may play a major role in the development of MOFS. The link between these two patient groups may be the presence of portal and systemic endotoxemia. The relationship between increased intestinal permeability to bacteria and endotoxin and organ failure is outlined in Figure 4–1. In this chapter, the clinical and experimental evidence supporting the concept that failure of gut barrier function results in a septic state that ultimately results in MOFS due to the uncontrolled escape of bacteria or endotoxin, or both, from the intestine will be reviewed.

Clinical Evidence for the Gut as a Reservoir for Systemic Infections and Endotoxemia

Since most bacterial infections occur, in critically ill or immunocompromised patients, when the patient's microflora successfully breach the host's local mechanical defenses, most infections originate at sites of integumentary damage, ciliary dysfunction, or mucosal damage. Examples of failure of local mechanical defenses range from loss of the skin barrier to bacteria in the burn patient to loss of the gut mucosal barrier in the patient with a perforated viscus. In fact, many of our therapeutic manuevers facilitate bacterial penetration across these mechanical barriers and consequently increase the risk of infection. Invasive monitoring lines and intravenous catheters may serve as conduits that allow bacteria colonizing the skin surface direct access to the bloodstream, whereas endotracheal tubes and urinary catheters promote infections by breaching the host's normal mechanical barriers. The intestinal mucosal barrier is no different from the body's other mechanical antibacterial barriers.

Normal intestinal function is frequently altered in the patient who is stressed, septic, or critically ill, often prior to the development of MOFS. Gut failure takes many forms in these patients, including stress gastritis, ileus, and intolerance to enteral feedings, any or all of which may weaken gut mucosal barrier function. Although it is widely recognized that intestinal motility, absorption, and secretion are altered in the critically ill patient, it has only been recently recognized that the gut's immunologic and barrier functions may also fail after injury or during stress.

Some of the earliest clinical studies documenting that bacteria and endotoxin originating in the gut may gain access to the systemic circulation were performed in the 1960s.[13,14] However, these early studies were largely ignored, and the concept that the gut can be a reservoir for systemic bacteria or endotoxin lay dormant for a decade. This concept was resurrected after several epidemiologic studies documented that the normal intestinal microflora was a clinically important reservoir for bacteria and fungi causing systemic infection in immunocompromised patients, such as bone marrow recipients,[15] or granulocytopenic patients with cancer or leukemia.[16] This relationship between gut-associated microorganisms and systemic infection was established in these patient populations when surveillance cultures documented that the bacterial serotypes causing systemic infections were the same as those contained in the patient's stool samples. Once the gut was identified as a reservoir for bacteria causing systemic infections, several groups of investigators attempted to reduce the incidence of infection in these high-risk patients by prophylactically treating these patients with oral nonabsorbable antibiotics. In most studies, the use of prophylactic oral antibiotics to sterilize or selectively decontaminate the gut in neutropenic cancer and leukemia patients significantly reduced the incidence of systemic infections, although their effect on improving survival was less consistent.[17,18] Recent studies in trauma patients also indicate that selective antibiotic decontamination of the gut in combination with topical hypopharyngeal antibiotics will reduce the incidence of primary bacteremias, respiratory tract, urinary tract, and wound infections.[19] The results of these clinical trials suggest that it is possible to reduce the incidence of systemic infections in selected patient populations by preventing intestinal overgrowth and hypopharyngeal colonization with gram-negative enteric bacilli.

Whether or not the use of prophylactic oral and/or topical nonabsorbable antibiotics to decontaminate the hypopharynx and intestine selectively will prevent infection or improve survival in patients with MOFS has not been clinically investigated. However, as previously mentioned, life-threatening infection with gut-associated bacteria, in which no infective focus can be identified, is a relatively common event in patients developing MOFS.[3,10]

Systemic endotoxemia was proposed as a cause of disease in man more than 20 years ago;[14] however, this concept fell into disfavor because of the inability of other investigators to verify consistently the presence of endotoxin in the blood of their patients. Today, with the development of improved methods of measuring endotoxin and the appreciation of the fact that plasma may contain high levels of factors that mask the presence of circulating endotoxin,[20] it is clear that endotoxemia does occur in patients at risk of developing MOFS.[21,22] Most studies on the effects of endotoxin have concentrated on its ability to modulate the immune response and induce a shock state. Yet, endotoxin exerts a profound effect on many other organ systems, including the lung, kidney, and liver, as well as the immune and cardiovascular systems.[23] In fact, endotoxin has been documented to mediate many of the pathophysiologic changes associated with sepsis in both experimental animals and man.[23,24] Endotoxin appears to exert its toxic effects by triggering the release of endogenous mediators and cytokines, such as tumor necrosis factor, interleukin-1, platelet activating factor, and the prostanoids.

The underlying mechanisms of how bacteria or endotoxin contained within the gut cross or translocate the mucosal barrier are poorly understood. Nonetheless, there is a clear clinical association between the presence of an immunocompromised state and bacterial translocation or endotoxemia. This is especially true in patients with altered intestinal perfusion or function, as well as in patients whose normal intestinal microflora has been overgrown with enteric bacilli. The goal of our research has been to investigate potential relationships between the gastrointestinal microflora, systemic host defenses, and trauma in order to clarify the mechanisms responsible for gut barrier failure.

Normal Intestinal Antibacterial Defense Systems

It is necessary to understand the mechanisms by which the gut maintains its barrier function both in health and disease, in order to develop effective therapeutic strategies to combat gut failure, bacterial translocation, and endotoxemia. In some respects, it is surprising that infections with intestinal microorganisms are not more common. The gut contains high concentrations of bacteria and endotoxin that must be excluded, while at the same time it contains nutrients that must be selectively absorbed. Thus, the host has developed multiple defense mechanisms that function together to prevent intestinal bacteria and endotoxin from reaching systemic organs or tissues. These defenses include the stabilizing

**Table 4–1 Intestinal Antibacterial and Antiendotoxin
Host Defenses**

Bacterial	Immunological
1. Bacterial antagonism	1. Secretory immunoglobulins
2. Colonization resistance	2. GALT system
Mechanical	Hepatobiliary
1. Intestinal peristalsis	1. Bile salts
2. Mucous production	2. RES function
3. Epithelial desquamation	
4. Epithelial barrier	

influence of a normal intestinal microflora, plus mechanical and immunologic defenses (Table 4–1).

The first step in the translocation of bacteria from the intestinal tract begins with the association and then adherence of the translocating bacteria to the epithelial cell surface or to ulcerated areas of the intestinal mucosal surface. However, direct bacterial adherence to the intestinal wall is not sufficient to cause translocation, since for bacterial translocation to occur the adherent bacteria also must cross the mucosal barrier and reach the lamina propia in a viable state. Once the bacteria have reached the lamina propria, they have technically translocated out of the intestinal tract; however, unless these bacteria can successfully spread from the lamina propria to systemic organs or invade the bloodstream, the process is of no clinical significance. The normal intestinal tract of healthy persons is very resistant to the translocation of bacteria, although, even under normal circumstances, intestinal infections with viruses and enteropathogenic bacteria, such as Salmonella, *Vibrio cholerae*, or certain strains of *Escherichia coli* can occur.

The host has developed a wide spectrum of defense mechanisms to prevent bacteria colonizing the gut from adhering directly to the intestinal mucosa and translocating to systemic organs. The protective role of the normal intestinal microflora in preventing intestinal infections and bacterial translocation has received increasing attention, since van der Waaij et al.[25–27] documented that different oral nonabsorbable antibiotics will increase or decrease "colonization resistance" of the gut to infection by potential pathogens. This term "colonization resistance" was coined by van der Waaij et al.[25] to describe the protective role of the normal intestinal microflora. It is now clear that the obligate anaerobic bacteria are responsible for colonization resistance, since they associate closely with the intestinal epithelium and form a barrier that limits the direct attachment or intimate association of potential translocating bacteria to the mucosa. Thus, these obligate anaerobes act synergistically with the host's mechanical and immunologic defenses to limit directly and indirectly the growth and epithelial attachment of potential pathogens, such as the enteric bacilli. Under normal circumstances, there are generally 1000- to 10,000-fold more obligate anaerobes, such as Bacteroides sp., within the gut than gram-negative enteric bacilli or aerobic gram-positive bacteria. This anaerobic bacterial barrier is lost when broad-spectrum antibiotics are administered, since the obligate anaerobes are in general more sensitive to antibiotic suppression than the rest of the intestinal microflora.[28]

The exact mechanisms by which the normal gut microflora prevents the establishment of invading populations of microorganisms is not fully understood. However, the processes whereby the normal flora maintains communal stability has been termed "bacterial antagonism." This term includes such diverse processes as the production of antimicrobial factors, such as colicins or volatile fatty acids by the indigenous flora, as well as competition for nutrients or attachment sites. Although it is not known how the normal microflora maintains stability, it is clear that disruption of the normal ecology of the gut flora will promote colonization of the gut by potential pathogens and may lead to bacterial translocation and systemic infection. The understanding that the obligate anaerobes are necessary for colonization resistance has led to the clinical development of oral antibiotic regimens that kill aerobic bacteria and fungi but spare the obligate anerobic bacteria. The use of oral nonabsorbable antibiotics that preserve colonization resistance by selectively sparing the obligate anaerobes has been termed selective antibiotic decontamination of the gut. As previously mentioned, selective antibiotic decontamination of the gut has been effective in reducing infection in certain groups of patients.

The mechanical defenses of the intestine also limit the ability of bacteria to reach the epithelial mucosa as well as cross the epithelial mucosal barrier. In the small intestine, normal peristalsis prevents the prolonged stasis of bacteria in close proximity to the intestinal mucosa and thereby reduces the chance that any individual bacterium will have adequate time to penetrate the mucous layer and attach to the epithelium. If the peristaltic clearing of bacteria is altered, either by mechanical obstruction or due to the development of an ileus, bacterial stasis will occur. Under these circumstances, there is an increased likelihood that bacteria will be able to penetrate the mucous layer successfully and adhere directly to the epithelial mucosa.

Although, under normal circumstances, the combination of peristaltic waves and the mucous layer limits the direct attachment of bacteria to the epithelial mucosa, some bacteria do reach the mucosal surface and adhere to the epithelial cells at the villous tips. Since the epithelial cells at the villous tips are constantly being desquamated and replaced by younger cells migrating from the crypts, the few bacteria that have adhered to these epithelial cells are ejected back into the intestinal lumen with the sloughed cells. Epithelial migration and desquamation is a rapid and constant process that results in the complete replacement of the epithelium every 2 to 3 days in rodents and every 4 to 6 days in man. In this way, epithelial renewal serves to limit the number of bacteria that are attached to the epithelium at any one time.

The intestinal immune system known as gut-associated lymphoid tissue (GALT) consists of Peyer's patches, lymphoid follicles, lamina propria lymphocytes, intraepithelial lymphocytes, and cells of the mesenteric lymph nodes. The gut lymphoid tissue contains the same full repertoire of lymphocyte and macrophage subsets as the systemic immune system. These intestinal lymphocyte subsets regulate the local immune response to soluble and particulate oral antigens, such as endotoxin and bacteria. The exact role of the systemic and intestinal immune systems in preventing bacterial adherence and bacterial translocation has not been determined. However, secretory immunoglobulin A (IgA) produced by antigen-primed B cells lining all mucosal surfaces appears to play a major role in the defense against mucosal invasion by bacteria.[29] Secretory IgA is unique among the various classes of immunoglobulins, since it binds to bacteria but does not activate the effector arms of the immune system. In this way, secretory IgA can bind to bacteria and prevent their attachment to epithelial cells without creating a local inflammatory response, which might impair the normal absorptive processes of the gut. The importance of secretory IgA in preventing bacterial translocation is not clear, since persons with selective IgA deficiencies do not commonly develop intestinal infections.[30] However, IgA-deficient persons compensate for their IgA deficiency by producing increased amounts of secretory IgM.

Up to this point, most of the discussion has centered on antibacterial defenses of the gut, since much less is known about the antiendotoxin defenses of the gut. Most investigators believe that bile within the intestinal tract is the primary factor responsible for preventing the escape of endotoxin from the gut. Bile salts are thought to prevent portal endotoxemia by binding directly to intraluminal endotoxin and forming detergent-like complexes that are poorly absorbed.[31,32] Although portal endotoxemia appears to occur normally, systemic endotoxemia does not occur due to the reticuloendothelial system (RES) function of the liver.

Many, if not all, of the defenses that prevent bacterial translocation are impaired in patients at risk of developing MOFS. These patients are frequently immunosuppressed, and the antibiotic regimens they receive may disrupt the normal ecology of the gut microflora, resulting in impaired colonization leading to bacterial overgrowth with potential pathogens. Current therapeutic regimens, such as prophylactic and therapeutic H_2 blockers or antacid therapy, may result in the colonization of the stomach with bacteria due to the increased survival of orally ingested bacteria. Hyperosmolar enteral or parenteral feedings may disrupt not only the normal bacterial ecology of the gut, but may also result in mucosal atrophy and altered intestinal mechanical defenses. The hypoalbuminemia and capillary leak syndrome that commonly occurs in these patients can result in intestinal edema, impaired jejunoileal peristalsis, intestinal stasis, bacterial overgrowth, and altered intestinal permeability. These and other changes can easily be seen to promote the failure of the gut barrier to bacteria. Liver failure allows portal endotoxin to reach the systemic circulation where it may induce a septic state.

The next section will present the results of experimental studies designed to determine the relative importance of some of these defenses in the failure of the gut mucosal barrier to bacterial translocation.

Experimental Evidence for the Gut as a Reservoir for Systemic Infections

Although there is abundant indirect clinical evidence suggesting that gut failure and bacterial translocation may occur in critically ill or immunocompromised patients, the underlying mechanisms of how and under what circumstances bacteria contained within the gut translocate across the epithelial barrier to cause infection is poorly understood. In order to study the phenomenon of bacterial translocation, we have developed several in vivo rodent models. The results of these studies indicate that certain conditions that commonly occur in the patient at risk of developing MOFS will promote bacterial translocation in healthy rodents.

In these experiments, the animals are subjected to actual or sham injury, then sacrificed at various times postinjury. At sacrifice, the blood, peritoneal cavities, and organs (mesenteric lymph node complex, liver, and spleen) are harvested and quantitatively cultured for translocating bacteria. The mesenteric lymph node complex consists of an aggregated group of lymph nodes that drain the small intestine, cecum, and proximal colon. Since the mesenteric lymph nodes are normally sterile, the presence of bacteria in these nodes is a sensitive marker of bacterial translocation. To determine the effect of the experimental manipulation on the ecology of the indigenous gastrointestinal microflora, the population levels of resident bacteria within the cecum are quantitated. In selected experiments, sections of the ileum and cecum are examined histologically to determine whether the gut mucosa has been physically damaged.

Nonlethal burn injuries were chosen as the initial model to examine the relationship between trauma and bacterial translocation, since by altering the size of the burn injury, the effect of varying levels of trauma on gut barrier function could be assessed.[12,33,34] No bacteria were cultured from the blood or systemic organs of the control or sham-burned rats or mice. In contrast, 44% of the rats receiving 40% body surface area burns had bacteria cultured from their mesenteric lymph nodes, although their blood, livers, and spleens remained sterile. Since disruption of the ecology of the normal gut flora is common in severely ill patients as well as patients receiving certain systemic antibiotics, the effect of thermal injury on bacterial translocation also was tested in mice and rats whose normal gut flora had been disrupted resulting in overgrowth with gram-negative enteric bacilli. The burned animals could not prevent the systemic spread of translocating bacteria as well as control uninjured animals (Table 4–2). Furthermore, the mean number of bacteria surviving in the organs of the burned mice were 1000- to 10,000-fold higher than in the unburned mice (Table 4–2). These results indicate that the combination of trauma and intestinal overgrowth with gram-negative enteric bacilli results in the synergistic spread of bacteria from the gut to systemic organs.

Because of the clinical association between hypotension, infection, and the development of MOFS, we tested whether limited periods of hypotension would induce bacterial translocation from the gut in a rat model of hemorrhagic shock.[35] Three different periods of shock (30, 60, or 90 minutes) were tested so that the effect of increasing periods of hypotension on bacterial translocation and intestinal mucosal integrity could be measured. Bacteria translocated to the mesenteric lymph nodes of all three groups of shocked rats. The rats subjected to 90 minutes of shock had more mucosal damage and a higher incidence of translocating bacteria in their livers, spleens, and bloodstreams than rats subjected to the shorter periods of shock. Thus, hemorrhagic shock appears to promote

Table 4–2   Thermal Injury Promotes Increased Bacterial Translocation in Mice Whose Intestines are Overgrown with *E. coli*

	INCIDENCE OF TRANSLOCATION*				CFU[†]
Group	*MLN*	*Spleen*	*Liver*	*Blood*	*MLN*
Control—*E. coli*	77%	3%	49%	0%	5.3
	(27/35)	(1/35)	(17/35)	(0/35)	
15% burns—*E. coli*	90%	10%	60%	0%	4.3
	(27/30)	(3/30)	(18/30)	(0/30)	
30% burns—*E. coli*	100%	60%	90%	25%	73,000
	(20/20)	(12/20)	(18/20)	(5/20)	
p value[‡]	0.11	0.0001	0.007	0.002	0.0002

*Incidence expressed as number of positive organs over number tested.
[†]Mean colony forming units (CFU) of bacteria per gram of mesenteric lymph nodes.
[‡]p values are 30% burns versus controls.

bacterial translocation by injuring the intestinal mucosa (Fig. 4–2). Furthermore, the histologic appearance of the mucosa of the shocked rats was similar to that documented in humans experiencing periods of hypotension.[36]

Since protein malnutrition and endotoxemia are common in many groups of patients, we measured the effects of protein malnutrition and endotoxin on bacterial translocation, individually and in combination.[3,37] Endotoxin and protein malnutrition were chosen for study, since they both impair host defenses and are associated with conditions leading to MOFS.[38,39] Nonlethal doses of endotoxin promoted bacterial translocation in a dose-dependent fashion; however, the translocating bacteria remained localized to the mesenteric lymph nodes and did not spread to other organs. Although bacterial translocation did not occur in protein-malnourished animals, protein-malnourished mice challenged with endotoxin were more susceptible to lethal sepsis from translocating bacteria than were normally nourished mice. The duration of protein malnutrition correlated directly with the number of organs containing translocated bacteria and endotoxin-induced mortality (Fig. 4–3). Similar results were found when we challenged burned mice with endotoxin.[40] The mortality rate of mice receiving only endotoxin or only a thermal injury was less than 10%, whereas the combination of a nonlethal dose of endotoxin plus a nonlethal thermal injury increased the mortality rate to 100%. Therefore it appears that neither protein-malnourished nor thermally injured mice can control the systemic spread of bacteria translocating from the gut as well as normally nourished mice receiving endotoxin. Thus, the combination of endotoxin plus a protein-malnourished state or a thermal injury results in a rapidly fatal septic syndrome due to bacteria translocating from the gut.

The histologic appearance of the ilea and ceca of the mice challenged with endotoxin was identical to that found in rats subjected to 30, but not 90, minutes of hemorrhagic shock (Fig. 4–2). These findings suggest that these two different insults may have damaged the mucosal barrier through a common pathway.

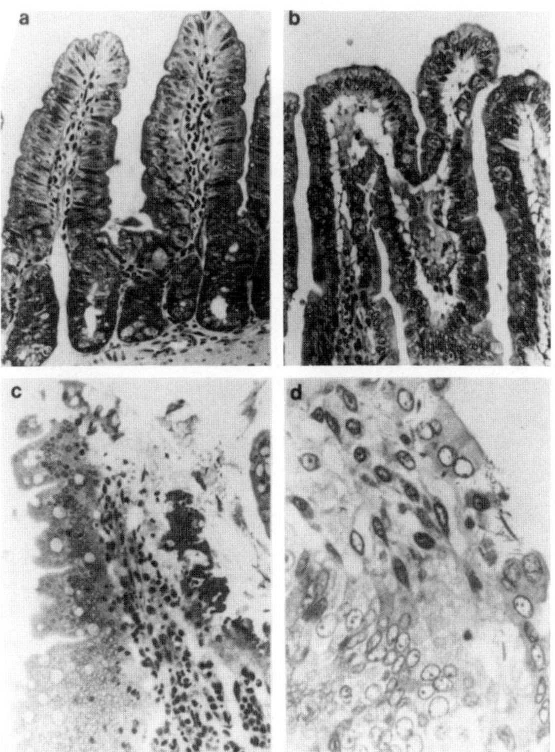

Figure 4–2.   a: Normal rat ileal villi ($\times$240). b: Ileal villi of a rat sacrificed 24 hours after 30 minutes of shock ($\times$240). The lamina propria is edematous and there are localized areas of submucosal edema lifting the epithelial mucosa off the lamina propria at the villous tips. c: Ileal villus of a rat sacrificed 24 hours after 90 minutes of hemorrhagic shock ($\times$260) that has diffuse necrosis of distal villous. d: High-power magnification of area of epithelial injury and site of bacterial translocation.

Thus, experiments were performed to determine whether the mucosal injury and subsequent bacterial translocation were due to an intestinal reperfusion injury mediated by xanthine oxidase-generated oxidants (Fig. 4–4). The incidence of bacterial translocation after endotoxin challenge or 30 minutes of hypotension was significantly reduced by agents that inactivated (tungsten diet) or inhibited (allopurinol) intestinal xanthine oxidase activity.[41,42] Furthermore, both xanthine oxidase inactivation or inhibition largely prevented the mucosal injury in both models (Fig. 4–5).

Gram-negative enteric bacilli, such as *E. coli*, Proteus, Klebsiella, and Enterobacter, are the most common translocating bacteria in our animal models as well as the most common bacteria recovered clinically. Therefore an important question to answer is whether various members of the normal gut microflora translocate at similar rates or whether certain species are especially adept at translocating from the gastrointestinal tract. To answer this question, we measured the translocation rates of several species of normal gut flora bacteria using a germ-free mouse model.[43] The results of these experiments indicate that gram-

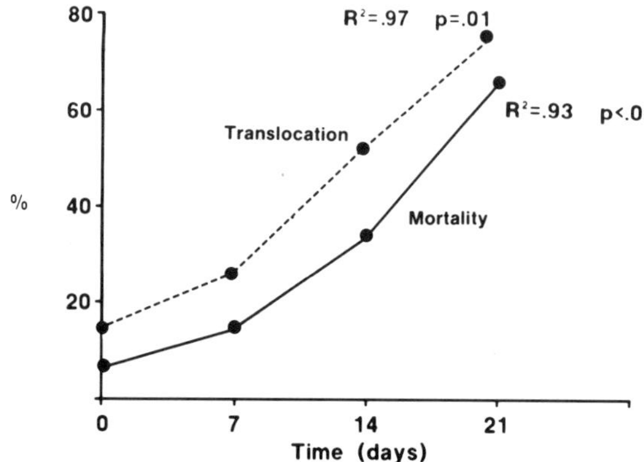

Figure 4–3. There was a strong association both between the duration of protein malnutrition and endotoxin-induced bacterial translocation (p = 0.01) and mortality (p <0.05).

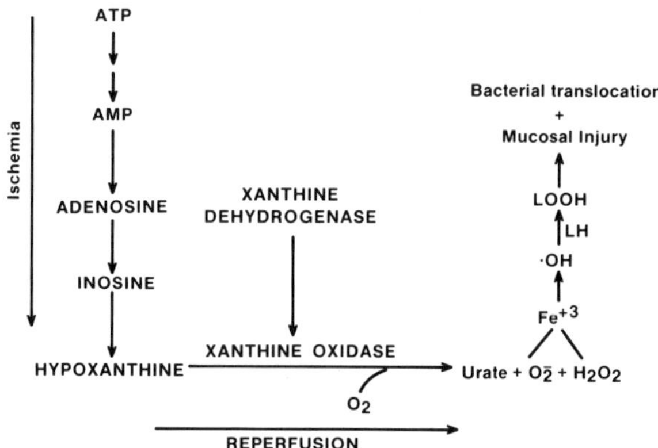

Figure 4–4. Schematic illustration of the relationship between intestinal ischemia and oxidant-mediated mucosal injury resulting in bacterial translocation.

negative, enteric bacilli are the most common bacteria isolated from the organs of our experimental animals and the blood of debilitated patients, because these bacteria translocate more efficiently from the gastrointestinal tract than other bacterial species.

The routes by which the translocating bacteria reach the mesenteric lymph nodes, liver, spleen, and bloodstream are not known with certainty. Wells and coworkers[44,45] have shown that bacteria present within the mesenteric lymph nodes are associated with macrophages and have proposed that the macrophage plays a pivotal role in the transport of bacteria from the intestine. At this time, it appears likely that translocating bacteria reach systemic organs via the lymphatics, since the mesenteric lymph nodes are the first and may be the only tissue to contain translocating bacteria. However, these facts do not prove that translocating bacteria reach the systemic circulation only by the lymphatic sys-

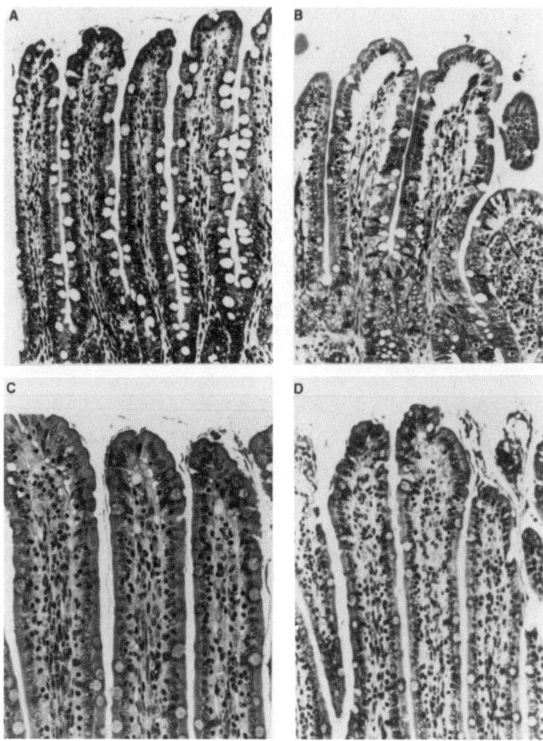

Figure 4–5.   a: Normal mouse ileum. b: Ileum 24 hours after endotoxin challenge. The lamina propria is edematous and the epithelial mucosa has separated from the basal lamina. c: Photomicrograph documenting that inhibition of xanthine oxidase activity (allopurinol) prevents endotoxin-induced ileal damage. d: Ileum of rat sacrificed 24 hours after 30 minutes of hemorrhagic shock, illustrating that inactivation of xanthine oxidase activity (tungsten diet) prevents shock-induced mucosal damage. (All, original magnification × 190.)

tem. It is possible that bacteria do invade the intestinal capillaries, but that the bactericidal defenses of the liver are superior to those of the mesenteric lymph nodes and thus the translocating bacteria that reach the liver are killed. Further studies are needed to determine how bacteria that have crossed the intestinal barrier reach the mesenteric lymph nodes, systemic organs, and bloodstream.

There is also evidence that bacteria can translocate into experimental abdominal abscesses[46] or sterile abdominal inflammatory lesions,[47] even in the absence of a direct communication between the intestinal tract and the abscess or sterile fluid cavity. From these and other studies, it appears that intestinal bacteria can colonize or infect extraintestinal, abdominal fluid collections in the presence of a grossly intact intestinal barrier.

Human data on bacterial translocation to the mesenteric lymph nodes is extremely limited. We recently documented that mesenteric lymph nodes obtained at laparotomy from patients undergoing elective surgery rarely contain bacteria (1 of 25 patients).[48] In contrast, 10 of 17 (59%) patients operated on for simple intestinal obstruction had viable bacteria in their mesenteric lymph nodes, although none of these patients had a necrotic bowel and cultures of their peritoneal cavities were sterile. The results of our study are similar to those reported by Ambrose et al.,[49] who sampled ileal serosa and mesenteric lymph nodes from patients with and without Crohn's disease. They found that only 5% of the patients without Crohn's disease had viable bacteria in their mesenteric lymph nodes, whereas 33% of the lymph nodes from the Crohn's patients contained bacteria. Thus, the limited clinical information that is available supports the concept that bacteria can translocate from the intestine to the mesenteric lymph nodes under certain circumstances.

Relationship of Gut Failure to Multiple Organ Failure

The exact relationship of gut failure, bacterial translocation, or endotoxemia to clinical infection, the septic state, or MOFS is not known with certainty. However, it is clear that gut failure and the translocation of intestinal bacteria or endotoxin to the portal or systemic circulation is part of the MOFS. Normal gastrointestinal function is unquestionably altered in patients at risk of developing MOFS and many, if not all, of the defense mechanisms that normally contain bacteria or endotoxin within the intestinal tract are impaired in these patients. These patients are immunosuppressed, and the antibiotic regimens they receive frequently disrupt the normal ecology of the gut microflora, resulting in impaired colonization resistance and intestinal overgrowth with potential pathogens. Gut failure can take many forms in these patients, including stress ulcers, ileus, and intolerance to enteral feedings; all of which may weaken the gut mucosal barrier to luminal bacteria and endotoxin. Episodes of hypotension or decreased regional perfusion of intestinal segments may lead to gastric or intestinal erosions,[50,51] which could act as portals of entry for intestinal bacteria or endotoxin. Although these clinical studies do not establish a cause and effect relationship between gut failure, systemic sepsis, or MOFS, our experimental studies clearly document that trauma, impaired host antibacterial defenses, shock, malnutrition, intestinal obstruction, or disruption of the normal gut flora will promote gut barrier failure and bacterial translocation.

Furthermore, it appears reasonable to assume that in some circumstances gut barrier failure can become self-sustaining. For example, the endotoxemic or bacteremic states can become self-sustaining when they lead to the further absorption of intestinal endotoxin or bacteria (Fig. 4–1). Since endotoxemia occurs in patients at risk of developing MOFS[21,22] and experimentally endotoxin increases intestinal permeability, promotes bacterial translocation, and in combination with other nonlethal insults will induce the development of a lethal septic syndrome, it appears that endotoxemia may be an important link between gut failure and MOFS. Additionally, it appears that the gut can fuel the septic process in endotoxemic or bacteremic patients, since endotoxemia or bacteremia can induce gut barrier failure leading to the further absorption of intestinal endotoxin or bacteria.

In putting the phenomena of gut failure and bacterial translocation into perspective, it is important to realize that neither is an all or none phenomenon. Although many of the factors associated with the care of the critically ill patient predispose to gut barrier failure, if the host's immune defenses are intact, the translocating bacteria are killed and their products, such as endotoxin, are cleared or inactivated. Thus, although disruption or impairment of a single major intestinal defense system consistently promotes bacterial translocation, the translocating bacteria are usually limited to the mesenteric lymph nodes and do not spread systemically. Instead, these translocating bacteria are locally contained and eventually eradicated as the animal or patient recovers. However, if the host's systemic defenses are impaired, the translocating bacteria multiply in the mesenteric lymph nodes and spread to invade systemic organs and may induce distant organ failure and a lethal septic syndrome.

It appears that the state of RES function of the liver may be especially important in determining whether translocating bacteria or endotoxin are neutralized or cause organ dysfunction. Endotoxin is present at low levels in human portal but not systemic blood in patients with a normal functioning liver.[52,53] However, in patients with liver disease, endotoxin is present in both portal and systemic venous blood. These results suggest that Kupffer cells may be important in preventing intestinal exdotoxin entering the portal circulation from reaching the systemic circulation. In addition, the in vitro and in vivo studies of Simmons, Cerra, and their coworkers indicate that gut-derived endotoxin may regulate Kupffer cell activity and the subsequent liberation of endogenous mediators that modulate hepatocyte function.[54,55] Therefore a clinically important relationship may exist between the state of the intestinal barrier, Kupffer cell function, and distant organ dysfunction.

Thus, there is abundant clinical and extensive experimental evidence to support the hypothesis that gut failure may promote or potentiate the development or progression of MOFS. This is not to say that gut failure is the only cause of MOFS. It is clear that in many patients who develop MOFS, gut barrier failure is not the inciting cause. Rather, it is the failure to diagnose and adequately treat septic foci in the lung, abdomen, or elsewhere. Nonetheless, there is a distinct group of patients who develop MOFS and in whom no septic focus is ever found either clinically or at autopsy.

Therapeutic Options

The development of infection requires a susceptible host, a break in local mechanical defenses, and the presence of a bacterial pathogen. This is true whether the infection is manifested as pneumonia or bacterial translocation. Clearly, the best treatment of gut failure and its potential sequelae is prevention. For example, it is now clear that the stomach can be a reservoir for gram-negative bacteria that may colonize the hypopharynx and ultimately cause pneumonia in patients treated with prophylactic antacids or cimetidine. Since sucralfate is as effective as antacids or H_2 blockers in preventing stress-induced gastric bleeding, while minimizing the risk of pneumonia,[56,57] sucralfate appears to be the drug of choice for the prevention of stress bleeding in ICU patients.

Furthermore, the classic studies of Border and coworkers[1] have clearly established that a policy of early definitive surgery in trauma patients will improve survival by reducing the incidence of organ failure and sepsis associated with gut dysfunction. As early as 1977, Eiseman et al.[58] stressed that intraoperative and postoperative errors in technique and judgment were contributing factors in more than 50% of their patients who developed MOFS. These reports highlight the fact that there is no substitute for mature clinical judgment and good operative technique in the prevention of MOFS. By debriding necrotic tissue, controlling bacterial contamination, and preventing the development of postoperative seromas and hematomas, the surgeon not only removes the milieu in which bacteria multiply, but also improves the delivery of host antibacterial defense factors to sites of injury and infection. In fact, early definitive primary or reoperative surgery leading to the removal of necrotic tissue, the drainage of abscesses, and the control of peritoneal soilage may bolster host defenses both by reducing the circulating levels of various putative suppressive factors, such as interleukin-1, tumor necrosis factor, and prostaglandin E_2, as well as by limiting the period of stress. Thus, early definitive surgery by reducing the incidence or magnitude of gut failure and enhancing host systemic defenses may prevent the development of a vicious cycle of gut failure leading to the escape of bacteria or endotoxin from the gut, which further impairs gut function.

The role of selective intestinal malnutrition in the evolution of gut failure has received increasing attention, since Kudsk et al.[59,60] documented that animals fed enterally survive a septic insult better than animals fed an identical diet parenterally. Wilmore et al.[61] recently reviewed the concept that gut barrier failure may occur in critically ill patients due to the fact that current methods of parenteral nutrition do not support mucosal structure or function. Thus, intestinal starvation frequently occurs in parenterally fed ICU patients due to the fact that many of the essential nutrients required for normal enterocyte growth and repair are not present in adequate quantities in these parenteral feedings. Enteral feeding may have beneficial systemic metabolic effects as well as beneficial effects on mucosal structure and function, since Mochizuki et al.[62] have documented, in a guinea pig model, that immediate enteral feeding prevents the hypermetabolic response to thermal injury by maintaining gut mass and preventing the excessive secretion of catabolic hormones.

The exact reasons why enteral feedings maintain gut mass and function better than parenteral feedings is not fully known, although it appears that maintenance of mucosal mass and perhaps mucosal integrity requires the presence of specific intraluminal nutrients, such as glutamine.[63] This conclusion is based on in vitro and in vivo studies documenting that intestinal enterocytes preferentially utilize glutamine as their major energy source.[61] Other major fuels of the gut are the ketone bodies. In contrast to other tissues, glucose and free fatty acids contribute relatively little to the energy needs of the intestine. The ability of high protein enteral feedings to improve outcome was conclusively shown by Alexander et al.[64] in a prospective randomized study of burned children. In this study, burned children were randomized to receive nutritional support either enterally or parenterally. The enterally fed children had less impairment of their systemic immune defenses, fewer infections, and an increased survival rate compared with the parenterally fed children.

Thus, a major therapeutic option in the prevention and treatment of gut failure is early enteral feeding of a high protein diet. This is not to say that parenteral alimentation is not beneficial. Many patients receiving enteral alimentation also require parenteral nutrition to meet their metabolic needs. Recent studies indicate that specific growth factors and hormones, such as epidermal growth factor or growth hormone, have trophic effects on the intestinal mucosa.[61] Thus, in the future, the optimal therapy to maintain or restore intestinal mucosal structure and function may be a combination of specific enterally administered nutrients and mucosal trophic factors. Currently, it is my practice to administer 60 ml of a high protein enteral diet every 2 hours to all high-risk patients. Since gastric motility may be impaired in these patients, the stomach is aspirated every 2 hours just prior to the enteral feeding. In this way, the risk of aspiration of gastric contents is significantly reduced. These enteral feedings are begun in nonoperative patients as soon as the patients are hemodynamically stable and in operative patients immediately postoperatively. In my opinion the presence of an ileus is not an absolute contraindication to enteral feeding.

Another area of importance is the judicious use of oral and systemic antibiotics to prevent or limit the incidence of intestinal overgrowth with enteric bacilli. To minimize antibiotic-mediated intestinal bacterial overgrowth, perioperative antibiotics should be stopped shortly after surgery and the narrowest spectrum antibiotic regimen possible should be administered for the shortest time possible when treating established infections. The use of selective antibiotic decontamination of the gut to maintain colonization resistance has been documented to decrease the incidence of systemic infections in several groups of patients. However, since it is not clear whether selective antibiotic decontamination of the gut will improve survival, more information is needed before this approach can be recommended for all patients at risk of developing MOFS.

Conceptually, there are several general approaches that can be taken to reduce the risk or biologic consequences of systemic endotoxemia. These include attempts to prevent the development of endotoxemia and the use of drugs or vaccines to neutralize the deleterious effects of endotoxin, either by binding directly to the endotoxin molecule, or by preventing the release or blocking the activity of endotoxin-induced endogenous mediators.[23] Since endotoxemia generally originates from the gut or from areas of localized infection, to prevent endotoxemia it is necessary to maintain gut barrier function and to prevent or treat infections. In general, therapeutic manuevers to neutralize endotoxin have concentrated on the use of vaccines, monoclonal antibodies against endotoxin or drugs, such as polymyxin B, that bind directly to the endotoxin molecule.[23,65] The use of specific drugs to block or neutralize endotoxin-induced mediators from activated macrophages is in its infancy.[24] However, this approach may be more widely used in the future. The role of immunomodulators in the treatment of endotoxemia is not clear, since experimentally most drugs that augment the immune response activate macrophages and thus predispose the host to en-

Table 4–3 Potential Therapeutic Options

Maintain normal gut microflora
  1. Selective antibiotic decontamination with oral antibiotics
  2. Judicious use of systemic antibiotics to maintain colonization resistance

Support gut barrier function
  1. Early enteral feeding
  2. Use of trophic hormones, such as growth hormone

Limit stress state
  1. Early definitive surgery
  2. Prompt diagnosis and control of systemic infections

Therapeutic agents
  1. Antioxidants to prevent mucosal damage
  2. Use of agents to neutralize or block endotoxin

dotoxic shock.[3,23] A summary of the potential clinical options available to prevent or treat gut barrier failure is presented in Table 4–3.

Summary and Conclusions

The initial status of the gut in MOFS may range from that of an innocent bystander organ to that of the motor of MOF. Gut failure may contribute to MOF by allowing bacteria or endotoxin, or both, to pass into the portal or systemic circulations where they may serve to fuel the septic process. Whether maintenance of mucosal integrity and the preservation of the mucosal barrier to bacterial translocation and endotoxin will prevent the development or progression of MOF is unknown. It is also unknown whether the restoration of mucosal integrity and barrier function in the patient with MOF will result in improved survival.

It is known that, under normal circumstances, the normal gut flora acts in concert with the host's mechanical and immunologic defenses to prevent directly and indirectly intestinal colonization or overgrowth with potential pathogens. Although many factors may influence the gut flora, including intestinal motility, diet, and antibiotics, attempts must be made to maintain the normal ecology of the patient's intestinal microflora. This consideration does not mean that appropriate antibiotics should not be used to treat established infections, but it does highlight an additional potential risk of antibiotic therapy. Since the starved gut loses mucosal mass, villous height, and becomes more permeable to intraluminal bacteria and endotoxin, early enteral feeding may be important in maintaining gut mucosal integrity.

Nonintestinal factors may also impair gut function and lead to gut-mediated distant organ dysfunction. Hypotension, hemodynamic instability, or vasoactive agents that decrease intestinal perfusion may promote bacterial translocation or systemic endotoxemia by increasing intestinal permeability. Systemic insults or drugs that decrease intestinal motility may be deleterious, since ileus is associated with bacterial overgrowth and loss of colonization resistance. Uncontrolled distant infections, such as pneumonias, or the presence of endotoxemia may alter intestinal permeability and promote the translocation of intestinal bacteria or the escape of endotoxin from the gut. Thus, attention should be paid to systemic factors that may influence intestinal function, as well as factors that directly affect the gut.

Does gut failure promote or potentiate MOFS? I believe that the answer to this question is yes.

References

1. Border JR, Hassett J, LaDuca J, et al. Gut origin septic states in blunt multiple trauma (ISS = 40) in the ICU. Ann Surg 1987;206:427–446.
2. Carrico CJ, Meakins JL, Marshall JC, et al. Multiple organ failure syndrome. Arch Surg 1986;121:196–203.
3. Deitch EA, Berg R, Specian R. Endotoxin promotes the translocation of bacteria from the gut. Arch Surg 1987;122:185–190.
4. Fry DE, Pearlstein L, Fulton RL, et al. Multiple system organ failure: the role of uncontrolled infection. Arch Surg 1980;115:136–140.
5. Baue AE. Multiple, progressive, or sequential systems failure: a syndrome of the 1970s. Arch Surg 1975;110:779–781.
6. Polk HC, Shields CL. Remote organ failure: a valid sign of occult intra-abdominal infection. Surgery 1977;81:310–313.
7. Ferraris VA. Exploratory laparotomy for potential abdominal sepsis in patients with multiple-organ failure. Arch Surg 1983;118:1130–1133.
8. Meakins JL, Wicklund B, Forse RA, et al. The surgical intensive care unit: current concepts in infection. Surg Clin North Am 1980;60:117–132.
9. Norton LW. Does drainage of intra-abdominal pus reverse multiple organ failure? Am J Surg 1985;149:347–350.
10. Goris RJ, Beokhorst PA, Nuytinck KS, et al. Multiple organ failure: generalized autodestructive inflammation. Arch Surg 1985;120:1109–1115.
11. Berg RD, Garlington AW. Translocation of certain indigenous bacteria from the gastrointestinal tract to the mesenteric lymph nodes and other organs in a gnotobiotic mouse model. Infect Immun 1979;23:403–411.
12. Deitch EA, Maejima K, Berg R. Effect of oral antibiotics and bacterial overgrowth on the translocation of the GI-tract microflora in burned rats. J Trauma 1985;25:385–392.
13. Woodruff PW, O'Carroll DE, Koizumi S, et al. Role of the intestinal flora in major trauma. J Infect Dis 1973;128:S290–S294.
14. Ravin HA, Fine J. Biological implications of intestinal endotoxins. Fed Proc 1962;21:65–68.
15. Wells CL, Podzorski RP, Peterson PK, et al. Incidence of trimethoprim-sulfamethoxazole-resistant Enterobacteriaceae among transplant recipients. J Infect Dis 1984;150:699–706.
16. Tancrede CH, Andremont AO. Bacterial translocation and gram-negative bacteremia in patients with hematological malignancies. J Infect Dis 1985;152:99–103.
17. Gurwith MS, Burnton JL, Lank BA, et al. A prospective controlled investigation of prophylactic trimethoprim/sulfamethoxazole in hospitalized granulocytopenic patients. Am J Med 1979;66:248–256.
18. de Vries-Hospers HG, Sleijfer DR, Mulder NH, et al. Bacteriological aspects of selective decontamination of the digestive tract as a method of infection prevention in granulocytopenic patients. Antimicrob Agents Chemother 1981;19:813–820.
19. Stoutenbeek CP, van Saene HKF, Miranda DR, et al. The effect of oropharyngeal decontamination using topical nonabsorbable antibiotics on the incidence of nosocomial respiratory tract infections in multiple trauma patients. J Trauma 1987;27:357–364.
20. Warren HS, Knights CV, Siber GR. Neutralization and lipoprotein binding of lipopolysaccharides in tolerate rabbit serum. J Infect Dis 1986;154:784–791.
21. Rush BF Jr, Sori AJ, Murphy TF, et al. Endotoxemia and bacteremia during hemorrhagic shock: the link between trauma and sepsis? Ann Surg 1988;207:549–554.
22. Winchurch RA, Thepari TN, Munster AM. Endotoxemia in burn patients: levels of circulating endotoxins are related to burn size. Surgery 1987;102:808–812.

23. Deitch EA. Endotoxin-induced impairment of host defenses. In: Symposium on immune consequences of trauma, shock, and sepsis, Feist G (ed). Heidelberg: Springer-Verlag, 1989.
24. Revhaug A, Michie HR, Manson J McK, et al. Cyclooxygenase blockade attenuates the metabolic response to endotoxin in humans. Arch Surg 1988;123:162–170.
25. van der Waaij D, Berghuis-de Vries JM, Lekkerkerk-van der Wees JEC. Colonization resistance of the digestive tract in conventional and antibiotic-treated mice. J Hyg (Camb) 1971;69:405–411.
26. van der Waaij D, Berghuis-de Vries JM, Lekkerkerk-van der Wees JEC. Colonization resistance of the digestive tracts and the spread of bacteria to the lymphatic organs in mice. J Hyg (Camb) 1972;70:335–342.
27. van der Waaij D, Berghuis JM, Lekkerkerk JEC. Colonization resistance of the digestive tract of mice during systemic antibiotic treatment. J Hyg (Camb) 1972;70:605–609.
28. Berg RD. Promotion of the translocation of enteric bacteria from the gastrointestinal tracts of mice by oral treatment with penicillin, clindamycin, or metronidazole. Infect Immun 1981;33:854–861.
29. Tomasi TB. Mechanisms of immune regulation at mucosal surfaces. Rev Infect Dis 1983;5:S784–S792.
30. Brown WR, Savage DC, Dubois RS, et al. Intestinal microflora of immunoglobulin-deficient and normal human subjects. Gastroenterology 1972;62:1143–1152.
31. Cahill CJ, Pain JA, Bailey ME. Bile salts, endotoxin and renal function in obstructive jaundice. Surg Gynecol Obstet 1987;165:519–522.
32. Bertok L. Physico-chemical defense of vertebrate organisms: the role of bile acids in defense against bacterial endotoxins. Perspect Biol Med 1977;21:70–76.
33. Maejima K, Deitch EA, Berg RD. Bacterial translocations from the gastrointestinal tracts of rats receiving thermal injury. Infect Immun 1984;43:6–10.
34. Maejima K, Deitch EA, Berg RD. Promotion by burn stress of the translocation of bacteria from the gastrointestinal tracts of mice. Arch Surg 1984;119:166–172.
35. Baker JW, Deitch EA, Li M, et al. Hemorrhagic shock induces bacterial translocation from the gut. J Trauma 1988;28:896–906.
36. Sorenson FH, Vetner M. Hemorrhagic mucosal necrosis of the gastrointestinal tract without vascular occlusion. Acta Chir Scand 1969;135:439–448.
37. Deitch EA, Winterton J, Li M, et al. The gut as a portal of entry for bacteremia: role of protein malnutrition. Ann Surg 1987;205:681–692.
38. Morrison DC, Ryan JL. Bacterial endotoxins and host immune responses. Adv Immunol 1979;28:293–450.
39. Chandra RK. Nutrition infection and immunity: present knowledge and future directions. Lancet 1983;1:688–691.
40. Deitch EA, Berg RD. Endotoxin but not malnutrition promotes bacterial translocation from the gut. J Trauma 1987;27:161–166.
41. Deitch EA, Bridges W, Baker J, et al. Hemorrhagic shock-induced bacterial translocation is reduced by xanthine oxidase inhibition or inactivation. Surgery 1988;104:191–198.
42. Deitch EA, Ma L, Wen J, et al. Inhibition of endotoxin-induced bacterial translocation in mice. J Clin Inv 1989;84:36–42.
43. Steffen EK, Berg RD, Deitch EA. Comparison of the translocation rates of various indigenous bacteria from the gastrointestinal tract to the mesenteric lymph node. J Infect Dis 1988;157:1032–1038.
44. Wells CL, Maddaus MA, Simmons RL. The role of the macrophage in the translocation of intestinal bacteria. Arch Surg 1987;122:48–53.
45. Wells CL, Maddaus MA, Erlandsen SL, et al. Evidence for the phagocytic transport of intestinal particles in dogs and rats. Infect Immun 1988;56:278–282.
46. Wells CL, Rotstein OD, Pruett TL, et al. Intestinal bacteria translocate into experimental intra-abdominal abscesses. Arch Surg 1986;121:102–107.
47. Schwinburg FB, Seligman AM, Fine J. Transmural migration of intestinal bacteria. N Engl J Med 1950;242:747–751.
48. Deitch EA. Simple intestinal obstruction causes bacterial translocation in man. Arch Surg 1989;124:699–701.
49. Ambrose NS, Johnson M, Burdon DW, et al. Incidence of pathogenic bacteria from mesenteric lymph nodes and ileal serosa during Crohn's disease surgery. Br J Surg 1984;71:623–625.
50. Haglund U, Hulten L, Ahren C, et al. Mucosal lesions in the human small intestine in shock. Gut 1975;16:979–984.
51. Richardson, RS, Norton LW, Sales JEL, et al. Gastric blood flow in endotoxin-induced stress ulcer. Arch Surg 1973;106:191–195.
52. Jacob AI, Goldberg BS, Bloom N, et al. Endotoxin and bacteria in portal blood. Gastroenterology 1977;72:1268–1270.
53. Prytz H, Holst-Christensen J, Korner B, et al. Portal venous and systemic endotoxaemia in

patients without liver disease and systemic endotoxaemia in patients with cirrhosis. Scand J Gastroenterol 1976;11:857–863.

54. West MA, Keller GA, Cerra FB, et al. Killed *E. coli* stimulate macrophage-mediated alterations in hepatocellular function during *in vitro* coculture. Infect Immun 1985;49:563–570.
55. Billiar TR, Maddaus MA, West MA, et al. The role of intestinal flora on the interactions between nonparenchymal cells and hepatocytes in coculture. J Surg Res 1988;44:397–403.
56. Tryba M. Risk of acute stress bleeding and nosocomial pneumonia in ventilated intensive care patients: sucralfate versus antacids. Am J Med 1987;83(Suppl 3B):117–124.
57. Driks MR, Craven DE, Celli BR, et al. Nosocomial pneumonia in intubated patients given sucralfate as compared with antacids or histamine type 2 blockers: the role of gastric colonization. N Engl J Med 1987;317:1378–1382.
58. Eiseman B, Beart R, Norton L. Multiple organ failure. Surg Gynecol Obstet 1977;144:323–326.
59. Kudsk KA, Stone JM, Carpenter G, et al. Enteral and parenteral feeding influences mortality after hemoglobin E coli peritonitis in normal rats. J Trauma 1983;23:605–609.
60. Kudsk KA, Stone JM, Carpenter G. Effects of enteral versus parenteral feeding on body composition of malnourished animals. J Trauma 1982;22:904–906.
61. Wilmore DW, Smith RJ, O'Dwyer ST, et al. The gut: A central organ after surgical stress. Surgery 1988;104:917–923.
62. Mochizuki H, Trocki O, Dominioni L, et al. Mechanism of prevention of postburn hypermetabolism and catabolism by early enteral feeding. Ann Surg 1984;200:297–310.
63. Souba WW, Smith RJ, Wilmore DW. Glutamine metabolism by the intestinal tract. JPEN 1985;9:608–617.
64. Alexander JW, MacMillan BG, Stinnet JD, et al. Beneficial effects of aggressive protein feeding in severely burned children. Ann Surg 1980;192:505–517.
65. Ziegler EJ, McCutchan JA, Fierer J, et al. Treatment of gram-negative bacteremia and shock with human antiserum to a mutant *Escherichia coli*. N Engl J Med 1982;307:1225–1230.

5

Role of the Macrophage and Endogenous Mediators in Multiple Organ Failure

ROGER W. YURT
STEPHEN F. LOWRY

The peptides, polypeptides, and lipids that appear to play a central role in the pathophysiologic changes associated with multiple organ failure (MOF) have a broad spectrum of activity. In fact, the intrinsic activity of many of these mediators has been shown to be sufficient to account for the disruption of homeostasis that occurs with major injury or sepsis. The real difficulty at the present time is to ascertain how these mediators work in concert to produce the clinical syndrome of MOF.

Some insight into the overall process can be gained through the recognition that the endogenous mediators appear under normal conditions to regulate cellular function and interaction. For example, the minor perturbations of homeostasis that occur on a regular basis are counterbalanced by the action of these mediators. It is only when excessive activation or loss of control occurs that the clinical manifestations of mediator activity are recognized. These concepts were illustrated by the pioneering work of Burke.[1] He documented that in the case of bacterial contamination of a wound small numbers of bacteria are localized and controlled, whereas larger numbers lead to the clinical expression of mediators, that is, the erythema, cellular infiltration, and edema associated with infection. If the process is not localized, then systemic manifestations of an exaggerated response occur. Furthermore, when the systemic response is uncontrolled, a malignant process develops that leads to cellular injury and ultimately to organ damage that presents as MOF.

Each of the mediator pathways will be reviewed from the perspective of their contribution to disruption of homeostasis in multiple organ failure; however it should be kept in mind that the pathways do not function in isolation. The corollary to such an approach is that control of one pathway is not likely to return the organism to a normal balance. Furthermore, therapeutic intervention that is directed at disrupting a pathway is not likely to be successful, since in doing so a basic homeostatic mechanism will be totally eliminated. It is more likely that the process will be controlled by modulation of the most proximal mediator pathway or elimination of the initiating factor or factors.

Plasma Cascades

The plasma cascades are composed of proteins or polypeptides that usually circulate in an inactive form. Activation of a cascade occurs when an inactive or proenzyme is converted to its active state. Therefore, active enzymes sequentially activate additional proteins that may yield products with mediator activity or activate an additional step in the pathway. As will be seen in some pathways, the elimination of a controlling factor, such as an inhibitor or an inactivator, may be just as significant a stimulus to initiation of the pathway as is direct activation of the pathway.

Coagulation

The coagulation pathway is traditionally considered as a mechanism of hemostasis. However, activation of the pathway via the Hageman factor leads to generation of other mediators as well. Bradykinin is generated when a trimolecular complex of plasma kininogen, Hageman factor, and prekallikrein forms after activation of the Hageman factor. Bradykinin, in addition to being vasoactive, contributes to the pain associated with the inflammatory response. During this trimolecular interaction, prekallikrein is activated as well, and the kallikrein that is generated is a chemoattractant for neutrophils. Fibrinolysis also may occur when the Hageman factor is activated, since plasmin is produced when kallikrein cleaves plasma plasminogen.

The Hageman factor-dependent pathway is activated when plasma is exposed to damaged endothelium, collagen,[2] negatively charged surfaces, and lipopolysaccharides.[3] Proteases released in tissue can activate this pathway and enzymes from circulatory cells, such as elastase from neutrophils, have been shown to activate the Hageman factor. The coagulation pathway is activated via tissue factor at a later step in the cascade that leads to coagulation but bypasses the kallikrein-generating Hageman factor activation step.

Evidence is available to support interaction of the coagulation pathway with other pathways and cells. Both kallikrein and plasmin can activate the classic complement pathway via activation of complement protein C1. Elastase is known to be present in bronchoalveolar lavage fluid of patients with adult respiratory distress syndrome (ARDS)[4] and therefore the Hageman factor is likely to be activated in this syndrome. Pulmonary mast cells are exposed to bradykinin during this activation sequence and bradykinin is known to activate mast cells.

Complement

The complement cascade is made up of at least 20 plasma proteins that ultimately interact in sequence to cause lysis of susceptible cells.[5] Several biologically active products are generated during activation of the complement pathway that contribute significantly to the inflammatory process. There are two major pathways of complement activation. The classical pathway is composed of a series of proteins that are named by number, whereas the alternative pathway proteins have letter designations. The third component of complement, C3, is a central protein to both pathways. The classical pathway is usually initiated by activation of C1 in association with antigen interaction with one molecule of immunoglobulin M (IgM) or two adjacent molecules of IgG. Activation of C3 via the alternative pathway is not antibody dependent and appears to be the most common pathway of activation of the complement cascade in injury and sepsis. Burn injury, microbial polysaccharides, lipopolysaccharides, and teichoic acid from pneumococci activate complement via the alternative pathway.

Lysis of target cells occurs when the terminal complement sequence, C5b-9, inserts itself into the cell membranes and forms a "cylinder" through the membrane (see review by Frank[5]). Since membrane integrity is lost, the cell swells and ruptures. Prior to generation of the C5b-9 "attack complex," a number of biologically active products are generated from cleavage of C3. These include C3a, which is an anaphyloxin that activates mast cells, and C3b, which binds to cell membranes via the C3b receptor, termed CR1. The presence of C3b on a surface serves as a recognition protein for further fluid phase attack of the particle or for attachment by neutrophils, macrophages, or monocytes. Following C3 activation, C5 is cleaved to yield C5a, which like C3a is an activator of mast cells. In addition, C5a is a potent chemoattractant for neutrophils and can cause degranulation of these cells. Recent evidence indicates that C5a attracts macrophages and fibroblasts as well. Furthermore, C5a appears to modulate the neutrophil response to injury and infection. When a cell has many molecules of C5a attached to it, it becomes deactivated, that is, unable to respond to a C5a stimulus again.[6,7] With lesser degrees of activation, the neutrophil appears to become hyperresponsive to additional stimulation.[8] Clinical study of the role of the complement system in MOF is hampered by the inability to detect reproducibly changes in plasma complement levels during this syndrome. This is in part due to the fact that only small amounts of activated complement protein are needed to produce an effect. Nevertheless, some studies support a substantial role for the complement system in the pathogenesis of MOF.

Angiotensin System

For a number of years, a neutral peptide mediator that caused smooth muscle contraction was known to be generated from plasma by a neutrophil enzyme. More recently, that peptide has been identified as angiotensin II (A II), the substrate as angiotensinogen, and the enzyme as neutrophil cathepsin G.[9] That this system is active during inflammation and infection is supported by studies that show that when neutrophils phagocytose particles, they release sufficient enzyme to generate A II. Of note is the finding that enzymes that generate A II are also found in mast cells, endothelial cells, and macrophages. In addition, a chymotrypsin-like enzyme, chymase, has been isolated from myocytes of the rat.[10] This enzyme, identical to the chymase of rat mast cells that generates A II from angiotensin I (A I), apparently is a source of A II-generating capacity in muscle.

Since kallikrein not only generates bradykinin from kininogen but also converts prorenin to renin, there is a second renal independent system to generate A II during inflammation. When this system is balanced, the bradykinin generated may offset the activity of A II; however, the relative contributions of each to vasomotor control on a local level are unknown. Overall, it is clear that several pathways are available to lead to intense vasoconstriction of the microvasculature during sepsis and MOF.

Cell-Derived Mediators

The mediators derived from cells can be classified in several ways. Some, such as the cytokines interleukin-1 (IL-1) and tumor necrosis factor (TNF), function to facilitate cell-cell interaction and function, whereas others, for example, histamine, act primarily to promote changes in tissue. When the mediators are separated by mechanism of cell activation and their subsequent release, they can be divided into preformed and generated mediators. The clinical importance of this classification lies in the fact that preformed mediators may be released in the absence of specific cellular activation. In this case, direct injury to the cell or cytolysis will lead to release of mediators. When a cell is specifically activated, the preformed mediators are released either by exocytosis, an active process of extruding the mediators into the microenvironment, or during phagocytosis, when they appear to passively "leak" into the extracellular space. Generated mediators, such as prostaglandins, require cellular activation to occur prior to their release.

The generation of mediators appears to coincide with membrane rearrangement that occurs after membrane perturbation. The lipid rearrangement that occurs via the action of phospholipases A and C leads to the release of arachidonic acid. The arachidonic acid is further metabolized to yield prostaglandins

Table 5–1   Mediators from Mast Cells

Histamine	Prostaglandin D_2
Proteases	Leukotrienes C_4, D_4, E_4
Heparin	PAF
Eosinophil chemotactic factor-anaphylaxis	Tumor necrosis factor
Neutrophil chemotactic factor	

and thromboxane via the cyclooxygenase pathway or to generate leukotrienes via the lipoxygenase pathway. Another generated mediator, superoxide, and its more active product, the hydroxyl radical, is produced during the respiratory or oxidative burst that occurs when cells are activated. Each cell type appears to have the capability to produce these generated mediators; however, they vary in which product predominates.

Mast Cells

The mast cell was originally characterized histologically as an unusual cell based on its property of metachromatic staining. Although it was subsequently reported that the metachromasia was due to the presence of heparin in the mast cell granules, it has now been shown that heparin is not the only glycosaminoglycan present in these cells.[11] Studies in both rat and man suggest that there are at least two types of mast cells. The connective tissue mast cell primarily contains heparin and a chymotrypsin-like enzyme and has large amounts of histamine. These cells are found in peritoneal and pleural spaces and skin. The mast cells that predominate in the mucosa of the gastrointestinal tract have chondroitin sulfates rather than heparin, a trypsin-like enzyme, and contain less histamine than other mast cells. These cells appear to be derived from the bone marrow and are dependent on interleukin-3 (IL-3) as a growth factor. Patients with T-cell deficiencies have few of this type of mast cell. However, recent studies have shown that mucosal-type, IL-3 dependent, mast cells convert to a connective tissue type cell when they are cocultured with fibroblasts. Thus, the amount and type of mediators in mast cells appear to be dependent on the location of the cell and its microenvironment.

The mast cell has been found in virtually every tissue of the body; it resides adjacent to blood vessels and at the interfaces of the body with the external environment. As such, it serves as a sentinel cell in the acute response to injury, but also participates in a late-phase response as well. The concentration of mediators in the cell is sufficient not only to affect the local environment, but also to spill over into the circulation in quantities large enough to cause hypotension and degradation of circulating proteins.

That the mast cell participates in the response to sepsis is supported by its mechanisms of activation.[12] The preformed mediators (Table 5–1) in the granule are released by exposure of the cell to direct injury, endotoxin, C3a, C5a, or bradykinin. In addition, the arachidonic acid metabolites leukotriene C_4, leukotriene B_4 (LTB_4), and prostaglandin D_2 are generated on stimulation of the

Table 5–2 Mediators from Neutrophils

Leukotriene B_4
Elastase
Acid hydrolases
Lysozyme
Hydroxyl radicals
Prostaglandin E_2
Cathepsin G
Collagenase

mast cell. Platelet activating factor (PAF) is also released from mast cells. Studies of the late-phase response to injury indicate that mast cell granules cause infiltration of neutrophils and monocytes into tissues. Although it is not well documented, it is likely that the mast cell mediators contribute to the changes seen in MOF.

The Neutrophil

The circulating neutrophil, much like the tissue-based mast cell, serves as a sentinel cell for tissue injury and invasion by microorganisms. The classic response of the neutrophil to infection results in accumulation of neutrophils at the site of invasion with continued concentration of neutrophils leading to localization of infection via the formation of an abscess. Studies of neutrophils in the setting of sepsis or uncontrolled local infection have provided evidence that the function of this cell is modulated by circulating mediators. There is in vitro evidence that the neutrophil is less responsive compared with normal after major injury[13,14] and during infection.[15] However, neutrophils appear to be more sensitive to stimulation early after injury when studied in vivo.[8] This paradox may explain the clinically observed increased susceptibility to infection and systemic tissue destruction that occurs during overwhelming infection and MOF.

The preformed mediators of the neutrophil (Table 5–2) include the enzymes elastase, cathepsin G, collagenase, and lysozyme. On activation of the cell, these enzymes are released into the microenvironment in concentrations sufficient to degrade the extracellular matrix. Under controlled conditions, the process remains localized; however, the capacity to destroy large amounts of tissue exists when neutrophils continue to accumulate, the activation process is sustained, or enzyme inhibitors are unable to control the enzymatic process.

On activation of the neutrophil, a membrane bound reduced nicotinamide-adenine dinucleotide phosphate oxidase is activated that generates the short-lived superoxide anion. Two molecules of superoxide react spontaneously to form hydrogen peroxide (H_2O_2). Although H_2O_2 can cause tissue damage, it appears that it is present for only a brief time in the microenvironment.[16] The fate of H_2O_2 is not entirely clear, but it seems unlikely that it is converted to the highly reactive ·OH radical, since iron does not appear to be available to catalyze this reaction.[17] It is more likely that H_2O_2 is converted to hypochlorous acid by

Table 5–3   Mediators from Macrophage or Monocyte*

Lysozyme	Arginase
Prostaglandins	Fibronectin
Leukotrienes	Complement
Lipoprotein lipase	Interleukin 1
Elastase	Tumor necrosis factor (cachectin)
Plasminogen activator	Interferon $\propto$ and β
Collagenase	Angiogenesis factor

*As outlined by Johnston.[53]

myeloperoxidase of the neutrophil. The biologic reactivity of hypochlorous acid is sufficient to cause damage to tissues and proteins.[16]

An additional mediator pathway is activated on perturbation of the neutrophil to generate products of the metabolism of arachidonic acid. The primary product of the cyclooxygenase pathway of arachidonic acid metabolism appears to be prostaglandin E_2 (PGE_2), whereas arachidonate that is metabolized via the lipo-oxygenase pathway results in the generation of LTB_4.

Monocyte or Macrophage

A family of endogenous proteins or glycoproteins, now commonly known as cytokines, exists in both nascient and rapidly transcribable form within mono-cytes or macrophages (Table 5–3). When presented with the appropriate stimulus, such cells produce these proteins in membrane-bound as well as secretory forms. The cytokines subsequently diffuse or interact locally on target cells in minute concentrations. These mediators are capable of influencing a wide range of biologic effects, many of which are essential to normal or beneficially adaptive host responses.[18] It is now appreciated that a complex interaction exists between the cytokines and other inflammatory mediators as well as with classic neuro-humoral hormones. It can be presumed that overlapping stimulatory and in-hibitory functions between these mediators serve to regulate the host response to injury, at least initially, in a manner beneficial to survival and repair. However, it is also increasingly clear that excessive or prolonged influence of these me-diators can adversely influence critical organ function and survival.[19,20]

One cytokine that has received widespread recent attention as a critical me-diator of tissue injury is cachectin/TNF-alpha. This cytokine, which exists in a circulating form of molecular weight 17,000 and in a transmembrane-bound form of molecular weight 29,000, is the dominant protein initially produced by ap-propriately stimulated macrophages.[21] A variety of cells derived from the mye-loid line, such as blood monocytes, pulmonary macrophages, liver Kupffer cells, peritoneal macrophages, mast cells, and natural killer cells, have been shown to be capable of producing this protein. The secretion of cachectin is elicited by a large assortment of infectious and inflammatory stimuli, including bacterial cell wall membranes (LPS), parasite membranes, and viral particles. The secre-tion of TNF is inhibited at the transcriptional and translational level by prophy-lactic glucocorticoid administration.[22]

Many tissues, including adipocytes, myocytes, macrophages, hepatocytes, and osteocytes, are known to possess receptors for TNF. The tissue-specific effects of TNF have been extensively reviewed and appear, in several instances, to mimic the cellular changes associated with injury.[23,24] Although the extent to which this, or any cytokine, may directly contribute to the progressive loss of cellular homeostasis observed in MOF remains speculative at this time, the anatomic proximity of TNF-secreting cells and the large number of high-affinity receptors for TNF within susceptible cell populations lends credence to the potential role of TNF as important effector mediators in MOF[25] (see Clinical Implications).

In addition to the purported role of TNF as an inducer of acute-phase protein synthesis, perhaps the roles most critical to the initiation or propagation of organ failure are the induction of neutrophil degranulation, superoxide production, lysozyme release, and increases in neutrophil adherence to endothelial cells. Certain endothelial cell surface antigens that are observed in delayed-type hypersensitivity reactions and enhanced endothelial cell procoagulant production are directly attributable to TNF. In addition, recent evidence suggests that TNF may also act as a growth factor, possessing not only angiogenic potential, but also serving as a stimulant to fibroblast proliferation. With the capacity to influence both acute injury responses as well as for remodeling of tissue, this cytokine may be necessary for the appropriate orchestration of host tissue responses throughout the recovery phase.

IL-1 is an additional monocyte-derived[26] cytokine mediator with potent biologic effects. This cytokine, which is transcribed in at least two intracellular forms, also influences host responses in both paracrine and endocrine fashion. Like TNF, IL-1 is bound to high-affinity receptors on a wide variety of somatic tissues, although the mechanism for postreceptor signal transmission is more clearly defined and appears to operate via calcium influx and altered cyclic adenosine monophosphate levels. Although early studies focused on the immunomodulatory role of IL-1 and suggested that this cytokine was an enhancing element in the host response to infection or inflammation, recent evidence also suggests a potential role for IL-1 in the early shock and injury phase.[27] This latter effect appears to be most evident in synergy with TNF. Another important attribute shared with TNF is the capacity of IL-1 to exhibit autocrine regulation of its own production. Hence, there appears to be the capacity for continued monocyte production of such cytokines under conditions of continuous or repetitive presence of the inciting stimulus. Whether this autocrine feedback loop is operative under clinical conditions consistent with MOF remains to be determined, although preliminary animal experiments have demonstrated the presence of messenger RNA for both IL-1 and TNF in liver and spleen during prolonged sepsis[28] (see Clinical Implications).

An additional group of macrophage cytokines, known as macrophage inflammatory proteins, have recently been identified and sequenced.[29] These heparin-binding proteins appear to act predominantly by activation of neutrophils, for which they are chemokinetic and chemotactic. Doubtless additional properties will be ascribed to these cytokines in the future.

Two additional cytokine groups, the transforming growth factors and interleukin-6 families, are also produced in macrophages as well as other tissue sites.[30] Although the role for these cytokines appears to be as promoters of healing and direct induction of acute-phase protein synthesis, respectively, they may also serve to modulate the influences of other cytokines. For example, tissue growth factor-beta may possess some properties that suppress the inflammatory effects of TNF and IL-1 such as reductions in the H_2O_2 production of neutrophils and direct inhibition of neutrophil-endothelial cell adherence.

Intrinsic Control of Pathways

There is evidence that all of the pathways of mediator generation are being constantly activated. However, each is immediately controlled by intrinsic mechanisms. Most commonly, these are in the form of circulating inhibitors or inactivators. In the case of cellular activation, most systems have a feedback control to moderate the sequential biochemical reactions involved in generation of mediators.

Recently, Weiss[16] has hypothesized that there is a complex interaction of inhibitors, inactivators, and enzymes that leads to moderation of the effects of neutrophil release of mediators. Although many investigators have proposed that oxidants play a primary role in tissue injury, this investigator has outlined another pathway for tissue injury. He has noted that the chlorinated oxidants that are produced by neutrophils can inactivate the plasma inhibitors of the enzymes that are released by the activated neutrophil. When this occurs, potent enzymes are free to degrade surrounding tissues. Conversely, when inhibitors are readily available, the oxidants are outstripped of their capacity to inactivate them and the enzymes are rendered inactive. This proposal suggests that control of the oxidant production limits tissue injury by an indirect mechanism.

Each of the pathways of mediator generation is regulated by mechanisms such as that previously mentioned. From a clinical perspective, it is important to recognize that loss of inhibition of a pathway is likely to have just as great a clinical effect as does overwhelming activation of the system.

Clinical Implications

The evidence for a central role for mediators in the development of MOF is primarily indirect. Nevertheless, there is solid support for this based on numerous observations of action of the pathways during sepsis and MOF. Immune response is suppressed after injury[31,32] and susceptibility to infection is increased.[33] Chemotactic factors such as C5a are generated during pulmonary failure,[34] and these factors have been shown to modulate the inflammatory response.[6,35] The proteolytic activity in plasma is increased after injury,[36] and increased amounts of elastase have been found in the bronchoalveolar fluid of patients with ARDS.[4] Activation of the complement system occurs[5] and may act primarily or cause secondary damage, as seen in hepatic damage mediated by toxic oxygen intermediates.[37] The prostaglandins and thromboxane A_2 are generated during sepsis and may account for both down-regulation of the response as well as lead to an increase in injury.[38,39] Lung injury is caused by PAF[40] and by interactions of catecholamines and kinins.[41] In each of these cases it is difficult to determine the relative contribution of the individual pathways, since activation of one pathway is sure to lead to activation of others. Furthermore, plasma levels of mediators do not reflect the activity and concentration that is present at the cellular level. Studies in this laboratory suggest that such is the case for mediators derived from macrophages and monocytes.[42]

Recent studies have identified detectable circulating levels of several cytokines during disease states.[43,44] However, given the well-established relationship between endotoxin or viral stimulation to the appearance of certain cytokines in vitro, it may appear somewhat surprising that a higher degree of correlation between infection and cytokine presence does not exist. We have been able to detect circulating TNF in only 40% of critically ill and presumptively infected burn patients.[45] Other investigators have reported consistently greater frequencies of TNF detectability in certain disease states, such as meningococcal septicemia and septic purpura.[20] The seeming discrepancy between the inability to detect this, or other cytokines, in the circulation in association with systemic or tissue-specific effects attributable to their activity may be related to the sensitivity of current assays, although certainly other factors may contribute. Perhaps most likely is the evidence that transmembrane or tissue-fixed cytokine products may be functional even at a time when detectable circulating products are not evident. Recent experimental data from peritoneal macrophages would support this hypothesis.[21] It is also likely that the appearance of circulating forms of several cytokines may be a transient phenomenon, as indicated by recent data from endotoxin-challenged subjects and in infected patients. In fact, as is the case for some cytokines, such as IL-1, circulating forms of the protein may rarely exist. Another potential mechanism by which the production of cytokines may be suppressed is the ability of glucocorticoids to suppress transiently transcription and translation of viable protein. This mechanism may explain, in part, the inability to detect circulating cytokines in some conditions associated with persistent hypercortisolemia whereas states associated with adrenal cortical injury may exhibit high levels.[19,20,45]

Attempts to understand better the pathophysiologic events associated with sepsis and MOF have centered on identifying the locus of activation of the systems and on modulating the mediator generation or its activity. Currently, it is not possible to determine whether the primary site of ongoing disruption of homeostasis is in the "black box" of the wound,[46] the gut,[47] or in the systemic circulation. Initial reports suggested that broad intervention with steroids to modulate the response might reverse the response to sepsis.[48] However, more recent data do not support these findings.[49,50] Initial clinical experiments by Slotman et al.[51] have, however, suggested that inhibition of the production of thromboxane A_2 may prevent respiratory failure in critically ill patients. Furthermore, the infusion of inhibitors of enzymes may assist in controlling organ injury, as has been shown in patients with alpha$_1$-antitrypsin-deficiency-associated emphysema.[52] Thus, there is some evidence that specific medical intervention to control mediator pathways may control organ damage. Nevertheless, at the present time the primary approach still remains a surgical one, that is, prompt tissue repair and removal of sites of infection. In so doing, the activating stimulus to the pathways is removed and homeostasis is maintained or restored.

References

1. Burke JF. The effective period of preventive antibiotic action in experimental incisions and dermal lesions. Surgery 1961;50:161–168.
2. Niewiarowski S, Bankowski E, Rogowicka I. Studies on the absorption and activation of Hageman factor (Factor XII) by collagen and elastin. Thromb Diath Haemorrh 1965;14:387–391.
3. Morrison DC, Cochrane CG. Direct evidence for Hageman factor (Factor XII) activation by bacterial lipopolysaccharides. J Exp Med 1974;140:797–802.
4. Spragg RG, Cochrane CG, McGuire WW. Enzymatic activity causing cleavage of Hageman factor system components in human bronchoalveolar lavage fluid. (Abstr.) Am Rev Respir Dis 1980;122:279.
5. Frank MM. Complement in the pathophysiology of human disease. N Engl J Med 1987;316:1525–1530.
6. Solomkin JS, Cotta LA, Ogle JD, Brodt JK, Ogle CK, Satoh PS, Hurst JM, Alexander JW. Complement-induced expression of cryptic receptors on the neutrophil surface: a mechanism for regulation of acute inflammation in trauma. Surgery 1984;96:336–343.
7. Solomkin JS, Nelson RD, Chenoweth DE, Solem LD, Simmons RL. Regulation of neutrophil migratory function in burn injury by complement activation products. Ann Surg 1984;200:742–746.
8. Yurt RW, Pruitt BA. Decreased wound neutrophils and indiscrete margination in the pathogenesis of wound infection. Surgery 1985;98:191–198.
9. Wintroub BU, Klickstein LB, Kaempfer CE, Austen KF. A human neutrophil-dependent pathway for generation of angiotensin II: purification and physiochemical characterization of the plasma protein substrate. Proc Natl Acad Sci USA 1981;78:1204–1210.
10. Heath R, Kay J, Kuehn L, Dahlmann B, Stauber WT, Mayer M. Immunochemical characterisation of the myofibrillar proteinase from cultured rat myocytes as chymase. Biochem Int 1987;14:675–683.
11. Stevens RL, Fox CC, Lichtenstein LM, Austen KF. Identification of chondroitin sulfate E proteoglycans and heparin proteoglycans in the secretory granules of human lung mast cells. Proc Natl Acad Sci USA 1988;85:2284–2287.
12. Yurt RW. Noncomplement mediators. In: Shires GT, Davis JM (eds): Host defenses in trauma, general surgery, and thermal injury. New York: Raven Press, 1986;19–36.
13. Davis JM, Dineen P, Gallin JI. Neutrophil degranulation and abnormal chemotaxis after thermal injury. J Immunol 1980;124:1467–1471.
14. Warden GD, Mason AD, Pruitt BA. Evaluation of leukocyte chemotaxis in vitro in thermally injured patients. J Clin Invest 1974;54:1001–1003.
15. Alexander JW, Dionigi R, Meakins JL. Periodic variation in the antibacterial function of human neutrophils and its relationship to sepsis. Ann Surg 1971;173:206–213.
16. Weiss SJ. Tissue destruction by neutrophils. N Engl J Med 1989;320:365–376.
17. Britigan BE, Cohen MS, Rosen GM. Hydroxyl radical formation in neutrophils. N Engl J Med 1988;318:858–859.
18. Nathan CF. Secretory products of macrophages. J Clin Invest 1987;79:319–326.
19. Waage A, Halstensen A, Espevik T. Association between tumor necrosis factor in serum and fatal outcome in patients with meningococcal disease. Lancet 1987;1:355–357.
20. Girardin E, Grau GE, Dayer JM, Roux-Lombard P, J5 Study Group, Lambert PH. Tumor necrosis factor and interleukin-1 in the serum of children with severe infectious purpura. N Engl J Med 1988;319:397–400.
21. Kriegler M, Perez C, DeFay K, et al. A novel form of TNF/cachectin is a cell surface cytotoxic transmembrane protein: ramifications for the complex physiology of TNF. Cell 1988;53:45–53.
22. Beutler B, Krochin N, Milsark IW, et al. Control of cachectin (tumor necrosis factor) synthesis: mechanisms of endotoxin resistance. Science 1986;232:977–980.
23. Tracey KJ, Lowry SF. The role of cytokine mediators in septic shock. Adv Surg 1989;21–56.
24. Fong Y, Tracey KJ, Lowry SF, Cerami A. Biology of cachectin. In: Sorg C, ed: Macrophage-derived cell regulatory factors. Cytokines. Basel: S. Karger. 1989;1:74–88.
25. Silen ML, Hesse DG, Felsen D, et al. Cachectin/tumor necrosis factor production by fetal and newborn rat hepatic macrophages. J Pediatr Surg 1989;24:34–38.

26. Dinarello CA. Biology of interleukin-1. FASEB J 1988;2:108–113.
27. Okusawa S, Gelfand JA, Ikejima T, et al. Interleukin-1 induces a shock-like state in rabbits. Synergism with tumor necrosis factor and the effect of cyclooxygenase inhibition. J Clin Invest 1988;81:1162–1172.
28. Marano M, Fong Y, Moldawer LL, et al. Infected burn injury alters hepatic monokine and albumin mRNA contents. Surg Forum 1988;39:6–7.
29. Davatelis G, Tekamp-Olson P, Wolpe SD, et al. Cloning and characterization of a cDNA for murine macrophage inflammatory protein (MIP), a novel monokine with inflammatory and chemokinetic properties. J Exp Med 1988;167:1939–1944.
30. Tatter SB, Santhanam U, Ray A, et al. Interferon-b$_2$ / B-cell differentiation factor BSF-2 / hepatocyte stimulating factor. In UCLA Symposium on Growth Inhibitory and Cytotoxic Polypeptides. In press.
31. Moss NM, Gough DB, Jordan AL, Grbic JT, Wood JJ, Rodrick ML, Mannick JA. Temporal correlation of impaired immune response after thermal injury with susceptibility to infection in a murine model. Surgery 1988;104:882–887.
32. Tchervenkov JI, Latter DA, Psychogios J, Christou NV. Altered leukocyte delivery to specific and nonspecific inflammatory skin lesions following burn injury. J Trauma 1988;28:582–588.
33. Yurt RW, McManus AT, Mason AD Jr, Pruitt BA Jr. Increased susceptibility to infection related to extent of burn injury. Arch Surg 1984;119:183–188.
34. Weigelt JA, Chenoweth DE, Borman KR, Norcross JF. Complement and the severity of pulmonary failure. J Trauma 1988;28:1013–1019.
35. Yurt RW, Shires GT. Increased susceptibility to infection due to infusion of exogenous chemotaxin. Arch Surg 1987;122:111–116.
36. Neely AN, Nathan P, Highsmith RF. Plasma proteolytic activity following burns. J Trauma 1988;28:362–367.
37. Schirmer WJ, Schirmer JM, Naff GB, Fry DE. Contribution of toxic oxygen intermediates to complement-induced reductions in effective hepatic blood flow. J Trauma 1988;28:1295–1300.
38. Oates JA, Fitzgerald GA, Branch RA, Jackson EK, Knapp HR, Roberts LJ. Clinical implications of prostaglandin and thromboxane A2 formation. N Engl J Med 1988;319:689–698.
39. Oates JA, Fitzgerald GA, Branch RA, Jackson EK, Knapp HR, Roberts LJ. Clinical implications of prostaglandin and thromboxane A2 formation: Part II. N Engl J Med 1988;319:761–767.
40. Chang SW, Feddersen CO, Henson PM, Voelkei NF. Platelet-activating factor mediates hemodynamic changes and lung injury in endotoxin-treated rats. J Clin Invest 1987;79:1498–1509.
41. de Oliveira GG, de Oliveira A. Adult respiratory distress syndrome (ARDS): the pathophysiologic role of catecholamine-kinin interactions. J Trauma 1988;28:246–253.
42. Marano MA, Moldawer LL, Fong Y, et al. Cachectin/tumor necrosis factor production in experimental burns and Pseudomonas infection. Arch Surg 1988;123:1383–1388.
43. Scuderi P, Lam KS, Ryan KJ, et al. Raised levels of tumor necrosis factor in parasitic infections. Lancet 1986;2:1364–1365.
44. Balkwill F, Osborne R, Burke F, et al. Evidence for tumor necrosis factor/cachectin production in cancer. Lancet 1987;1:1229–1232.
45. Marano MA, Fong Y, Moldawer LL, et al. Serum cachectin/TNF in critically ill burn patients correlates with infection and mortality. Surg, Gynecol Obstet. In press.
46. Yurt RW, Dolecek R, Brizio-Molteni L, Molteni A, Vaughan G, eds: Tissue hormones. In: Endocrinology of Burn. Philadelphia: Lea & Febiger. In press.
47. Wilmore DW, Smith RJ, O'Dwyer ST, Jacobs DO, Ziegler TR, Wang XD. The gut: a central organ after surgical stress. Surgery 1988;104:917–923.
48. Schumer W. Steroids in the treatment of clinical septic shock. Arch Surg 1976;184:333–341.
49. Bone RC, Fisher CJ, Clemmer TP, Slotman GJ, Metz CA, Balk RA. A controlled clinical trial of high-dose methylprednisolone in the treatment of severe sepsis and septic shock. N Engl J Med 1987;317:653–658.
50. Veterans Administration Systemic Sepsis Cooperative Study Group. Effect of high-dose glucocorticoid therapy on mortality in patients with clinical signs of systemic sepsis. N Engl J Med 1987;317:659–665.
51. Slotman GJ, Burchard KW, D'Arezzo A, Gann DS. Ketoconazole prevents acute respiratory failure in critically ill surgical patients. J Trauma 1988;28:648–654.
52. Wewers MD, Casolaro A, Sellers SE, Swayze SC, McPhaul KM, Wittes JT, Crystal RG. Replacement therapy for alpha-1-antitrypsin deficiency associated with emphysema. N Engl J Med 1987;316:1055–1062.
53. Johnston RB Jr. Current concepts: immunology of monocytes and macrophages. N Engl J Med 1988;747–752.

6

Reticuloendothelial System Failure

Marc Eric Lanser

The reticuloendothelial system (RES) is comprised of the resident macrophages in the liver, spleen, and bone marrow, as well as the more mobile and transient tissue macrophages that populate virtually all interstitial tissues. These macrophages are characterized principally by their marked phagocytic capacity. The RES plays a major role in the removal of circulating particulate and soluble antigens from the blood and may thus be viewed as a barrier to the systemic dissemination of bacteria, endotoxin, immune complexes, and fibrin degradation products.[1-5] This chapter will discuss the mechanisms involved in RES clearance and its role in maintaining peripheral organ integrity by preventing systemic spillover of endotoxin and particulate antigens.

Functional Anatomy of the Reticuloendothelial System

Eighty to 90% of the phagocytic capacity of the RES resides within the phagocytic cells lining the liver sinusoids.[6] This hepatic perisinusoidal unit[7] is comprised of the sinusoid, the lining endothelial and Kupffer cells, the space of Disse, and the adjacent vascular pole of the hepatocyte, all of which have been shown to contribute to the overall phagocytic capacity of the liver.

The hepatic sinusoid differs from capillaries in other tissues in that it is lined by endothelial and Kupffer cells and there is no contiguous basement membrane. Instead, a fenestrated sieve plate bounded by an endothelial membrane opens into the subjacent space of Disse. The fenestrations range from 0.1 to 1 μM in diameter, permitting entry of plasma proteins, macromolecules, and chylomicrons into this space. Destruction of Kupffer or endothelial cells, or both, enlarges or destroys these fenestrations and permits access to the space of Disse by viruses, cell fragments, and bacteria.

Endothelial cells account for the majority of nonparenchymal cells in the liver. These cells, originally thought to be much less active than Kupffer cells in regard to their endocytic capacity, have been shown to endocytose a number of different test particles as effectively as Kupffer cells.[1] Endocytosis by both endothelial and Kupffer cells takes place by both receptor-dependent and receptor-independent mechanisms.[8] Receptor-independent endocytosis consists of uptake of small amounts of plasma by pinocytosis[1] and is the mechanism by which polyvinyl-pyrrolidone, endotoxin, and other substances are removed from the circulation. Endothelial cells are as active as Kupffer cells in their ability to endocytose by this mechanism. Endothelial cells possess Fc receptors for immunoglobulin G (IgG), and avidly bind and endocytose soluble IgG-immune complexes.[9,10] Endothelial cells also possess receptors for insulin and transferrin.[11,12] In contrast to Kupffer cells, however, endothelial cells do not express receptors for the opsonin C3.[13]

Endothelial cells also contain membrane lectins that specifically bind glyco-proteins containing terminal N-acetylglucosamine or mannose residues.[14] This mannose receptor appears to be unique to endothelial cells, since neither Kupffer cells nor hepatocytes exhibit significant numbers of these receptors. It may play a role in removal of some lysosomal enzymes, antigen-antibody complexes, and bacteria.

Phagocytosis has been thought not to be a property of endothelial cells. This was due to the fact that ordinarily the phagocytic capacity of Kupffer cells overshadows that of endothelial cells. However, when Kupffer cells are damaged or are otherwise incapable of phagocytosis, endothelial cells may effectively phagocytose a variety of blood-borne particulates.[15]

Kupffer cells comprise nearly 50% of the nonparenchymal cells of the liver. They are derived from circulating monocytes and have a resident half-time of approximately 12 days in the liver. Although the ultimate fate of the resident Kupffer cells is unknown, these cells are capable of migrating to regional lymph nodes.[16] Such movement implies the capability of interacting with antibody-forming cells. Such an accessory function in antigen-stimulated lymphocyte proliferation has been shown,[17] as has the presence of Ia antigens on the Kupffer cell surface.[13]

Kupffer cells lie on and in between endothelial cells, with their membrane processus extending into the sinusoidal lumen. These cells are thereby in optimal position to sample sinusoidal blood; their main function being clearance of in-soluble and particulate antigens. These cells possess both Fc and complement (C3) receptors. Clearance of immune complexes, both IgG and IgA, occurs by binding to Fc receptors, while opsonized particles (including most bacteria) bind to Kupffer cell C3 receptors.[18] Although C3 receptors mediate binding, "activation" of these receptors is required in order for them to mediate ingestion. Endotoxin, fibronectin (FN) and other proteins activate C3 receptors to permit internalization of the bound ligand.[19,20] The activity of both Fc and C3 receptors is influenced by a number of physiologic and pathologic conditions, as will be discussed later.

Kupffer cells avidly bind and ingest endotoxin, both in vitro and in vivo.[3,21] Endotoxin clearance appears to be mediated by a process of absorptive pinocytosis. The capacity for endotoxin uptake by Kupffer cells is enormous and can be overcome only by severely depressing Kupffer cell phagocytic function. Uptake of ^{125}I-labeled endotoxin may be inhibited by a tenfold excess of unlabeled endotoxin, implying that endotoxin clearance is not a nonspecific phenomena and that there are a finite number of receptors on the cell membrane. Uptake is inhibited by 2-deoxyglucose, demonstrating that endotoxin uptake is at least partially energy dependent.

A fucose-binding lectin has recently been described that appears to be unique to Kupffer cells.[22] Although the exact physiologic significance of such a receptor is presently unknown, the possibility that it plays an important role in nonspecific phagocytosis of a variety of ubiquitous glycoproteins must be considered.

Macrophages secrete a number of important mediators of the inflammatory response. Interleukin-1, tumor necrosis factor, and interleukin-6 have received the most recent attention. These monokines regulate hepatocyte production of a number of acute-phase proteins. Kupffer cells have been shown to secrete monokines in response to endotoxin and fibrin split products.[23,24] It seems reasonable to assume that Kupffer cell monokines that are produced following injury or during inflammation may act in a paracrine fashion on neighboring hepatocytes to control acute-phase protein production.

To the extent that the vascular pole of the hepatocyte is in close proximity to the Kupffer cell and that hepatocytes are capable of endocytosing a variety of particles, these cells should be considered in any discussion of the RES.[7] The vascular pole of the hepatocyte is made up of a convoluted plasma membrane consisting of thousands of microvilli, which markedly increase the plasma membrane surface area. These cells possess receptors for a number of substances, including glycoproteins, growth factors, and antibiotics. In addition, hepatocytes possess a galactose-binding lectin. Uptake of autologous immune complexes by hepatocytes has also been shown to occur.[9,25] This uptake appears to be mediated by Fc receptors, which have been demonstrated on hepatocyte membranes.[9,26,27] Hepatocyte uptake of IgA complexes is particularly important and is mediated by IgA secretory component on hepatocyte membranes, which functions as a receptor for IgA.[27] Hepatocytes also endocytose a variety of colloidal particles, including colloidal albumin and antimony sulfur colloid.[1]

In addition to the normal uptake of numerous substances, hepatocyte uptake may increase in a number of pathologic conditions associated with destruction of Kupffer cell and endothelial cell phagocytic capacity. Such a phenomena may account for the hepatocyte injury following Kupffer cell destruction by agents such as frog virus 3.[28]

In summary, this perisinusoidal complex of endocytosing cells is well-situated and equipped to remove a wide variety of soluble and insoluble antigens effectively from the circulation. These cells function primarily as a filter to remove gut-derived antigens, circulating particulates, and antigen-antibody complexes from the portal circulation. Depression in the phagocytic capacity of the RES results in prolonged systemic circulation of these antigens and an increase in their uptake in peripheral organ vascular beds. Peripheral localization of endotoxin, platelet aggregates, and antigen-antibody complexes has in turn been postulated as being a major cause of peripheral organ dysfunction.

Modulation of RES Endocytic Function and the Phenomenon of RES Blockade

The phagocytic capacity of the RES is generally determined by injecting test substances known to be phagocytosed by the macrophages of the RES. These RES test particles include carbon, lipid emulsions, latex, antimony sulfur colloid, and aggregated albumin. The rate of disappearance of the test particles from the circulation (phagocytic index) is a reflection of the functional phagocytic capacity of the RES.

Clinically, microaggregated albumin and antimony sulfur colloid have been found to be the most useful agents to assess the phagocytic capacity of the RES.[29] Many of these substances are taken up by other nonparenchymal cells, so that clearance capacity cannot be taken to reflect only Kupffer cell phagocytic activity. The role of specific receptor-mediated uptake of many of these substances is also unknown. However, most of these test particles activate the alternative complement pathway, so that C3 receptor binding undoubtedly plays a role in their clearance. Specific activity of Fc and C3 receptors can be measured both experimentally and clinically by using IgG-immune complexes and complement-coated IgM complexes, respectively. The function of the mannose receptor can be assessed using mannose-derivatized glycoproteins.[30]

The phagocytic capacity of the RES is depressed following the intravenous injection of a large quantity of particles that are cleared by the cells of the RES.[31] This depression, or blockade is manifested by an increase in the half-time in the circulation of a subsequent test dose of the same particle. The duration of the blockade is variable, but typically it lasts from 6 to 12 hours in experimental animals. Both the duration and amount of depression are related to the particle dose.

RES blockade is actually due to a decrease in the number of receptors available to interact with the subsequently injected test particles. The number of Fc and C3 receptors correlates with the capacity of the liver to clear particles that bind to these receptors. For example, the number of Fc receptors on the surface of the sinusoidal lining cells following injection of IgG complexes markedly decreases.[32] This is followed by a return to the baseline number of receptors after approximately 24 hours. Depression of Fc-mediated clearance of immune complexes following the injection of a large dose of such complexes does not affect C3-mediated clearance of complement-coated particles.

Both the transient nature of the blockade and the necessity for the injection of an extremely large particle load in order to achieve blockade should be emphasized. Although RES blockade remains an excellent model in which to investigate the mechanisms involved in RES clearance, it remains to be determined whether acute RES blockade actually occurs clinically.

Experimentally, transient RES depression occurs following burn, mechanical trauma, surgery, and even anesthesia.[5,33–38] This depression lasts 12 to 18 hours, is followed by a rapid recovery, and does not seem to be due to a decrease in the hepatic blood flow, since a similar reduction in hepatic blood flow by hemorrhage does not depress the RES to the same degree.[35] C3-mediated liver localization of opsonized red blood cells is depressed approximately 50% after trauma,[35] although eventually the test particles do localize to the liver, albeit with an increased circulating half-time. The effect of RES depression on the clearance of trauma-generated endogenous particles cannot be discerned from the experimental data, since the identity of such a particle and the amount that is discharged into the circulation by trauma remains speculative.

Although the exact reason for the decrease in C3-mediated clearance following trauma is unknown, it would seem that a likely explanation for post-traumatic RES depression may be an alteration in the number or activity of C3b or C3bi (or both) receptors. Whether the decrease in the number of receptors is due to antigenic or particle overload at the time of injury remains an open question.

Neutrophil exposure to phorbol esters, which directly activate protein kinase C (PKC), results in an eventual decrease in the number of C3b receptors.[39] In an analogous manner, activation of macrophage PKC by endogenous mediators or complement products generated by trauma could conceivably increase and then reduce complement receptor expression. Tissue debris, immune complexes, or cell aggregates discharged into the circulation at the time of injury could also result in macrophage PKC activation after interacting with specific cell receptors.

Down-regulation of Fc receptors occurs following exposure to IgG immune complexes and even monomeric IgG.[2,40,41] Down-regulation is reversible and transient, with recovery of Fc function occurring within 1 hour of removal of the immune complexes. In this regard, Fc recovery appears to occur a bit faster than recovery of C3 receptors. It appears that a constant exposure to high doses of either immune complexes or C3-opsonized particles is necessary to maintain suppression of these receptors. Such a prolonged, constant exposure of the RES to these complexes or particles after injury does not seem to occur, since RES depression resolves within 24 hours, indicating that any RES depressing substances generated at the time of injury are no longer circulating. This observation has a direct bearing on whether or not RES depression could explain the delayed multiple organ failure that occurs following severe injury. This will be discussed in greater detail later.

Effect of Endotoxin on RES Clearance Capacity

It has been observed that specific pathogen-free animals and animals treated with antibiotics have a lowered resistance to hemorrhagic shock.[33,42] This lowered resistance is associated with depression of RES phagocytic capacity in SPF and antibiotic-treated animals. It appears that stimulation of the liver RES by absorbed enteric pathogens may be important in maintaining RES phagocytic capacity and resistance to hemorrhagic shock.

Chronic endotoxin administration does in fact prime the RES by increasing its phagocytic capacity.[43,44] Repetitive injections of low doses of endotoxin increases RES phagocytic capacity almost two- to threefold in rats, while at the same time increasing the animal's resistance to a lethal dose of the endotoxin. The increase in RES phagocytic capacity may be related to the activating effect of portal vein endotoxin (or other activating factors) on C3 receptor function.[19,45] Endotoxin tolerance may not be entirely attributable to RES hyperactivity, however, because recent data suggest that monocyte production of inflammatory monokines and other enzymes is markedly reduced in endotoxin-tolerant animals.[46,47] An increase in RES phagocytic capacity has also been observed in patients with peritonitis.[48] Presumably, this increase in RES function is due to its stimulation by repetitive episodes of endotoxemia. It seems likely that gut-derived endotoxin plays an important physiologic role in maintaining RES phagocytic capacity.

A sublethal or lethal injection of endotoxin results in an immediate and transient decrease in RES phagocytic capacity.[43,44] This decrease is followed within 24 hours by a state of RES hyperphagocytosis. The immediate depression in phagocytic activity is related to the dose of injected endotoxin, and it lasts less than 24 hours regardless of the dose used. Similar results are obtained following intravenous or intraperitoneal injection of live bacteria. In each case an immediate RES depression is followed by a rebound hyperphagocytic state within 24 hours. These data are therefore not fully compatible with the notion that acute or chronic endotoxemia or bacteremia is responsible for protracted RES phagocytic depression. Furthermore, it seems unlikely that pure RES depression could be invoked as a cause of progressive multiple organ failure during prolonged sepsis.

Role of the RES in Preventing Antigen Spillover and Antibody Formation

Antibodies are produced in peripheral lymphoid tissues; predominantly lymph nodes and spleen. Exposure of peripheral B lymphocytes to macrophage-processed antigen and T-cell helper factors results in their clonal expansion and antibody production. Obviously, antigen must reach these lymphoid tissues in order to initiate antibody production. The functional state of the RES has a direct bearing on the amount of gut-derived antigen that reaches lymphoid tissue in order to initiate antibody production. Although Kupffer cells do possess Ia antigens and are capable of antigen-presenting activity,[17] it is generally believed that the liver itself is immunologically relatively unresponsive in order to inhibit the development of chronic inflammatory hepatic lesions.

Sequestration and metabolism of gut-derived antigen in the liver decreases the amount of antibody produced to the particular antigen.[49] Injection of soluble antigen into the inferior vena cava results in a far greater antibody response than does intraportal injection,[50] and blockade of the RES with colloidal carbon results in an augmented immune response to peripherally injected antigens.[51] Serum levels of antibodies against enteric bacteria, especially *Escherichia coli*, are elevated in patients with cirrhosis, chronic active hepatitis, and portacaval shunts.[52–55] Antibodies to dietary proteins are also elevated in cirrhosis. The cause of the increased antibody production is thought to be decreased hepatic uptake, with consequent spillover of antigen into the systemic circulation where it stimulates peripheral lymphoid tissue.[56] This hypothesis is further supported by the increased incidence of systemic (as opposed to portal) endotoxemia in patients with cirrhosis.[54,57] The decrease in hepatic uptake of endotoxin and other antigens in the stable cirrhotic patient appears to be due to shunting of portal blood flow away from endocytosing cells, rather than to a specific defect in the Kupffer cell's ability to take up antigen.[58] This is in contrast to cases of acute hepatic failure, where decreased RES uptake is due to individual cell dysfunction rather than intrahepatic shunting.[59] The degree to which spillover occurs in acute hepatic failure is determined by the severity of the hepatic necrosis.[59]

Endocytosis of endotoxin occurs by pinocytosis. Normal Kupffer cells have an enormous capacity for adsorbing endotoxin. In rabbits, in vivo clearance of intravenously injected endotoxin occurs rapidly, with a $t_{1/2}$ of less than 30 minutes.[3] Conversion of the remaining circulating endotoxin to a low molecular weight form results in a marked delay in its subsequent clearance, with a $t_{1/2}$ of approximately 12 hours. Approximately 80% of the cleared endotoxin is localized to Kupffer cells, where it is subsequently metabolized. Although uptake of endotoxin may occur independent of C3 and Fc receptor activity, endotoxin does activate complement, and animals do possess natural antibodies against a variety of gut organisms. It would therefore be expected that alteration in C3 and Fc receptor activity could influence the rate of endotoxin clearance.

Endotoxin is a normal constituent of human portal blood.[57] Severe liver disease, chronic or acute, compromises the ability of the liver to remove this gut-derived endotoxin.[54,57] Simultaneous portal vein and peripheral arterial blood sampling for endotoxin reveals the presence of endotoxin in 50 to 75% of portal blood samples taken from individuals without gastrointestinal or liver disease. Peripheral endotoxemia is rare, except in those patients with liver disease or gram-negative bacterial sepsis. Spillover of endotoxin into the systemic circulation cannot be demonstrated in hemodynamically stable patients without an overt septic focus, clinically evident liver necrosis, or cirrhosis. Unfortunately, no studies correlating the degree of RES depression with the presence of peripheral endotoxemia have been undertaken, so that the degree of RES depression that is required before endotoxin spills over into the systemic circulation is not known.

Alteration in endotoxin clearance occurs under a variety of acute experimental and clinical conditions. A 70% hepatectomy results in a 50% decrease in RES clearance of endotoxin[60] and in this circumstance endotoxin uptake by the spleen, lungs, and kidneys increases in a compensatory manner, without any obvious detrimental effect. The clinical significance of this increase in peripheral uptake of endotoxin is unclear.

During hemorrhagic or traumatic shock, RES function is transiently depressed,[33,37,61] and, during the shock period, experimental animals are more susceptible to bacteremia or endotoxemia.[62] Although gut-derived endotoxin becomes detectable in the peripheral circulation during shock,[63-65] and since RES depression is present only during shock and shortly thereafter RES returns to normal, it seems unlikely that peripheral endotoxemia of gut origin would persist following resuscitation from burn, trauma, or hemorrhage. Although the appearance of endotoxin in the peripheral circulation may be due to a decrease in the RES clearance of gut-derived endotoxin, some evidence suggests that gut-derived endotoxin may also enter the systemic circulation directly after translocating across the bowel wall into the peritoneal cavity.[66] Such a route of absorption would bypass the liver entirely.[67,68] In dogs, hemorrhagic shock does not result in peripheral bacteremia unless the RES is further depressed by blockading with colloidal carbon.[69] Although RES function in humans may be depressed enough during severe hypovolemic shock to permit systemic detection of endotoxin and even bacteria, this is undoubtedly a transient phenomenon. Severely burned patients, who present often in hypovolemic shock prior to resuscitation, do not manifest peripheral endotoxemia until a few days after injury, when RES function has returned to normal.[70,71] In one study,[70] peripheral endotoxemia could only be detected in patients with gram-negative bacterial colonization of the burn wound. Such studies indicate that for severe but initially survivable injuries, it is unlikely that RES depression and escape of gut endotoxin accounts for the relatively late clinical deterioration associated with multiple organ failure.[72]

Failure of RES function to become normal within 24 hours after severe ischemic liver injury is associated with death, whereas return of RES function to normal is associated with survival.[61] Early death in this case may be due in part to failure of the RES to remove circulating gut-derived endotoxin or bacteria, but it may also be due to associated irreversible ischemic injury to other vital organs. In critically ill but stable trauma patients, reticuloendothelial phagocytic function has been found to be initially depressed, but within 1 or 2 days RES function becomes normal or even elevated.[48] This is despite the fact that many such patients eventually succumb to their injuries. Patients who are critically ill with peritonitis have likewise been found to have normal or elevated RES phagocytic function throughout their course. Such clinical data correlates well with experimental studies showing transient RES depression after trauma and normal or elevated reticuloendothelial phagocytic function during chronic infection.

In contrast to the generally intact RES in diseases that primarily do not affect the liver, experimental or clinical liver destruction results in persistent peripheral endotoxemia and even bacteremia of gut origin.[73,74] This endotoxin, which is normally released from the gut into the portal vein, appears capable of having significant detrimental effects on peripheral organs if it is not cleared efficiently by the RES. Endotoxin has been implicated in the central nervous system (CNS) disturbances observed in Reye's syndrome,[73] and in the renal failure, coagulopathy, and CNS dysfunction seen with fulminant hepatic failure from many causes.[74] These findings are in accord with the known direct effects of endotoxin or renal function, the coagulation system, and the CNS. Although cholestatic jaundice is associated with some depression in reticuloendothelial phagocytic function,[75] the liver injury is apparently not severe enough to cause endotoxin spillover into the systemic circulation.[59,74] Extreme degrees of hepatic necrosis are necessary before RES depression results in endotoxin spillover.

Role of the RES in Host Defense Following Injury

The experimental and clinical evidence already discussed suggests that transient RES depression following injury is unlikely to result in prolonged, repetitive endotoxemia. Neither does the degree and duration of postinjury RES depression appear to be a likely cause of post-traumatic multiple organ failure. However, a role for RES failure in contributing to early death from injury seems plausible. RES depression is associated with early death from experimental trauma, and stimulation of the phagocytic capacity of the RES prior to injury is protective.[5,31,34,38,49,76–78] Repetitive, minor, whole body trauma results in resistance to more severe injury. This adaptive resistance to trauma is associated with an increase in both in vivo and in vitro RES phagocytic capacity.[79] Blockade of the RES at the time of injury increases early mortality.[37] The increased susceptibility to trauma only occurs if the blockading substance is given a few hours prior to the experimental injury. Since one of the functions of the RES is to clear platelet aggregates, fibrin degradation products, and immune complexes, it may be that RES depression at the time of injury results in prolonged circulation of such particulates, permitting their microembolization to peripheral vascular beds.[38,80]

Unfortunately, the cause of early death in experimentally traumatized animals is not precisely known. It is also not known whether alteration in RES phagocytic function would affect the amount of trauma-generated endogenous microaggregates embolizing in peripheral tissues. Trauma certainly increases the amount of exogenously injected test particles that localize in the lung, but this increase is relatively modest (about 70%) and it returns to normal about 6 hours after injury in surviving animals.[5] Thus, RES failure is associated with early death, but whether it is a significant contributing factor remains unclear.

Fibronectin, RES Function, and Pulmonary Microembolization

Plasma FN is a 440 kd glycoprotein that is synthesized predominantly by hepatocytes.[81] After an initial decline following experimental trauma or introduction of bacteria, FN levels increase two- or threefold and then slowly return to normal over a period of 1 to 2 days.[38,82,83] Levels of FN change similarly following severe burn injury in humans, although the increase is less striking than that seen experimentally.[84] In contrast to experimental infection, clinical infection is associated with consistently depressed levels of FN, which only return to normal after resolution of the sepsis.[84,85] Hepatic synthesis of FN is stimulated by interleukin-6,[86] which is produced by macrophages during inflammation. FN should therefore be considered an acute-phase protein, at least in some animals. The prolonged depression of human FN levels during clinical sepsis may be due to accelerated peripheral consumption at the site of inflammation. Alternatively, FN may not be an acute phase protein in humans. Measurement of FN mRNA in human liver during sepsis should resolve this question.

FN binds to a wide variety of proteins, including fibrin and denatured collagen, and cells such as platelets, bacteria, and macrophages.[81] This property of FN has been cited as evidence that FN functions as a nonspecific opsonin in vivo, mediating the RES clearance of tissue debris, platelet aggregates, and fibrin.[38,87]

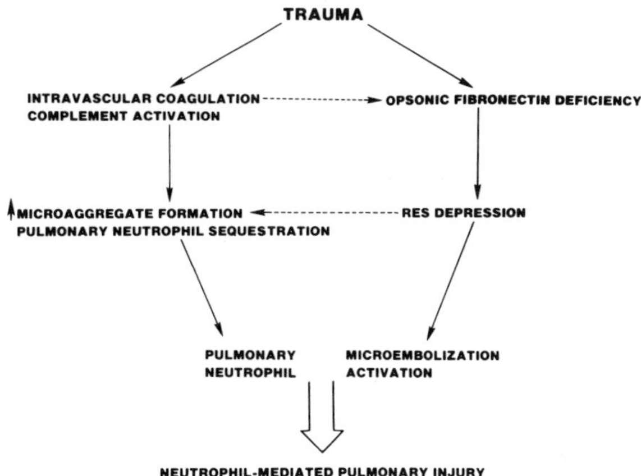

Figure 6–1. Hypothesized relationship between fibronectin-mediated RES failure and neutrophil-induced ARDS.

The function of FN as a nonspecific opsonin has implications for its potential role as a modulator of RES clearance of microaggregates. Embolization of platelet aggregates and tissue debris in the pulmonary microvasculature after injury or during inflammation has been hypothesized to be a major cause of adult respiratory distress syndrome (ARDS).[38,87] Depression of FN-mediated RES clearance could permit the debris to embolize in the pulmonary microcirculation. In situ activation of neutrophils during phagocytosis of such debris in the pulmonary microvasculature could then result in neutrophil-mediated endothelial injury. Such an hypothesis is outlined in Figure 6–1. Unfortunately, it is unclear what role such aggregates play in the development of ARDS, or whether such aggregates even circulate in vivo in amounts sufficient to cause peripheral organ dysfunction after injury. Perhaps due to the lack of clear evidence for the endogenous generation of this debris, attention has recently been turned to the generation of soluble factors as a cause of ARDS. These factors are discussed in detail elsewhere in this book.

The importance of FN as a modulator of RES function is currently being reevaluated. Although macrophages have receptors for FN,[88] they also have receptors for C3b/bi and the Fc portion of immunoglobulins.[20] These receptors and their regulation have already been discussed. It is difficult if not impossible to separate FN receptor activity from C3b/bi receptor activity. It is therefore unclear whether FN is the sole or even the major opsonin for circulating particulates in vivo.

Much of the evidence that FN mediates RES clearance of particulates is based on RES blockade experiments, whereby injection of a particulate load simultaneously depresses FN levels and RES clearance of a subsequent particle challenge.[87] Experimental trauma has the same effect as a particle load.[5,82] Pulmonary uptake of the particle challenge increases during the period of RES depression. However, C3-mediated clearance is also depressed under these same experimental conditions.[35] The 50 to 80% reduction in FN levels that occurs following blockade or trauma seems unlikely to affect in vivo opsonization, since in general opsonins such as C3 are normally present in considerable excess, and reduction of this magnitude typically has no effect on in vitro opsonization.

FN levels do not always correlate with in vivo RES phagocytic activity. In critically ill septic patients, FN levels are consistently depressed,[84,85] and yet RES function remains normal.[48] In patients with hepatic failure, plasma FN levels are poorly correlated with RES clearance of microaggregated albumin.[89] Experimentally, discrepancies between FN levels and in vivo RES clearance function are observed following induction of tolerance to endotoxin or traumatic shock.[44,79,90] In these models, RES activity is markedly increased, whereas FN levels are normal. Administration of FN to animals following trauma normalizes their FN plasma levels, but does not normalize their reticuloendothelial function.[82,90,91] In fact, FN administration actually increases the amount of test colloid that is trapped in the lung during RES depression.[82,84] The paradoxical increase in lung localization following bolus FN administration is probably due to the increased intravascular aggregation of the colloid caused by the high plasma concentration of FN during bolus infusion.

The evidence for FN-mediated RES depression following injury is therefore rather weak, and most of the RES depression that occurs following injury can be accounted for by decreases in C3 and Fc receptor activity. In contrast, FN appears to be important in regulating the biologic activity of cells within the area of tissue injury. FN is capable of activating macrophages, triggering phagocytosis by C3b/bi receptors.[20,92] Ordinarily, these receptors mediate binding but not ingestion of C3b-opsonized particles. In the presence of FN, binding to these receptors results in their ingestion. FN also mediates ingestion of non-opsonized particles that activate the alternative complement pathway.[93] In this way, FN could increase the phagocytic activity of macrophages in the area of injury. Thus, rather than acting as an opsonin in the systemic clearance of particulates, FN may play an important local role in wound biology.

Summary and Conclusions

The RES removes endotoxin, bacteria, platelet aggregates, and fibrin from the portal circulation, thus preventing their spillover into the systemic circulation. Removal occurs via both receptor-dependent and receptor-independent mechanisms. FN may not be an important modulator of RES phagocytic activity. RES phagocytic capacity may be transiently depressed following trauma, hemorrhagic shock, or endotoxemia. This RES depression is most likely mediated by a decrease in number or activity of C3b/bi receptors on hepatic nonparenchymal cells. Since RES depression is so transient, it appears unlikely that it plays a major role in the late clinical deterioration seen after injury or during persistent sepsis. RES function in critically ill patients with trauma or sepsis has been shown to be relatively normal, a fact that supports the hypothesis that RES failure is not a potential cause of delayed multiple organ failure. In contrast, transient RES phagocytic depression during and after trauma may contribute to the early mortality seen following lethal injury. In this case it remains difficult to ascribe death to RES failure alone, since massive associated injuries to vital structures also occurs.

RES failure seems to have a more defined role in the systemic endotoxemia and multiple organ failure associated with hepatic necrosis. In these cases, gut-derived endotoxin is frequently detected in the peripheral circulation, and its effects on the CNS, kidney, and coagulation system may be pronounced.

Acknowledgment. This work was supported in part by National Institutes of Health GM36258 and Research Career Development Award GM00511.

References

1. Dalen DP, Brouwer A, Knook DL. Clearance capacity of rat liver Kupffer, endothelial, and parenchymal cells. Gastroenterology 1981;81:1036–1044.
2. Laan-Klamer SM, Atmosoerodjo-Briggs JE, Harms G, Hoedermaeker PJ, Hardonk MJ. A histochemical study about the involvement of rat liver cells in the uptake of heterologous immune complexes from the circulation. Histochemistry 1985;82:477–482.
3. Mathison JC, Ulevitch RJ. The clearance, tissue distribution, and cellular localization of intravenously injected lipopolysaccharide in rabbits. J Immunol 1979;123:2133–2143.
4. Nolan JP. Endotoxin, reticuloendothelial function, and liver injury. Hepatology 1981;1:458–465.
5. Saba TM. Reticuloendothelial systemic host defense after surgery and traumatic shock. Circ Shock 1975;2:91–108.
6. Biozzi G, Stiffel C. The physiopathology of the reticuloendothelial cells of the liver and spleen. Prog Liver Dis 1965;2:166–191.
7. David H, Reinke P. The concept of the "perisinusoidal function unit" of the liver—importance to pathological processes. Exp Pathol 1987;32:193–224.
8. Silverstein SC, Steinman RM, Cohn ZA. Endocytosis. Annu Rev Biochem 1977;46:669–722.
9. Laan-Klamer SM, Harms G, Atmosoerodjo JE, Meijer DK, Hardonk MJ, Hoedemaeker PJ. Studies on the mechanism of binding and uptake of immune complexes by various cell types of rat liver *in vivo*. Scand J Immunol 1986;23:127–133.
10. Muro H, Shirasawa H, Maeda M, Nakamura S. Fc receptors of liver sinusoidal endothelirum in normal rats and humans Gastroenterology 1987;93:1078–1085.
11. Soda R, Tavassoli M. Distribution of insulin receptors in liver cell suspensions using a minibead probe. Highest density is on endothelial cell. Exp Cell Res 1983;145:389–395.
12. Soda R, Tavassoli M. Insulin uptake by rat liver endothelium studied in fractionated liver cell suspensions. Mol Cell Biochem 1985;65:117–123.
13. Pulford K, Souhami RL. The surface properties and antigen-presenting function of hepatic non-parenchymal cells. Clin Exp Immunol 1981;46:581–588.
14. Steer CJ, Ashwell G. Hepatic membrane receptors for glycoproteins. Prog Liver Dis 1986;8:99–123.
15. Steffan AM, Gendrault JL, McCuskey RS, McCuskey PA, Kirn A. Phagocytosis, an unrecognized property of murine endothelial liver cells. Hepatology 1986;6:830–836.
16. Hardonk MJ, Dijkhuis WJ, Grond J, Koudstaal J, Poppema S. Evidence for a migratory capability of rat Kupffer cells to portal tracts and hepatic lymph nodes. Virchows Arch [Cell Pathol] 1986;51:429–442.
17. Richman LK, Klingenstein RJ, Richman JA, Strober W, Berzofsky JA. The murine Kupffer cell. I. Characterization of the cell serving accessory functions in antigen-specific T cell proliferation. J Immunol 1979;123:2602–2609.
18. Munthe-Kass AC, Kaplan G, Seljelid R. On the mechanism of internalization of opsonized articles by rat Kupffer cells in vitro. Exp Cell Res 1976;103:201–212.
19. Steffan AM, Kirn A. C3-mediated phagocytosis induced in murine Kupffer cells by *in vitro* activation with endotoxin. Gastroenterol Clin Biol 1986;10:117–121.
20. Wright SD, Craigmyle LS, Silverstein SC. Fibronectin and serum amyloid P component stimulate C3b- and C3bi-mediated phagocytosis in cultured human monocytes. J Exp Med 1983;158:1338–1343.
21. Ruitter DJ, van der Meulen J, Brouwer A, Hummel MJ, Mlauw J, Ploeg JC, Wisse E. Uptake by liver cells of endotoxin following its intravenous injection. Lab Invest 1981;45:38–45.

22. Haltiwanger RS, Lehrman MA, Ekhardt AE, Hill RL. The distribution and localization of the fucose-binding lectin in rat tissues and the identification of a high affinity form of the mannose/N-acetylglucosamine-binding lectin in rat liver. J Biol Chem 1986;261:7433–7439.
23. Kurokawa S, Ishibashi H, Shirahama M, Hayashida K, Tsuchiya Y, Sakaki Y, Niho Y. Production of hepatocyte stimulating factor of rat Kupffer cells induced by lipopolysaccharide: partial characterization and effects on alpha 2 macroglobulin gene expression in cultured adult rat hepatocytes. J Clin Lab Immunol 1988;25:131–137.
24. Sanders KD, Fuller GM. Kupffer cell regulation of fibrinogen synthesis in hepatocytes. Thromb Res 1983;32:133–145.
25. Hopf U, Schaefer HE, Hess G, Meyer Zum Buschenfelde KH. In vivo uptake of immune complexes by parenchymal and nonparenchymal liver cells in mice. Gastroenterology 1981;80:250–259.
26. Frommel D, Rachman R. Receptor for the Fc portion of IgG on the plasma membrane of the hepatocyte. Ann Immunol (Paris) 1979;130C:553–560.
27. Sancho J, Gonzalez E, Egido J. The importance of the Fc receptors for IgA in the recognition of IgA by mouse liver cells: its comparison with carbohydrate and secretory component receptors. Immunology 1986;57:37–42.
28. Jones EA, Summerfield JA. Functional aspects of hepatic sinusoidal cells. Semin Liver Dis 1985;5:157–174.
29. Ito M, Wagner HN Jr. Studies of the reticuloendothelial system (RES). I. Measurement of the phagocytic capacity of the RES in man and dog. J Clin Invest 1963;42:417–426.
30. Furbish FG, Steer CJ, Krett NL, Bananger JA. Uptake and distribution of placental glucocerebrosidase in rat hepatic cells and effects of sequential deglycosylation. Biochim Biophys Acta 1981;673:425–434.
31. Zweifach BW, Benacerraf B, Thomas L. The relationship between the vascular manifestations of shock produced by endotoxin, trauma, and hemorrhage. II. The possible role of the reticuloendothelial system in resistance to each type of shock. J Exp Med 1959;110:547–569.
32. Nishi T, Bhan AK, Collins AB, McCluskey RT. Effect of circulating immune complexes on Fc and C3 receptors of Kupffer cells in vivo. Lab Invest 1981;44:442–448.
33. Altura BM. Hemorrhagic shock and reticuloendothelial system phagocytic function in pathogen-free animals. Circ Shock 1974;1:295–300.
34. Altura BM, Hershey SG. RES phagocytic function in trauma and adaptation to experimental shock. Am J Physiol 1968;215:1414–1419.
35. Loegering DJ. Kupffer cell complement receptor clearance function and host defense. Circ Shock 1986;20:321–333.
36. Lofgstrom B, Schildt B. Reticuloendothelial function under general anaesthesia. Acta Anaesth Scand 1974;18:34–40.
37. McKenna JM, Zweifach BW. Reticuloendothelial system in relation to drum shock. Am J Physiol 1956;187:263–268.
38. Saba TM, Jaffe E. Plasma fibronectin (opsonic glycoprotein): its synthesis by vascular endothelial cells and role in cardiopulmonary integrity after trauma as related to reticuloendothelial function. Am J Med 1980;68:577–594.
39. Changelian PS, Jack RM, Collins LA, Fearon DT. PMA induces the ligand-independent internalization of CR1 on human neutrophils. J Immunol 1985;134:1851–1858.
40. Kelton JG, Singer J, Rodger C, Gauldie J, Horsewood P, Dent P. The concentration of IgG in the serum is a major determinant of Fc-dependent reticuloendothelial function. Blood 1985;66:490–495.
41. Kurlander RJ. Reversible and irreversible loss of Fc receptor function of human monocytes as a consequence of interaction with immunoglobulin G. J Clin Invest 1980;66:773–781.
42. Altura BM, Gebrewold A. Prophylactic administration of antibiotics compromises reticuloendothelial system function and exacerbates shock mortality in rats. BR J Pharmacol 1980;68:19–21.
43. Loegering DJ, Schneidkraut MJ. Effect of endotoxin on alpha-2-SB-opsonic protein activity and reticuloendothelial system phagocytic function. J Reticuloendothel Soc 1979;26:197–204.
44. Richards PS, Saba TM. Effect of endotoxin on fibronectin and Kupffer cell activity. Hepatology 1985;5:32–37.
45. Holdstock G, Hammond PG, Iles S, Smith JL, Tanner AR, Wright R. Activation of monocytes by portal serum and its relationship to immunoglobulin, immune complex and endotoxin content. Liver 1982;2:222–229.
46. Greisman SE, Hornick RB. Mechanisms of endotoxin tolerance with special reference to man. J Infect Dis 1973;128 (suppl):S265–S276.
47. McCuskey RS, Urbaschek R, McCuskey PA, Sacco N, Stauber WT, Pinkstaff CA, Urbaschek B.

Deficient Kupffer cell phagocytosis and lysosomal enzymes in the endotoxin-low-responsive C3H/HeJ mouse. J Leuk Biol 1984;36:591–600.
48. Schildt B, Gertz I, Wide L. Differentiated reticuloendothelial system (RES) function in some critical surgical conditions. Acta Chir Scand 1974;140:611–617.
49. Thomas HC, MacSween RN, White RG. Hyperglobulinaemia in liver disease. Lancet 1973;2:104–105.
50. Triger DR, Cynamon MH, Wright R. Studies on hepatic uptake of antigen I. Comparison of inferior vena cava and portal vein routes of immunization. Immunology 1973;25:941–950.
51. Souhami RL, Addison IE, Bradfield JW. Increased antibody production following depression of hepatic phagocytosis. Clin Exp Immunol 1975;20:155–159.
52. Bjorneboe M, Prytz H, Orskov F. Antibodies to intestinal microbes in serum of patients with cirrhosis of the liver. Lancet 1972;1:58–60.
53. Galbraith RM, Eddleston AL, Williams R, Webster AD, Pattison J, Doniach D, Kennedy LA, Batchelor JR. Enhanced antibody responses in active chronic hepatitis: relation to HLA-B8 and HLA-B12 and porto-systemic shunting. Lancet 1976;1:930–934.
54. Prytz H, Holst-Christensen J, Korner B, Liehr H. Portal venous and systemic endotoxaemia in patients without liver disease and systemic endotoxaemia in patients with cirrhosis. Scand J Gastroenterol 1976;11:857–863.
55. Triger DR, Wright R. Hyperglobulinaemia in liver disease. Lancet 1973;1:1494–1496.
56. Bradfield JW. Control of spillover. The importance of Kupffer-cell function in clinical medicine. Lancet 1974;2:883–885.
57. Jacob AI, Goldberg PK, Bloom N, Degenshein GA, Kozinn PJ. Endotoxin and bacteria in portal blood. Gastroenterology 1977;72:1268–1270.
58. Cooksley WG, Powell LW, Halliday JW. Reticuloendothelial phagocytic function in human liver diseases. Gut 1970;11:979.
59. Canalese J, Gove CD, Gimson AE, Wilkinson SP, Wardle EN, Williams R. Reticuloendothelial system and hepatocyte function in fulminant hepatic failure. Gut 1982;23:265–269.
60. Shirai M, Nishioka M, Shiga J, Mori W, Fukuda I, Kanegasaki S. Fate of ^{3}H-labeled endotoxin in partially hepatectomised rats. Hepatogastroenterology 1988;35:107–110.
61. Holper K, Oleay I, Kitahama A, Miller RH, Brettschneider L, Drapanas T, Trejo RA, DiLuzio NR. Effect of ischemia on hepatic parenchymal and reticuloendothelial function in the baboon. Surgery 1974;76:423–432.
62. Kaplan JE, Scovill WA, Bernard H, Saba TM, Gray V. Reticuloendothelial phagocytic response to bacterial challenge after traumatic shock. Circ Shock 1977;4:1–12.
63. Cuevas P, Fine J. Route of absorption of endotoxin from the intestine in nonseptic shock. J Reticuloendothel Soc 1972;11:535–538.
64. Ravin HA, Rowley D, Jenkins C, Fine J. On the absorption of bacterial endotoxin from the gastro-intestinal tract of the normal and shocked animal. J Exp Med 1960;112:783–792.
65. Rush BF, Sori AJ, Murphy TF, Smith S, Flanagan JJ Jr, Machiedo GW. Endotoxemia and bacteremia during hemorrhagic shock. The link between trauma and sepsis? Ann Surg 1988;307:549–555.
66. Nolan JP, Hare DK, McDevitt JJ, Ali V. In vitro studies of intestinal endotoxin absorption. I. Kinetics of absorption in the isolated everted gut sac. Gastroenterology 1977;72:434–439.
67. Cuevas P, Fine J. Role of intraintestinal endotoxin in death from peritonitis. Surg Gynecol Obstet 1972;134:953–957.
68. Gans H, Matsumoto K. The escape of endotoxin from the intestine. Surg Gynecol Obstet 1974;139:395–402.
69. Pardy BJ, Spencer RC, Dudley HA. Hepatic reticuloendothelial protection against bacteremia in experimental hemorrhagic shock. Surgery 1977;81:193–197.
70. Jones RJ, Roe EA. Measurement of endotoxins with the limulus test in burned patients. J Hyg (Camb) 1979;83:151–156.
71. Winchurch RA, Thupari JN, Munster AM. Endotoxemia in burn patients: levels of circulating endotoxins are related to burn size. Surgery 1987;102:808–812.
72. Goris RJ, Boekhorst TP, Nuytinck KS, Gimbrere JS. Multiple-organ failure. Generalized auto-destructive inflammation? Arch Surg 1985;120:1109–1115.
73. Cooperstock MS, Tucher RP, Baubelis JV. Possible pathogenic role of endotoxin in Reye's syndrome. Lancet 1975;1:1272–1274.
74. Wilkinson SP, Arroyo V, Gazzard BG, Moodie H, Williams R. Relation of renal impairment and hemorrhagic diathesis to endotoxaemia in fulminant hepatic failure. Lancet 1974;1:521–524.
75. Drivas G, James O, Wardle N. Study of reticuloendothelial phagocytic capacity in patients with cholestasis. Br Med J 1976;1:1568–1569.
76. Filkins JP, Lupitz JM, Smith JJ. The effect of zymosan and glucan on the reticuloendothelial

system and resistance to traumatic shock. Angiology 1964;15:465–472.

77. Loegering DJ, Garrett LJ. Reticuloendothelial system depression with hemolyzed blood and susceptibility to endotoxin shock and thermal injury. Circ Shock 1981;8:473–482.
78. Schneidkraut MJ, Loegering DJ. Effect of hemolyzed blood on reticuloendothelial function and susceptibility to hemorrhagic shock. Proc Soc Exp Biol Med 1978;159:418–423.
79. Richards PS, Saba TM. Alterations of fibronectin and reticuloendothelial phagocytic function during adaptation to experimental shock. Circ Shock 1983;10:189–198.
80. Kaplan JE, Moon DG, Minnear FL, Saba TM. Depressed reticuloendothelial clearance of platelets in rats after trauma. Am J Physiol 1984;246:H180–H188.
81. Hynes RO, Yamada KM. Fibronectins: multifunctional nodular glycoproteins. J Cell Biol 1982;95:369–383.
82. Saba TM, Cho E. Reticuloendothelial systemic response to operative trauma as influenced by cryoprecipitate or cold-insoluble globulin therapy. J Reticuloendothel Soc 1979;26:171–186.
83. Velky TS, Kagawa F, Greenburg AG, Yang JC. Plasma fibronectin response to *Escherichia coli* and hemoglobin. Arch Surg 1985;120:142–145.
84. Lanser ME, Saba TM, Scovill WA. Opsonic glycoprotein (plasma fibronectin) levels after thermal injury: relationship to extent of burn and development of sepsis. Ann Surg 1980;192:776–782.
85. Stevens LE, Clemmer TP, Laub RM, Miya F, Robbins LM. Fibronectin in severe sepsis. Surg Gynecol Obstet 1986;162:222–228.
86. Lanser ME, Brown GE. Stimulation of rat hepatocyte fibronectin production by interleukin 6. J Exp Med 1989;170:1781–1786.
87. Niehaus GD, Schumacker PR, Saba TM. Reticuloendothelial clearance of blood-borne particulates. Ann Surg 1980;191:479–487.
88. Wright SD, Meyer BC. Fibronectin receptor of human macrophages recognizes the sequence Arg-Gly-Asp-Ser. J Exp Med 1985;162:762–767.
89. Imawari M, Hughes RD, Gove CD, Williams R. Fibronectin and Kupffer cell function in fulminant hepatic failure. Dig Dis Sci 1985;30:1028–1033.
90. Loegering DJ, Daplan JE, Vincent PA, Saba TM. Kupffer cell complement receptor clearance function after surgical injury and phagocytosis of immune complexes: effect of changes in plasma fibronectin. J Lab Clin Med 1988;111:504–510.
91. Lanser ME, Saba TM. Correction of serum opsonic defects after burn and sepsis by opsonic fibronectin administration. Arch Surg 1983;118:338–342.
92. Sorvillo JM, Gigli I, Pearlstein E. The effect of fibronectin on the processing of C1q- and C3b/bi-coated immune complexes by peripheral blood monocytes. J Immunol 1986;136:1023–1026.
93. Czop JK, Kadish JL, Austen KF. Augmentation of human monocyte opsonin-independent phagocytosis by fragments of human plasma fibronectin. Proc Natl Acad Sci USA 1981;78:3649–3653.

7

Oxygen Delivery and Multiple Organ Failure

JAMES M. HARKEMA
IRSHAD H. CHAUDRY

Extensive tissue injury and sepsis can cause significant alterations in tissue function remote from the primary insult. If the primary insult is not controlled, multiple organ failure (MOF) frequently follows and has a high mortality. Although the mechanism of this cellular injury appears to be multifactorial, inadequate tissue oxygenation appears to be a predictor of outcome in patients with MOF.[1,2] Whether tissue hypoxia is present early in the septic process or becomes a manifestation of other pathophysiologic processes is poorly understood. The process of oxygen delivery and its relationship to oxygen consumption and tissue function in sepsis has thus become an area of marked interest, since abnormalities of almost every variable in the regulation of oxygen delivery have been described.[3,4]

To establish a framework for subsequent discussion, a brief overview of the normal mechanisms of oxygen delivery will be presented. Evidence from whole body studies indicating that oxygen consumption may not meet tissue demand in patients with MOF, despite adequate oxygen delivery, will be discussed. In addition, the alterations in oxygen delivery that could account for this apparent disturbance in the normal relationship of oxygen delivery to oxygen consumption will be examined. In view of this, we will examine the role of hypoxia in the dysfunction of individual organs that could lead to organ failure. Since sepsis is the most common cause of MOF and the experimental prototype used to

87

simulate the high cardiac output and hypermetabolic states of MOF, this review will primarily address the effects of sepsis, although references to nonseptic causes of MOF and endotoxin animal studies will be provided as appropriate.

Oxygen Delivery

Oxygen Transport Function

Aerobic organisms are dependent on the delivery of oxygen from the atmosphere to peripheral tissues for the production of energy by mitochondria. Substrates enter the Kreb's tricarboxylic acid cycle and energy released from the transfer of electrons is captured in the high-energy bonds of adenosine triphosphate (ATP). Oxygen is the terminal electron acceptor in this process of oxidative phosphorylation.[5] When oxygen is not available in sufficient amounts, energy is derived initially from limited stores of high energy bound phosphate in creatine phosphate.[6] Subsequently, glycolysis ensues, but it is an inefficient process and leads to lactic acidosis.[7]

Thus, the function of the oxygen delivery system is to ensure an intracellular oxygen supply at a rate that meets metabolic demand. The delivery of oxygen involves the diffusion of oxygen into pulmonary capillaries, cardiovascular transport of oxygen, and the diffusion of oxygen from systemic capillaries into the cell. Under normal conditions, these processes are coupled to cellular oxygen consumption by spontaneous circulatory changes and autonomic reflexes that control ventilation, cardiac output, and individual organ flow.[8] This results in regional distribution of flow to match oxygen delivery with individual tissue oxygen demand.

The volume of oxygen delivered from the heart each minute is determined by the cardiac output and the arterial oxygen content (CaO_2). The whole body oxygen delivery (DO_2) equals the product of cardiac output (CO) and CaO_2 ($DO_2 = CO \times CaO_2 \times 10$). As such, DO_2 is dependent on the variables that determine oxygen content and the factors that regulate cardiac output.

Blood Oxygen Content

Oxygen exists in blood dissolved in plasma and bound to hemoglobin. The partial pressure of oxygen (PO_2) determines the level of dissolved oxygen in plasma and is calculated from the product of the PO_2 and the solubility coefficient of oxygen in blood (0.003 ml/dl/mmHg). Dissolved oxygen is approximately 1% of total oxygen content. The amount of oxygen bound to hemoglobin is determined by the saturation of hemoglobin (SO_2) and the concentration of hemoglobin (gm/dl) in blood: 1.39 ml of oxygen combines with 1 g of hemoglobin (Hb) per dl at 37°C. Thus, oxygen content = $1.39 \times Hb \times SO_2 + (0.003 \times PO_2)$ ml/dl blood.

Hemoglobin because of its spatial molecular configuration has a greater affinity for oxygen when oxygenated than when reduced.[9] This ability of hemoglobin to alter its affinity is suitably adapted to the needs of oxygen transport, since the binding of hemoglobin is facilitated in the pulmonary capillaries and dissociation occurs readily in the systemic capillaries where oxygen tension is lower.

Several factors can alter the affinity of hemoglobin for oxygen. Hydrogen ion, carbon dioxide, temperature increase, and 2,3-diphosphoglycerate decrease hemoglobin's affinity for oxygen and shift the oxyhemoglobin dissociation curve to the right. Oxyhemoglobin dissociation is best indexed by P_{50}, which is the partial pressure of oxygen at which hemoglobin is half saturated. A shift to the right makes more oxygen available at a given tension. The more freely oxygen dissociates, the more oxygen can be consumed.

Cardiovascular Role in Oxygen Delivery

Cardiac output requires intrinsic cardiac function but flow is primarily determined by the peripheral vasculature, which alters venous return and left ventricular afterload.[10] The anatomy and physiology of the peripheral vasculature is particularly well designed for the local control of blood flow. The largest decrease in pressure occurs between the arteriole and capillary bed.[11] This allows local autoregulation to determine flow by varying arteriolar resistance. Two basic mechanisms appear to be operative in local autoregulation.[11,12] Any imbalance in oxygen supply and metabolic demand results in the accumulation of metabolites or a decrease in tissue oxygen tension, which relax precapillary sphincters and thus increase oxygen extraction by increasing the number of nutritive capillaries perfused. Also, vascular smooth muscle responds to changes in luminal pressure by contraction or relaxation, which alters local resistance and local flow.[11,12] The myogenic mechanism is directed more toward normalization of capillary pressure, whereas the metabolic mechanism is directed toward maintaining adequate blood flow and oxygen delivery.

The local vasculature anatomy has particular characteristics that allow maximal diffusion of oxygen within the tissues. The cross-sectional area of the capillaries and venules is 250 times that of the terminal arterioles.[13] This results in a large surface area available for diffusion. The large numbers of capillaries reduces the distance between the blood and cell, and in particular there is an increased number of capillaries on the venous side where the oxygen tension is reduced, thereby favoring uniform oxygen delivery. The recruitment of nonperfused capillaries appears to be the primary process of local autoregulation.[11]

Oxygen Diffusion from Systemic Capillaries

The diffusion of oxygen from the capillary to the mitochondria is determined by the pressure gradient of oxygen in the capillary and the resistance of the tissue to diffusion. The proximity of the capillary to the cell and the amount of surface area both influence tissue diffusion. Autoregulation of the microcirculation increases the numbers of capillaries perfused as well as increasing the surface area available for oxygen diffusion. The resistance to oxygen diffusion involves the blood configuration in the capillaries, the interstitial space, and the cell interior. The fact that the hematocrit of capillary vessels is reduced compared with the systemic hematocrit and that the plasma between the cells has a low

PO_2 may result in a reduced level of total capillary PO_2.[14] In addition, the orientation of the red cells in the center of the capillary bloodstream, where the flow is greatest, may create a further resistance to diffusion by the relatively slow-moving plasma.[15] Since the major decrease in PO_2 occurs between the blood and the interstitium, this indicates that the major resistance to diffusion occurs in the interstitium.[16] A relatively high capillary PO_2, as reflected by the venous PO_2, is necessary to provide the necessary diffusion gradient.

Oxygen Consumption

Oxygen consumption (VO_2) is the volume of oxygen consumed by tissue per minute and is derived from the product of the arteriovenous oxygen content difference and flow. Whole body consumption is determined from arterial and mixed venous oxygen content and cardiac output. The fraction of the delivered oxygen that is consumed designates the oxygen extraction ratio (VO_2/DO_2). Normal values are approximately 0.25. Over a wide range of DO_2, VO_2 remains unchanged, since local control increases oxygen extraction. At some point, the reduction in DO_2 is incapable of meeting energy demand and VO_2 decreases. This level of oxygen delivery is called the critical oxygen delivery and the extraction ratio at this level is the critical extraction ratio.[17,18]

Although these measurements are readily obtained in critically ill patients, they have definite limitations as indicators of adequate tissue oxygenation. The placement of a pulmonary arterial catheter and an arterial catheter allows simultaneous measurement of arterial and mixed venous oxygen and cardiac output. From these values DO_2, VO_2, and oxygen extraction can be monitored. Oxygen delivery is a good indicator of oxygen availability but does not give specific information concerning individual organ oxygen supply. In addition, the levels of hypoxemia necessary to reduce DO_2 to a critical level rarely are present. Although VO_2 is a good measure of the oxygen utilized, it does not measure tissue oxygenation nor does it determine the adequacy of oxygen consumption in individual organs. Since MOF and sepsis are hypermetabolic states, an increase in VO_2 does not necessarily indicate adequate tissue oxygenation. The relationship between DO_2 and VO_2 may be a better indicator of adequate tissue oxygenation and will be discussed in greater detail. The failure of tissue to extract oxygen despite an inadequate DO_2 indicates failure of local control to increase extraction. Similarly, a narrow arteriovenous oxygen difference could indicate failure of tissue to utilize the delivered oxygen.

Oxygen Delivery and Consumption in Multiple Organ Failure

Although multiple organ failure (MOF) occurs in clinical pathologic states without identifiable infection, sepsis remains the most common cause of MOF.[19,20] The septic state is typically hypermetabolic with accompanying increased oxygen consumption.[21,22] The expected response to this increased metabolic demand would be an increase in oxygen delivery (DO_2) and adjustment in the integrated regulatory process to match local DO_2 with individual tissue metabolic demand. Indeed, accompanying this hypermetabolic response is a hyperdynamic cardiovascular response characterized by an increased cardiac output and a decreased systemic vascular resistance (SVR).[23,24] Despite the resultant increase in DO_2, if arterial oxygenation is maintained, the systemic oxygen arteriovenous concentration difference narrows and the extraction ratio (ER) decreases.[23] Since under normal conditions an increase in VO_2 results in widened arteriovenous difference and an increase in the ER,[10] these findings strongly suggest a disruption in the normal integration of oxygen delivery and oxygen demand.[25]

An apparent uncoupling of the normal DO_2 and VO_2 relationship during sepsis and nonseptic-associated MOF supports this hypothesis.[25–29] Despite the finding that DO_2 exceeds the experimental critical DO_2 level, VO_2 changes in a linear fashion to changes in DO_2 over a wide range. In addition, attempts to increase DO_2 have not resulted in a plateau of VO_2 normally found when VO_2 is independent of oxygen supply.[27] With decreasing DO_2, these patients are unable to increase their ER as well.[28]

Although it has been suggested that supply-dependent VO_2 consumption is more likely to be present in patients with increased blood lactate levels, the relationship has been observed in patients with no evidence of metabolic acidosis.[2,27,30] These findings suggest that inadequate tissue oxygenation may occur in patients with sepsis despite an apparently adequate systemic blood flow, blood pressure, and PaO_2.

Several observations suggest that correction of this apparent tissue hypoxia may have clinical significance. Bihari et al.[27] were able to distinguish survivors from nonsurvivors on the basis of VO_2 response to increasing DO_2 with prostacyclin. A significantly greater increase in VO_2 was demonstrated in nonsurvivors. The ER increased but mixed venous oxygen concentration was unchanged. In contrast, survivors had a decrease in the ER and a narrowing of the arteriovenous oxygen content. Shoemaker and associates[31,32] have demonstrated that maintaining oxygen transport and oxygen uptake at supranormal levels improved the survival of critically ill patients. In patients with acute respiratory failure associated with trauma and sepsis a 7-day infusion of the vasodilator prostaglandin E reduced the incidence of MOF and improved survival.[33]

Nelson has demonstrated an increase in the critical DO_2 and decreased ER in bacteremic and endotoxin dog models.[34,35] These findings were not evident at higher levels of DO_2. Similar studies have not been done in animal models that simulate the hyperdynamic septic response seen in humans. These whole body studies in humans and animals do not identify what organs are oxygen supply dependent. Nor do these studies identify the specific mechanism to explain the abnormalities of oxygen extraction and utilization. The oxygen requiring reactions that respond to the increased oxygen supply also have not been identified. It seems unlikely that a mitochondrial deficit would account for these alterations in oxygen extraction and utilization in the absence of lactic acidosis unless local tissue acidosis can occur without elevated systemic lactate levels. Bihari et al.[27] proposed that an extramitochondrial oxygen debt could occur before any interference with ATP production, since oxygen is a rate-limiting substrate for mitochondrial reactions. This extramitochondrial oxygen deficit might account for early and reversible forms of organ dysfunction.

Possible Mechanisms for Abnormalities in the VO₂ and DO₂ Relationship

Several hypotheses have been proposed to explain the apparent failure of tissue to utilize oxygen despite a normal whole body DO_2. An abnormality of mitochondrial function resulting in an inability to utilize delivered oxygen could explain the abnormal oxygen extraction and utilization. Although mitochondria from animals in endotoxin shock have impaired function,[36,37] no compromise in oxidative capability was found in mitochondria from animals with hyperdynamic sepsis.[38,39] In addition the increase in utilization of oxygen with the increased delivery provides indirect evidence that mitochondria can utilize oxygen if available. However, the mitochondrial hyperfunction observed in livers of septic rats with decreased hepatic blood flow suggests a compensatory mechanism to local hypoxia.[40]

The redistribution of flow between organs could result in flow-dependent oxygen consumption, if some tissues are overperfused relative to their metabolic needs. Increased blood flow and increased fraction of cardiac output to the heart and splanchnic circulation have been reported in sepsis.[41,42] These changes appear to be appropriate responses to the increase in metabolic demand. Increased blood flow to the muscle also has been reported and muscle could be a candidate for overperfusion.[43] Based on the available data, no conclusion can be made concerning the distribution of flow, since flow-dependent oxygen consumption has not been determined for individual organs.

Although the decrease in systemic vascular resistance is a normal response to ensure increased flow to meet increased metabolic demand, it is evident that impaired vascular responsiveness also contributes to the decrease in systemic vascular resistance. This decrease in systemic vascular resistance could contribute to a mismatch between DO_2 and oxygen need. Chernow and Roth[44] suggested that circulating opioids, prostanoids, and inflammatory mediators could act as possible vasodilators. Carcillo et al.[45] found a down-regulation of alpha receptors. Prostacyclin may cause vasodilation in sepsis, since levels of phospholipase A_2, an enzyme that converts phospholipids to arachidonic acid, correlates with the degree of vasodilation.[46] Ibuprofen, a cyclooxygenase inhibitor, improved hemodynamics both in patients with acute respiratory distress as well as in a septic dog model.[47] This agent could exert its effects on prostanoids at the local tissue level or antagonize the effect of prostanoids on the adrenergic nervous system, allowing greater neurohumoral control.

Evidence also exists that increased vascular tone, which may also be present, interferes with the local autoregulation of blood flow. Infusion of prostacyclin and thromboxane A_2 inhibitors have been documented to improve flow in sepsis.[27,28] This apparent contradiction, the beneficial effect of the antagonism of certain prostanoids that dilate and others that constrict vessels, is best explained by differences in individual intraorgan prostanoid ratios and differences in local prostanoid concentrations. The inhibition of thromboxane A_2-induced platelet aggregation could also explain the beneficial effects of prostanoid synthetase inhibitors.[48,49] Elevated levels of angiotensin II, a potent vasoconstrictor, have been found in septic sheep.[50] Increased levels of epinephrine, a counterregulatory hormone and vasoconstrictor, are also found in sepsis.[51] Increased vascular tone due to these factors could counteract local metabolic control when a local oxygen deficit is present and thus prevent local vasodilation. Clinical studies have correlated the decrease in systemic vascular resistance with the ability of tissues to extract oxygen.[52] In addition a reduction in cardiac output and an increase in peripheral resistance, indicating restoration of local regulatory control, predicted survival in patients with sepsis.[53]

Maldistribution of local tissue blood flow could result if obstruction of capillaries were present. Some capillaries and tissue would receive inadequate flow, whereas other areas would have more flow than necessary. Microembolization in an experimental model caused a reduced oxygen uptake at all levels of DO_2.[54] Asher et al.[55] found coincident reductions in hepatic flow with the presence of increased levels of intrasinusoidal neutrophil aggregates. This same group demonstrated a pattern of reduced effective hepatic blood flow and function in a septic model that was consistent with vascular occlusion resulting in the exclusion of tissue from metabolic exchange.[56] They have subsequently demonstrated similar findings with activation of the complement system and propose that activated neutrophils release oxygen radicals and proteases that damage endothelial cells. This leads to fibrin and platelet aggregation.[57] Fibrin thrombi are a common finding in pathologic studies of late sepsis in human and nonhuman primates.[58] Kupffer cell swelling may occlude sinusoids as well.[59]

The obstruction of capillaries reduces the surface area available for oxygen diffusion and the reduction in the number of capillaries further affects diffusion by increasing the distance between the capillaries and the tissue. Increased permeability and tissue edema has been observed in sepsis.[60] Edema could increase the diffusion distance from capillary to the cell, but this has not been studied. In the hyperdynamic state an increased capillary transit time could decrease release of oxygen from hemoglobin.[16]

Discussion of possible mechanisms for flow-dependent oxygen consumption must include arteriovenous shunting, but no anatomic shunts have ever been demonstrated. However, the parallel position of arteries and veins could account for a physiologic shunt with oxygen diffusing directly from arteries to veins.[61]

Knowledge of local organ blood flow and its regulation during sepsis remains insufficient to elucidate fully the pathophysiology of flow-dependent oxygen consumption. The weight of the evidence points to microvasculature injury and subsequent loss of local autoregulatory control as the common mediator. The individual organ response will also depend heavily on the specific organ's metabolic demands and neurohumoral reactivity. An examination of the relationship of organ function and oxygen delivery will be examined next.

Individual Organ Blood Flow and Dysfunction in Sepsis

Whether local blood flow to specific organs is modified appropriately in sepsis depends on several factors. If there are, as previously discussed, alterations in the normal central and peripheral regulation of cardiovascular transport of oxygen, a potential intraorgan mismatch of DO_2 and tissue demand exists. In particular, if the abnormality of local regulation is generalized, then organs with greater metabolic demand would be at more risk for tissue hypoxia. Although the redistribution of flow in sepsis appears to be directed to organs with expected increases in metabolism, there is little data to determine if local organ flow is sufficient. Indeed, the finding that tissue dysfunction occurs with apparent normal blood flow raises the issue of occult tissue hypoxia or some other mechanism as the cause. To investigate the possibility of tissue hypoxia as the etiology for organ dysfunction, the relationship of organ blood flow and dysfunction in sepsis will be presented.

Liver

The liver plays a central role in the hypermetabolic response to massive tissue injury and sepsis. Indeed the transition from a clinical hypermetabolic response to frank MOF is accompanied by the failure of hepatic metabolic functions.[62] Frank hepatic failure in the setting of MOF is an ominous event and has a very high mortality.[19] Although hepatic failure in sepsis is generally considered to be a late complication, there is considerable evidence that hepatocellular dysfunction occurs in the early stages of sepsis.[63] Hypoxia secondary to a marked decrease in blood flow appears to be the cause for the reduction in ATP levels and increased lactate to pyruvate ratio in the liver in late sepsis.[41] The contribution of DO_2 and resultant tissue hypoxia to hepatic dysfunction in early sepsis is less well defined, since these markers of anaerobic metabolism are not present.[38,64]

The marked increase in hepatic metabolic activity and resultant oxygen demand in early sepsis is reflected in an increase in hepatic VO_2, hepatic DO_2, and total hepatic blood flow. An increased total hepatic blood flow and splanchnic blood flow has been a consistent finding in septic animal models and patients with sepsis and with hyperdynamic cardiovascular states.[65–72]

Not only does an absolute increase in splanchnic blood flow exist, but the splanchnic flow accounts for a greater fraction of cardiac output.[42,67,72,73] Accompanying this increase in blood flow is a marked increase in splanchnic VO_2.[67–71] In several studies, the extraction fraction of oxygen remained unchanged, suggesting that the increased oxygen demand was met by increasing blood flow rather than extraction.[68,70] Dahm et al.[67] found similar increases in splanchnic blood flow and VO_2 but observed an increased extraction fraction, suggesting an inadequate increase in DO_2 to meet hepatic metabolic demand. Wilmore et al.[69] had similar observations in a subgroup of burn patients with bacteremia who had increased hepatic oxygen extraction but reduced hepatic blood flow compared with uninfected burn patients. Leevy et al.[73] reduced hepatic DO_2 in normal subjects and demonstrated an increase in oxygen extraction.

Whether hepatic VO_2 is dependent on DO_2 in these patients with sepsis cannot be determined from these studies, since no manipulations were made to increase systemic or hepatic DO_2. To confirm flow-dependent hypoxia, it is necessary to demonstrate an increase in hepatic VO_2 when DO_2 is increased. These experiments have not been conducted in patients or experimental animals.

Further evidence for a hypoxic contribution to hepatic cellular dysfunction has been proposed by Schirmer, Fry, and associates[57,74,75] who have measured effective hepatic blood flow by galactose clearance in a hyperdynamic septic rat model. A decrease of approximately 20% in effective hepatic blood flow was reported. This correlated to a similar reduction in maximal clearance of galactose in the same model. The kinetics of the reduction in clearance showed that noncompetitive inhibition was present, indicating that there was a decrease in functional enzyme mass. Anatomic shunting could account for these findings, but anatomic shunts have not been demonstrated in the liver. Thus, these investigators[74] propose an intrahepatic redistribution of flow on the basis of microcirculatory obstruction. They propose endothelial damage with subsequent platelet and fibrin deposition as the mechanisms for the obstruction of the microvessels.[58] These studies suggest that early hepatic dysfunction may be due to intrahepatic redistribution of flow. Support for a microcirculatory maldistribution of flow comes from several different lines of experiments. Several studies support an intrahepatic redistribution of blood flow despite an increase in total hepatic blood flow. Comparison of indocyanine green (ICG) clearance and total hepatic blood flow measured by hydrogen polarography indicated an increase in hepatic flow and a decrease in ICG clearance.[66] Similar results were obtained in a septic dog model with direct measurement of total flow and ICG clearance.[65] Pathologic examination of the liver in sepsis shows microvascular thrombi, congestion, and hemorrhage consistent with microvascular or sinusoidal obstruction.[58] Kupffer cell swelling has also been proposed as a factor in microcirculatory obstruction.[59]

Although it appears that microcirculatory redistribution occurs and results in focal ischemia, evidence has not been provided that DO_2 is inadequate to meet the metabolic needs of the liver. Measurements of normal lactate and ATP levels in early sepsis suggest adequate oxygen delivery, but these measurements may not be sensitive enough to identify early hypoxic changes.[38,64] Indeed, the hyperfunctioning of mitochondria in early sepsis may indicate local hypoxia.[40] However, the depolarization of hepatic cells does not appear to be ischemic-induced, since hepatic cells in sepsis accumulate potassium, whereas ischemia causes a loss of potassium.[76,77] Similarly, the alterations in gluconeogenesis and its resistance to insulin are not oxygen dependent, suggesting other mechanisms.[78,79] Interventions to increase DO_2 and determination of its effect on VO_2, effective hepatic blood flow, and other hepatic functions are necessary to determine if cellular dysfunction is secondary to other causes.

In late sepsis hepatic blood flow is decreased and ATP levels decrease and the lactate to pyruvate ratio increases.[41] These changes indicate that hypoxia may play a significant role in late sepsis leading to organ failure.

Intestinal

The countercurrent exchange system within the intestinal villi makes the mucosa quite susceptible to ischemia.[80] In fact, transient episodes of mucosal ischemia, identified by acidosis in the mucosa, occur in 80% of patients with MOF.[81]

The splanchnic circulation normally reduces flow to preserve DO_2 to the heart and brain when a systemic oxygen deficit exists. In contrast, the redistribution of flow in the septic state preserves or increases intestinal and splanchnic blood flow in animals [43,82,83] and in patients.[67–69] The splanchnic flow in sepsis accounts for a significantly greater fraction of the cardiac output as well.[43,67,82,83] Accompanying the resultant increase in DO_2 is an increase in splanchnic VO_2.[67–69] Dahm et al.[67] found that an increase in oxygen extraction accounted for the majority of the increase in consumption. This finding suggests that local microcirculatory control did not increase flow to meet metabolic demand. Bacteremic burn patients, on the other hand, did not demonstrate a widened arterial-hepatic venous oxygen content except in a small subset of bacteremic patients with complications.[69] Gump et al.[68] also reported that flow accounted for the increased splanchnic VO_2 in patients with sepsis.

Abnormalities in intestinal DO_2 and VO_2 have not been investigated in animal models of hyperdynamic sepsis. Nelson et al.[34,35] demonstrated in bacteremia and endotoxin models that the intestine reaches the critical oxygen level when systemic DO_2 is above its critical level. Endotoxin produced a significant reduction in the critical intestinal oxygen extraction, indicating that the tissue was less able to increase oxygen extraction.[35] In addition, no further increase in blood flow occurred, indicating a loss of reactive hyperemia. These findings suggest a loss of local microcirculatory regulation.

Cyclooxygenase inhibition increased intestinal blood flow in an endotoxin model in sheep, suggesting vasoconstrictor prostanoids may prevent intestinal vasodilation.[84] Prostacyclin increased intestinal blood flow in an endotoxin model and attenuated the release of lysosomal hydrolase.[85] Angiotensin II is an especially potent vasoconstrictor in the splanchnic circulation and abnormal amounts were released in a hyperdynamic sheep model.[51]

Further studies in hyperdynamic septic models are needed to determine the DO_2 and VO_2 relationship in the splanchnic circulation, and its contribution to the hepatic and systemic flow-dependent states.

Renal

To meet the needs of filtration, the kidney normally has a blood flow and DO_2 greater than metabolic demand.[86] Despite this apparent reserve, the kidney remains very susceptible to ischemic damage. Indeed, acute renal failure is principally a consequence of ischemia. In particular, a marked reduction in medullary blood flow plays a critical role in the initiating of acute tubular necrosis.[87] In clinical acute renal failure 30% occur secondary to sepsis. Since the clinical picture is not dissimilar from acute renal failure that follows hypoperfusion, speculation on the pathogenesis in sepsis has centered primarily on ischemic changes.

Several investigators have reported increased renal blood flow and decreased renal vascular resistance in hyperdynamic patients with sepsis.[69,88,89] A number of hyperdynamic septic animal models have also been evaluated. An increase in renal blood flow has been reported by several investigators,[90–94] whereas others have reported normal blood flow.[43,51] Townsend et al.[75,95] described a decrease in effective renal blood flow in a septic rat model, indicating that apparent elevated or normal blood flow may not be sufficient to meet renal functional and energy needs. In a septic sheep model, adequate fluid resuscitation prevented an increase in plasma renin and a decrease in creatinine clearance that occurred in animals receiving only maintenance fluids.[51]

In a follow-up study in which the septic insult was more severe, an increase in plasma renin, a high urine osmolality, and a decrease in free-water clearance occurred despite normal arterial perfusion and an increase in cardiac output.[96] Lucas et al.[88] suggested that adequate fluid resuscitation can attenuate several renal effects of sepsis in man.

Thus, in the presence of apparent normal to increased renal blood flow, functional studies indicate renal dysfunction. However, little is proved concerning the pathogenesis leading to this dysfunction. In particular, there is little information concerning the adequacy of DO_2 for metabolic demand in either man or experimental models. Wilmore et al.[69] noted a narrowing of the renal arteriovenous oxygen content and diminished VO_2 in bacteremic burn patients compared with uninfected burn patients. This occurred despite a marked increase in renal blood flow.

In models of renal hypoperfusion a relative reduction of flow occurs in the outer cortex. However, when the degree of hypoperfusion is more severe, medullary blood flow is reduced and appears to initiate acute tubular necrosis.[87] Cronenwett and Lindenauer[92] documented a shift of flow from the outer cortex to inner cortex following live bacterial infusion, whereas Ravikant and Lucas[91] showed an increase in cortical blood flow. The direct infusion of *Escherichia coli* into an isolated kidney preparation produced polyuria associated with acute renal failure during sepsis but did not affect cortical flow.[97] Hayborn and associates observed a disproportionate decrease in glomerular filtration rate and effective renal blood flow, suggesting a cortical redistribution of flow.[95] Brenner et al.[89] noted a similar marked decrease in some patients with marked increase in renal blood flow. No studies have investigated medullary blood flow or the pathogenesis of changes in cortical flow in sepsis.

Vasoconstriction secondary to eicosanoid activity may alter microcirculatory blood flow in the kidney. Both a thromboxane-synthetase inhibitor and a leukotriene antagonist prevented the decrease of renal blood flow in an endotoxin model.[98] In a septic sheep model, a thromboxane-synthetase inhibitor prevented oliguria and a decrease in glomerular filtration rate.[99]

In summary, renal blood flow remains normal or increases in patients who demonstrate high output sepsis as well as in several septic animal models. Since renal dysfunction occurs despite this apparent adequate flow, it can be concluded that regional ischemia is present and that this regional ischemia leads to acute renal failure. Adequate fluid resuscitation appears to prevent renal failure during sepsis in patients and some animal models.

Heart

The heart plays a unique role in sepsis and MOF. As a major determinent of whole body DO_2 cardiac dysfunction could contribute to tissue hypoxia if cardiac output did not meet tissue oxygen demands. Also, the heart may be viewed as an end organ and subject to the same abnormalities of DO_2 that could affect its function.

In the absence of cardiac disease, such as myocardial infarction, the cardiac response in the early stages of sepsis appears adequate to maintain organ function. This early phase of sepsis is characterized by an increased cardiac output, DO_2, and a decrease in peripheral vascular resistance. These patients demonstrate no clinical evidence of cardiovascular dysfunction. If hypotension is present in this stage of sepsis, it is usually due to inadequate fluid resuscitation and not to intrinsic cardiac dysfunction that limits cardiac output.[23] In late sepsis it appears that increased cardiac output persists but systemic lactic acidosis is present, suggesting cardiac output is inadequate. If frank cardiovascular insufficiency with hypotension or septic shock occurs, it is a preterminal event.

Despite what appears to be adequate cardiac reserve with increased cardiac output and DO_2, cardiac dysfunction has been identified early in sepsis. Dilation of ventricles, depressed ejection fractions, and alterations of the Frank-Starling and diastolic pressure-volume relationships are present within 48 hours of the onset of sepsis.[100–102] Other factors compensate for this dysfunction and stroke volume is typically maintained. Explanations for this cardiac dysfunction include cytotoxic myocardial depression and ischemia due to a reduced or maldistributed coronary blood flow.

A decrease in myocardial blood flow and the resultant decrease in DO_2 do not appear to be an explanation for the observed early cardiac dysfunction. Cunnion et al.[103] measured coronary blood flow, arteriovenous oxygen difference, and oxygen extraction in patients with sepsis and transient myocardial dysfunction. These patients manifested elevated coronary blood flow, and the increased rate of myocardial VO_2 was calculated to be appropriate for the increase in cardiac output. In addition, a decrease in coronary vascular resistance was found. These findings suggest that an appropriate increase in coronary blood flow has occurred to meet the increased oxygen demands of the heart. This process appears to be regulated by the coronary vasculature. The increase in coronary blood flow was confirmed by Dhainant et al.[104] who found increased coronary flow in patients with sepsis when investigating myocardial substrate utilization. Arteriovenous lactate differences remained normal, supporting the observation that DO_2 is adequate and global ischemia does not occur.[103] Supporting this are normal myocardial ATP levels in sepsis.[105]

Other findings suggest that regional microvasculature abnormalities may alter local DO_2. During sepsis, arteriovenous oxygen difference was noted to be narrowed and oxygen ER decreased despite increased VO_2 in both human and animal studies.[103,104,106] Explanation for this finding must include arteriovenous shunting or obstruction of capillaries leading to maldistribution of flow. The changes in substrate utilization indicate that lactate extraction increases and thus any local lactate increase could be masked by increased lactate uptake in normally perfused myocardium.[104]

Findings of regional dysfunction in cardiac functions are common in patients with sepsis and are consistent with regional ischemia.[107] Pathologic studies, in a septic dog model with similar cardiac dysfunctions as documented in patients with sepsis, has shown endothelial swelling, aggregates of fibrin in the capillaries, myocardial interstitial edema, and neutrophil infiltration.[108] Unfortunately no measurements of coronary flow and DO_2 have been carried out to correlate these findings. Autopsy studies in patients with sepsis document the presence of myocardial edema, hemorrhage, subendocardial hemorrhage, and vascular thrombi and emboli.[58]

In summary, myocardial DO_2 and blood flow do not appear to limit the ability of the heart to maintain whole body DO_2. Yet, clinically occult myocardial dysfunction can be demonstrated in early sepsis. This dysfunction is best explained by changes in the microcirculatory response that produces areas of ischemia or dysfunction. Further experimentation is necessary to determine if flow-dependent oxygen consumption to the myocardium is impaired during sepsis. This necessitates more experimental studies measuring coronary artery flow and DO_2.

Summary and Conclusion

The systemic response to sepsis involves the activation of multiple mediator systems. The resultant metabolic, physiologic, and immunologic responses initially appear to support host defense. If this process is not interrupted, it appears to be counterproductive and MOF ensues. The complexity and interaction of the various mediator systems preclude a unifying hypothesis to explain the pathogenesis of MOF. However, the evidence that has been presented demands that any such hypothesis must include tissue hypoxia as contributing to cell injury and MOF.

The response to sepsis is characteristically a hypermetabolic response with increased oxygen demand. Several mediator systems contribute to these metabolic changes. Increases in adrenergic activity mediated by the central nervous system, the counterregulatory hormone, and cytokines, particularly the interleukins and tumor necrosis factor, have been implicated. An appropriate increase in cardiac output and decrease in SVR increases DO_2 to meet tissue oxygen demands. Tissue hypoxia does not appear to play a major role in this phase of sepsis, since tissue ATP levels are unchanged. However, as sepsis progresses, despite adequate blood flow and oxygenation, tissue oxygenation appears to be dependent on DO_2. This failure of DO_2 to match tissue demand appears to be a failure of local regulation so that vasodilation now reflects both an appropriate response to increased oxygen demand but also a failure of the microcirculation to increase oxygen extraction.

The mechanisms responsible for this failure of autoregulation are not well defined. Certainly, the persistent effects of mediators that can influence regional and tissue blood flow are involved. These include increased sympathetic activity, vasoactive prostaglandins and thromboxanes, and the activated complement system, which could cause endothelial injury. The resultant tissue hypoxia and local tissue injury could perpetuate the process by activating local cellular mediator systems. One could hypothesize a vicious cycle in which inflammation mediates a complex mediator response, which, if persistent, results in tissue hypoxia and damage and further activation of local cellular mediators. The finding that the delivery of supranormal amounts of oxygen results in a better prognosis in this group of patients suggests that such a cycle may be interrupted by adequate tissue oxygenation.

These findings dictate the support of cardiac output and oxygenation to maximize DO_2. Before other therapeutic interventions can be attempted to improve tissue oxygenation, the pathogenesis of the DO_2 and VO_2 mismatch needs to be defined further. In the meantime, however, it could be concluded that, although we do not know for sure if there is a definitive relationship between inadequate DO_2 and MOF, it is important to pay attention to DO_2 in patients with sepsis.

Acknowledgments.   The authors express their sincere thanks to Sharon Waite for her skill and assistance in typing this manuscript. This work was supported in part by Departmental Research Support and by National Institutes of Health GM 39519.

References

1. MacLean LD, Mulligan W, McLean, et al. Patterns of septic shock in man—a detailed study of 56 patients. Ann Surg 1967;166:543–558.
2. Rashkin MC, Bosken C, Baughman RP. Oxygen delivery in critically ill patients: Its relationship to blood lactate and survival. Chest 1985;87:850–854.
3. Dantzker D. Oxygen delivery and utilization in sepsis. Crit Care Clin 1989;5:81–98.
4. Bryan-Brown CW, Ayers SM, eds. Oxygen transport and utilization. Fullerton, CA: Society of Critical Care, 1987.
5. Hatifi Y. The mitochondrial electron transport and oxidative phosphorylation system. Annu Rev Biochem 1985;54:1015–1016.
6. Piper J, DiPrampero PE, Gerretelli P. Oxygen debt and high energy phosphates in gastrocnemius muscle of the dog. Am J Physiol 1968;215:523.
7. Clark MC, Lardy HA. Regulation of intermediate carbohydrate metabolism. Int Rev Sci 1975;5:223–226.
8. Wasserman K. Coupling of external to internal respiration. Am Rev Respir Dis 1984;129:521–524.
9. Pirutz MF. Hemoglobin structure and respiratory transport. Sci Am 1978;239:92–125.
10. Shepherd AP, Granger JA, Smith E, et al. Local control of tissue oxygen delivery and its contribution to the regulation of cardiac output. Am J Physiol 1973;225:747–755.
11. Johnson P. Autoregulation of blood flow. Circ Res 1986;59:483–495.
12. Parks DA, Jacobsen ED. Physiology of the splanchnic circulation. Arch Intern Med 1985;145:1278–1281.
13. Taylor AE, Hernandez L, Perry M, et al. Overview of tissue oxygen utilization. In: Bryan-Brown CW, Ayers SM, eds: Oxygen transport and utilization. Fullerton, CA: Society of Critical Care, 1987;13–23.
14. Desjardins C, Duling BR. Microvessel hematocrit: measurement and implications for capillary oxygen transport. Am J Physiol 1987;252:H494–H503.
15. Federspiel W, Sarelius I. An examination of the contribution of red cell spacing to the uniformity of oxygen flux at the capillary wall. Microvas Res 1984;27:273–285.
16. Gayeski TEJ, Honig CR. O_2 gradients from sarcolemma to cell interior in red muscle at maximal VO_2. Am J Physiol 1986;H789–799.
17. Cain SM. Oxygen delivery and uptake in dogs during anemic and hypoxic hypoxia. J Appl Physiol 1977;42:228–234.
18. Shibutani K, Komatsu T, Kubal F, et al. Critical level of oxygen delivery in anesthetized man. Crit Care Med 1983;11:640–643.
19. Fry DE, Pearlstein L, Fulton RL, et al. Multiple system organ failure—the role of uncontrolled infection. Arch Surg 1980;115:136–140.
20. Pine RW, Wertz MJ, Lennard S, et al. Determinants of organ malfunction or death in patients with intraabdominal sepsis. Arch Surg 1983;118:242–249.
21. Cerra FB. Hypermetabolism, organ failure and metabolic support. Surgery 1987;101:1–14.
22. Houtchens BA, Westenkow DR. Oxygen consumption in septic shock: collective review. Circ Shock 1984;13:361–384.

23. Siegal JH, Cerra FB. Physiological and metabolic correlations in human sepsis. Surgery 1979;86:163–193.
24. Abraham E, Shoemaker WC, Cheng PH. Cardiorespiratory responses to fluid administration in peritonitis. Crit Care Med 1984;12:664–668.
25. Kaufman BS, Rackow EC, Falk JL. The relationship between oxygen delivery and consumption during fluid resuscitation of hypovolemic and septic shock. Chest 1984;85:336–340.
26. Wolf YG, Corter S, Perel A, et al. Dependence of oxygen consumption on cardiac output in sepsis. Crit Care Med 1987;15:198–203.
27. Bihari D, Smithies M, Ginson A, et al. The effects of vasodilation with prostacyclin on oxygen delivery and uptake in critically ill patients. N Engl J Med 1987;317:397–403.
28. Danek S, Lynch JP, Wey JG, et al. The dependence of oxygen uptake on oxygen delivery in adult respiratory distress syndrome. Am Rev Respir Dis 1980;122:387–395.
29. Kariman K, Burns SR. Regulation of tissue oxygen extraction is disturbed in adult respiratory distress syndrome. Am Rev Respir Dis 1985;132:109–114.
30. Haupt M, Gilbert E, Carlson R. Fluid loading increases oxygen consumption in septic patients with lactic acidosis. Am Rev Respir Dis 1985;131:912–916.
31. Shoemaker W, Appel P, Kram, et al. Clinical trial of an algorithm for outcome prediction in acute circulatory failure. Crit Care Med 1982;10:390–395.
32. Shoemaker W. Relation of oxygen transport patterns to pathophysiology and therapy of shock states. Intensive Care Med 1987;13:230–243.
33. Holcraft J, Vassar M, Weber C. Prostaglandin E_1 and survival in patients with the adult respiratory distress syndrome. A prospective trial. Am Surg 1986;203:371–378.
34. Nelson DP, King CE, Dodd SL, et al. Systemic and intestinal limits of oxygen extraction in the dog. J Appl Physiol 1987;63:387–394.
35. Nelson DP, Samsel RW, Wood LD, et al. Pathologic supply dependence of systemic and intestinal O_2 uptake during endotoxemia. Am J Physiol 1988;64:2410–2419.
36. Schumer W, Das Gupta T, Moss G, et al. Effect of endotoxemia on liver cell mitochondria in man. Ann Surg 1970;171:875–882.
37. Mela L, Bacaljo L, Miller L. Defective oxidative metabolism of rat liver mitochondria in hemorrhagic and endotoxin shock. Am J Physiol 1971;220:571–577.
38. Fry D, Siler B, Rink R, et al. Hepatic cellular hypoxia in murine peritonitis. Surgery 1979;85:652–661.
39. Clemens M, Chaudry IH, Baue AE. Oxidative capability of hepatic tissue in sepsis. Adv Shock Res 1980;6:55–64.
40. Ohkawa M, Chaudry IH, Clemens MG, et al. Hepatic mitochondrial responses to sepsis and septic shock. Circ Shock 1983;10:273–274.
41. Cunnion RE, Schaer GL, Parker MM, et al. The coronary circulation in human septic shock. Circulation 1986;73:637–644.
42. Lang CH, Bagby GJ, Ferguson, et al. Cardiac output and redistribution of organ blood flow in hypermetabolic sepsis. Am J Physiol 1984;246:R331–R336.
43. Bersten A, Hersch M, Troster M, et al. Skeletal muscle injury despite aerobic metabolism in hyperdynamic sepsis. Chest 1988;94:705.
44. Chernow B, Roth BL. Pharmocologic manipulation of the peripheral vasculature in shock: clinical and experimental approaches. Circ Shock 1986;18:141–155.
45. Carcillo JA, Suba EA, Roth BL. A biochemical mechanism for vasodilation in septic shock. Crit Care Med 1987;15:440.
46. Vadas P, Pruzanski W, Stefanski E, et al. Pathogenesis of hypotension in septic shock: correlation of circulating phospholysase A_2 levels with circulatory collapse. Crit Care Med 1988;16:1–7.
47. Bernard GR, Reines MD, Metz CA, et al. Effect of a short course of ibuprofen in patients with severe sepsis. Am Rev Respir Dis 1988;137:A138.
48. Fink MP, McVitte TJ, Casey LC. Inhibition of prostaglandin synthesis restores normal hemodynamics in canine hyperdynamic sepsis. Ann Surg 1984;200:619–626.
49. Schirmer WJ, Schirmer JM, Townsend BC, et al. Imedazole and indomethacin improve hepatic perfusion in sepsis. Circ Shock 1987;21:253–259.
50. Richmond JM, Walker JF, Avila, et al. Renal and cardiovascular response to non-hypotensive sepsis in a large animal model with peritonitis. Surgery 1985;97:205–214.
51. Bessey PQ, Watters JM, Aoki TT, et al. Combined hormone infusion simulates the metabolic response to injury. Ann Surg 1984;200:264–281.
52. Groenveld ABJ, Kester ADM, Nauta JJP, et al. Relation of arterial blood lactate to oxygen delivery and hemodynamic variables in human shock states. Circ Shock 1987;22:35–53.
53. Parker MM, Shelhamer JH, Natanson C, et al. Serial cardiovascular variables in survivors and non-survivors of human septic shock: heart rate as an early predictor of prognosis. Crit Care Med 1987;15:925.

54. Ellworth ML, Goldfarb RD, Alexander RS, et al. Microembolization induced oxygen utilization impairment in the canine gracilis muscle. Adv Shock Res 1981;5:89–99.
55. Asher EF, Rowe RL, Garrison RW, et al. Experimental bacteremia and nutrient blood flow. Circ Shock 1986;20:43–49.
56. Schirmer WJ, Townsend MC, Schirmer JM, et al. Galactose clearance as an estimate of effective hepatic blood flow: validation and limitations. J Surg Res 1987;41:543–556.
57. Schirmer WJ, Schirmer JM, Naff GB, et al. Contribution of toxic oxygen intermediates to complement-induced reductions in effective hepatic blood flow. J Trauma 1988;28:1295–1300.
58. Coalson JI. Pathology of sepsis, septic shock and multiple organ failure. In: Sibbald WJ, Sprung CL, eds: Perspectives on sepsis and shock. Fullerton, CA: Society of Critical Care Medicine, 1986, 27–59.
59. Vermillion SE, Gregg JA, Bagenstross AA, et al. Jaundice associated with bacteremia. Arch Intern Med 1969;124:611–618.
60. Avila A, Warshawski F, Sibbald W, et al. Peripheral lymph flow in sheep with bacterial peritonitis: evidence for increased peripheral microvascular permeability accompanying systemic sepsis. Surgery 1985;97:685–695.
61. Piper J, Meyer M, Scheid P. Dual role of diffusion in tissue gas exchange: blood tissue equilibrium and diffusion shunt. Respir Physiol 1984;56:113–118.
62. Cerra FB, Siegel JH, Border J, et al. The hepatic failure of sepsis: cellular vs substrate. Surgery 1979;86:409–422.
63. Chaudry IH, Clemens MG, Baue AE. Cellular and subcellular function of the liver and other vital organs in sepsis and septic shock. In: Sibbald J, Spring CL, eds: Perspectives on sepsis and septic shock. Fullerton, CA: Society of Critical Care, 1986, 41–76.
64. Chaudry IH, Wichterman KA, Baue AE. Effect of sepsis on tissue adenine nucleotide levels. Surgery 1979;85:205–211.
65. Nxumalo JL, Teranaka M, Schenk WG Jr. Hepatic blood flow measurement III. Total hepatic blood flow measured by ICG clearance and electromagnetic flowmetry in a canine septic shock model. Ann Surg 1978;187:299–302.
66. Cameron DE, Chaudry IH, Schleck S, et al. Hepatocellular dysfunction in early sepsis despite increased hepatic flow. Adv Shock Res 1981;6:65–74.
67. Dahm MS, Lange P, Lobdell K, et al. Splanchnic and total body oxygen consumption differs in septic and injured patients. Surgery 1987;101:69–80.
68. Gump FE, Price JB, Kinney JM. Whole body and splanchnic blood flow and oxygen consumption in patients with intraperitoneal infection. Ann Surg 1970;171:321–328.
69. Wilmore GW, Goodwin CW, Aulick LH, et al. Effect of injury and infection on visceral metabolism and circulation. Ann Surg 1980;192:491–504.
70. Imamura M, Clowes GH. Hepatic blood flow and oxygen consumption in starvation, sepsis and septic shock. Surg Gynecol Obstet 1975;141:27–34.
71. Gottlieb ME, Sarfeh IJ, Stratton H, et al. Hepatic perfusion and splanchnic oxygen consumption in patients post injury. J Trauma 1983;23:836–843.
72. Raper RF, Rutledge FS, Hobson S, et al. Organ blood flow in high output normotensive sepsis. Crit Care Med 1986;14:440–445.
73. Leevy CM, George W, Lesko W, et al. Observations on hepatic oxygen metabolism in man. JAMA 1961;178:565–567.
74. Schirmer WJ, Townsend MC, Schirmer JM, et al. Galactose elimination kinetics in sepsis: correlations of hepatic blood flow with function. Arch Surg 1987;122:349–354.
75. Townsend MC, Hampton WW, Haybron DM, et al. Effective organ blood flow and bioenergy status in murine peritonitis. Surgery 1986;100:205–213.
76. Clemens MG, Chaudry IH, Baue AE. Alterations in hepatic water and electrolyte balance in sepsis. Arch Surg 1984;119:44–48.
77. Sayeed MM, Adler RJ, Chaudry IH, et al. Effect of hemorrhagic shock on hepatic transmembrane potential and intracellular electrolytes in vivo. Am J Physiol 1981;240:R211–R219.
78. Clemens MC, Chaudry IH, McDermott PH, et al. Regulation of glucose production from lactate in experimental sepsis. Am J Physiol 1983;244:R794–R800.
79. Gullem JG, Clemens MC, Chaudry IH, et al. Hepatic gluconeogenic capability in sepsis is depressed before changes in oxidative capability. J Trauma 1982;22:723–729.
80. Todal M, Haglund U, Lundgren. Countercurrent exchange mechanisms in the small intestine. In: Shepherd AP, Grange DW, eds: Physiology of the intestinal circulation. New York: Raven Press, 1984;83–97.
81. Fiddian-Grein RG. Hypotension, splanchnic hypoxia and arterial acidosis in ICU patients. Circ Shock 1987;21:326–331.
82. Fish RE, Lang CH, Spitzer JA. Regional blood flow during continuous low-dose endotoxin infusion. Circ Shock 1986;18:267–275.
83. Fink MP, Fiallo V, Stein KL, et al. Systemic and regional hemodynamic changes after intra-

peritoneal endotoxin in rabbits: development of a new model of the clinical syndrome of hyperdynamic sepsis. Circ Shock 1987;22:73–81.

84. Schuette AH, Huttermeier PC, Hill RD, et al. Regional blood flow and pulmonary thromboxane release after sublethal endotoxin infusion in sheep. Surgery 1984;95:444–453.

85. Lefer AM, Tabas J, Smith EF. Salutary effects of prostacyclin in endotoxin shock. Pharmacology 1980;21:206–212.

86. Mellander S, Johansson B. Control of resistance and capacitance functions in the peripheral circulation. Pharmacol Rev 1968;20:117–196.

87. Mason J, Torhorst J, Welsh J. Role of the medullary perfusion defect in the pathogenesis of ischaemic renal failure. Kidney Int 1984;26:283.

88. Lucas CE, Rector FE, Werner, et al. Altered renal homeostasis with acute sepsis: clinical significance. Arch Surg 1973;106:444–449.

89. Brenner M, Schaer GL, Mallory DL, et al. Determination of renal blood flow in septic and critically ill patients using a newly designed renal vein catheter. (Abstr.) Crit Care Med 1987;15:435.

90. Hemreck AS, Thal AP. Mechanisms for the high circulatory requirements in sepsis and shock. Ann Surg 1969;170:677–694.

91. Ravikant T, Lucas CE. Renal blood flow distribution in septic hyperdynamic pigs. J Surg Res 1977;22:294–298.

92. Cronenwett JL, Lindenauer SM. Distribution of intrarenal blood flow during sepsis. J Surg Res 1978;24:132–141.

93. Rector F, Goyal S, Rosenberg IK, et al. Sepsis: a mechanism for vasodilation in the kidney. Ann Surg 1973;178:222–226.

94. Stone AM, Stein T, LaFortune J, et al. Changes in intrarenal blood flow during sepsis. Surg Gynecol Obstet 1979;148:731–734.

95. Hayborn DM, Townsend MC, Hampton WW, et al. Alterations in renal perfusion and renal energy charge in murine peritonitis. Arch Surg 1987;122:328–331.

96. Walker JF, Cumming AD, Lindsay RM, et al. The renal response produced by non-hypotensive sepsis in a large animal model. Am J Kidney Dis 1986;8:88–97.

97. Auguste LJ, Stone AM, Wise L. The effects of Escherichia coli bacteremia on in vitro perfused kidneys. Ann Surg 1980;192:65–68.

98. Badr KF, Kelley VE, Rennfe HF, et al. Roles for thromboxane A_2 and leukotrienes in endotoxin-induced acute renal failure. Kidney Int 1986;30:474–480.

99. Linton AL, Lindsay RM, McDonald JWD, et al. Thromboxane synthetase inhibition (TSI) preserves renal function in sepsis. Kidney Int 1985;29:305.

100. Parker MM, Shelhamer JH, Bacharad SL, et al. Profound but reversible myocardial depression in patients with septic shock. Ann Intern Med 1984;100:483–495.

101. Ognibene FP, Parker MM, Natanson C, et al. Depressed left ventricular performance: response to volume infusion in patients with sepsis and septic shock. Chest 1988;93:903–910.

102. Rackow ED, Kaufman BS, Falk IL, et al. Hemodynamic response to fluid repletion in patients with septic shock: evidence for early depression of cardiac performance. Circ Shock 1987;22:11–22.

103. Cunnion RE, Schaer GL, Parker MM, et al. The coronary circulation in human septic shock. Clin Res 1988;36:453A.

104. Dhainant JF, Huyghebaert MF, Monsaillie JF, et al. Coronary hemodynamics and myocardial metabolism of lactate, free fatty acids, glucose and betone in patients with septic shock. Circulation 1987;75:533–541.

105. Pasque MK, Murphy CE, Tright PV, et al. Myocardial adenosine triphosphate levels during early sepsis. Arch Surg 1983;1437–1440.

106. Shapiro R, Breslow MJ, Miller C, et al. Sepsis induced coronary vasodilation. Circ Shock 1985;16:79.

107. Ellrodt AC, Riedinger MS, Kinachi A, et al. Left ventricular performance in septic shock: reversible segmental and global abnormalities. Am Heart J 1985;110:402–409.

108. Natanson C, Cunnion RE, Barrett DA, et al. Reversible myocardial depression in a canine model of septic shock is associated with myocardial microcirculatory damage and focal neutrophil infiltration. Clin Res 1986;34:639A.

8

Metabolic Changes in Sepsis and Multiple Organ Failure

Paul Kispert
Michael D. Caldwell

Sepsis and multiple organ failure (MOF) are characterized by progressive alterations in the metabolism of substrates used for energy production and synthetic processes. Changes in protein, fat, carbohydrate, and oxygen utilization are well described. The trauma-sepsis-MOF sequence has been described by Seigel et al.[1] who have identified various states through which patients progress from uncomplicated trauma to the MOF syndrome. These states are useful conceptually because many of the metabolic alterations seem to correspond to these states.

The relationship of sepsis to the development of MOF is clearly established in most instances. The majority of patients developing the MOF syndrome have passed through a period of sepsis. However, as many as 30% of patients dying from MOF syndrome were found not to have an infected focus at autopsy.[2,3] Border[4] among others[5] has proposed that activated pulmonary and hepatic macrophages may be responsible for the MOF syndrome through release of monokines, such as tumor necrosis factor (TNF), interleukin-1 (IL-1) and other monokines. These monokines produce alterations in intermediary substrate metabolism both directly and in conjunction with the neuroendocrine response to sepsis.

104

It is difficult, if not impossible, to separate the metabolic changes of sepsis from those of MOF. The overlap is considerable and the transition from sepsis to MOF seems to be a continuum. Several metabolic changes are consistent findings in both sepsis and MOF:

1. Glucose utilization is progressively impaired as sepsis worsens and MOF develops.
2. Proteolysis, principally from skeletal muscle breakdown with increased urinary nitrogen excretion, is markedly increased.
3. Lipid appears to be an increasingly used fuel.

The end result of this process is a hyperglycemic, catabolic, immunosuppressed patient with marked muscle wasting and organ failure. Although the end results are well characterized, the initiating events are unclear.

In this chapter, we hope to present the metabolic changes occurring in the trauma-sepsis-MOF sequence in such a way that substrate utilization and cycling are made clear. Although some of the metabolic consequences of severe catabolism are injurious, other changes in substrate utilization seem to confer a survival advantage to the organism.

Amino Acid Metabolism

Protein degradation is a normal part of protein metabolism. Under normal conditions, protein degradation is balanced by the synthesis of new protein with the net result being maintenance of normal muscle mass and visceral protein.

In normal persons subjected to periods of starvation, protein conservation occurs after an initial catabolic period. Trauma, sepsis, and MOF upset the normal pattern of protein sparing usually seen in starvation. Instead, protein catabolism proceeds at a rate far exceeding synthesis at a time when nutritional intake is absent and metabolic demands are great.[6,7] Urinary nitrogen and 3-methylhistidine excretion are markedly enhanced secondary to accompanying muscle wasting. Energy production in sepsis becomes progressively protein based until death due to MOF is imminent. At this time, there is a failure to use protein-derived amino acids as a source of fuel and their plasma levels increase. This increase in plasma amino acid levels may reflect hepatic failure and inability of the liver to clear amino acids from the blood. Additionally, accelerated skeletal muscle protein breakdown further contributes to the increase in plasma amino acid levels. The amino acids that are released into the circulation reflect proteolysis, de novo amino acid synthesis, and amino acid interconversion within skeletal muscle. Amino acids not metabolized by muscle (proline, phenylalanine, tyrosine, and methionine) reach increased levels in the plasma.[8] Alanine and glutamine are produced in the muscle by transamination reactions involving pyruvate and glutamine (Fig. 8–1). These transamination reactions result in carbon skeletons being shuttled from the muscle to the liver and gut where they are utilized for glucose synthesis, energy production, and protein synthesis. In order for amino acids to be used by muscle for energy, the amino

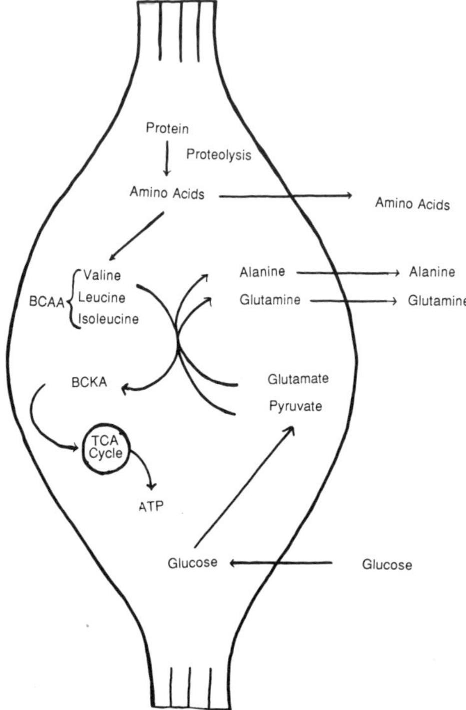

Figure 8–1.   Skeletal muscle proteolysis: Accelerated protein breakdown leads to elevated intracellular amino acid concentration. Some amino acids are directly released, whereas the branched chain amino acids (BCAA) are transaminated with pyruvate and glutamate, forming alanine, glutamine, and branched chain keto acids (BCKA). The BCKA enter the tricarboxylic acid cycle (TCA) for adenosine triphosphate (ATP) generation. Alanine and glutamine are released into the circulation in increased concentrations and subsequently extracted by the gut, liver, and kidney. Alanine and glutamine are released in concentrations exceeding those of skeletal muscle because of transamination and de novo synthesis.

groups must first be removed. The removed amino groups are transferred primarily to pyruvate and glutamate to form alanine and glutamine. This process contributes to the elevated plasma alanine and glutamine concentrations seen in trauma and sepsis (Fig. 8–1). As sepsis worsens and MOF develops, plasma amino acid profiles are further altered due to the development of progressive hepatic dysfunction. Under normal circumstances, the liver modulates against wide swings in plasma amino acid concentrations by removal or addition of amino acids to the plasma. Thus, either increased peripheral amino acid release or declining hepatic clearance can lead to altered amino acid profiles. As hepatic insufficiency develops, aromatic amino acid (AAA) clearance is impaired and consequently the plasma concentration of these amino acids increases. Branched chain amino acid (BCAA) clearance by muscle is well maintained even in late sepsis-MOF and BCAA levels therefore remain low, even when AAA levels are increasing. In this regard, the leucine (BCAA) to tyrosine (AAA) clearance ratio has been proposed as an index of hepatic function in trauma and sepsis.[9] The ratio increases as hepatic function deteriorates and AAA clearance fails with the continued clearance of BCAA by muscle.

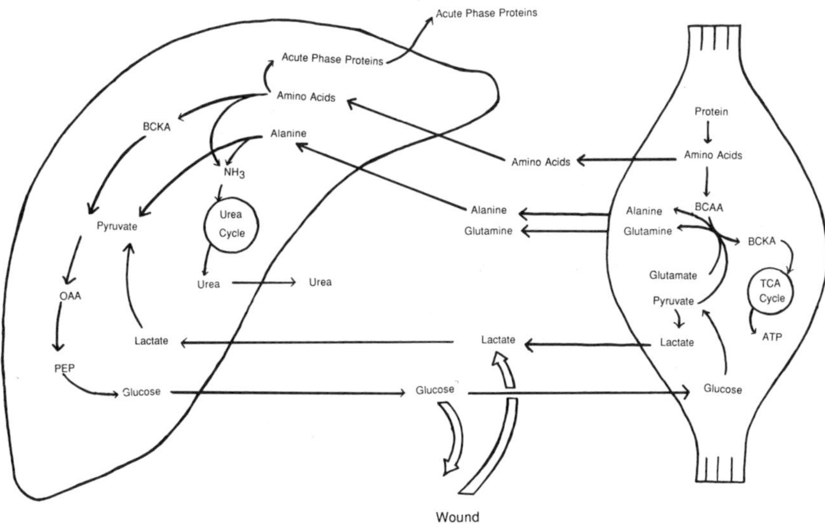

Figure 8–2. Skeletal muscle proteolysis leads to augmented alanine and glutamine release. Alanine and other amino acids are extracted by the liver. They are deaminated and the amino group is excreted as urea, accounting for the elevated urinary nitrogen loss seen in sepsis. The pyruvate and other alpha-keto acids generated are resynthesized into glucose, which is released into the circulation. Some amino acids extracted by the liver are used for acute-phase protein synthesis. Lactate derived from the wound is extracted by the liver and used for new glucose formation.

In summary, normally amino acid clearance increases as a function of the rate of amino acid delivery to most organs. However, despite elevated amino acid concentrations, the clearance of amino acids (other than the BCAA) is diminished in patients with sepsis. As sepsis worsens, branched chain amino acid clearance increases and aromatic amino acid clearance worsens, reflecting a deterioration of hepatic function. Exogenous amino acid administration (as with total parenteral nutrition [TPN]) also increases plasma amino acid levels. In addition, the gluconeogenic amino acids in TPN solutions may accentuate hyperglycemia in patients with sepsis.

Protein Metabolism

A key concept in understanding alterations in protein metabolism in sepsis if the concept of interorgan amino acid cycling. The most significant of these cycles are the skeletal muscle-liver (Fig. 8–2) and the muscle-gut interactions (Fig. 8–3).

Muscle-Liver Interactions

The negative nitrogen balance of sepsis and trauma is apparently due to breakdown of skeletal muscle protein. The urinary excretion of 3-methylhistidine is an indicator of skeletal muscle proteolysis and is markedly increased in sepsis.[6]

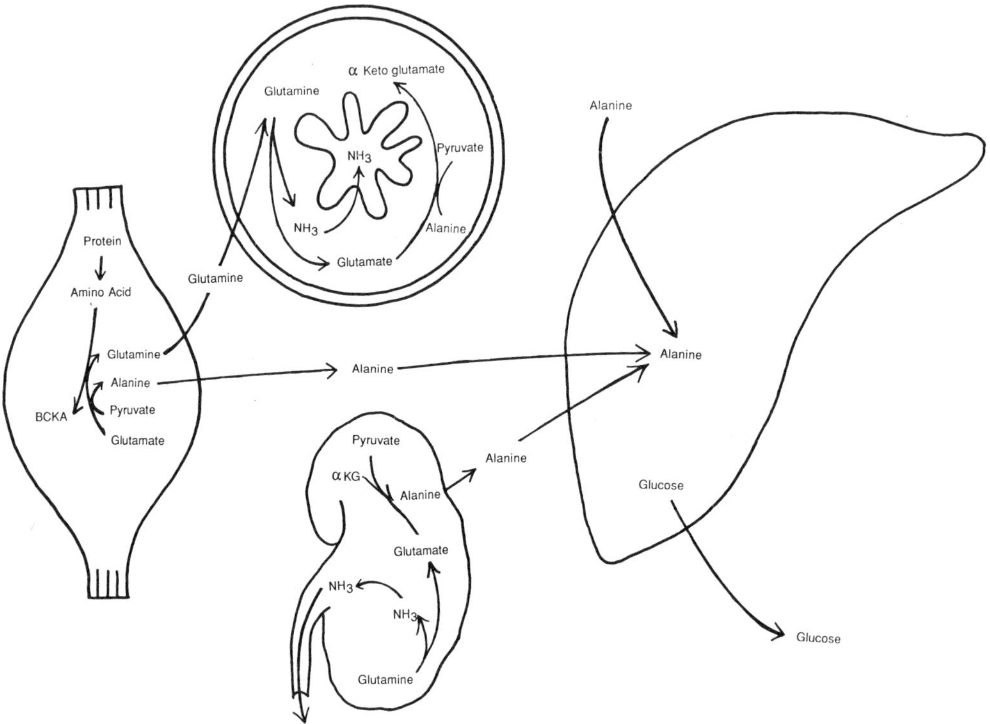

Figure 8–3. Skeletal muscle proteolysis leads to augmented alanine and glutamine release. Glutamine is extracted by the gut and kidney where deamination to glutamate occurs. The ammonia produced may be released into the gut lumen or urine to maintain acid-base balance. Glutamate is transaminated with pyruvate forming alanine and alpha-keto glutarate (α-KG). The α-KG may be used by the TCA cycle in the renal cells or enterocytes and the alanine formed is released and extracted by the liver where gluconeogenesis occurs.

It has been proposed that larger quantities of urinary nitrogen are lost for any given amount of muscle proteolysis in septic versus nonseptic trauma.[10] During septic states, amino acids may be released from skeletal muscle at three to five times the normal rate. Therefore the large nitrogen loss reflected in increased urea production is due to a compensatory increase in hepatic deamination reactions in response to increased plasma amino acid concentrations. These events form the basis of the muscle-hepatic interactions.

Ultimately, amino acid disposal requires removal of the amino group from the carbon skeleton of the amino acid. This amino group will generally enter the urea cycle or less frequently be excreted as ammonia. When the amino group is removed through transamination reactions with pyruvate and α-ketoglutarate, alanine and glutamate are generated. Glutamate can be further aminated in muscle to form glutamine. The alanine and glutamine formed in muscle are released into the circulation and travel principally to the liver and gut (Fig. 8–2).

In the liver, these amino acids are extracted from the plasma and undergo transamination and deamination reactions leading to the generation of pyruvate, glutamate, α-ketoglutarate, ammonia, and urea. In this way, the alpha-keto acid products of amino acids can be used by the liver for gluconeogenesis, oxidation, or ketogenesis. The glucose produced in the liver subsequently enters the circulation and travels to wounded or infected tissues as well as to the reticuloendothelial system where the glucose is utilized by inflammatory cells. This process is potentially very important, since inflammatory cells are obligate users of glucose.

Muscle-Gut Interactions

Glutamine is an amino acid that has received increasing attention recently. It contains two nitrogen moieties and functions as an important carrier of nitrogen and ammonia. The carbon skeleton of glutamine appears to be an important energy source, particularly for rapidly dividing cells (such as intestinal mucosa, dividing lymphocytes).

Glutamine is present in high concentrations in plasma as well as in the cells and serves as a major nitrogen carrier going from the skeletal muscle to the viscera. In skeletal muscle, glutamine, like alanine, is present in concentrations exceeding its normal content in muscle protein, suggesting de novo synthesis by the myocytes. Glutamine is synthesized in muscle from glutamate with the branched chain amino acids serving as a major nitrogen donor.

Plasma glutamine is extracted by the kidney, intestine, and the liver under certain circumstances (Fig. 8–3). In the kidney, glutamine is deaminated to glutamate and ammonia. The ammonia is released into the renal tubular lumen where it is eliminated, thereby maintaining acid-base balance, while the carbon skeleton (α-ketoglutarate) can be used for renal gluconeogenesis or for energy production in the Krebs cycle. Lastly, the glutamate produced from glutamine may be transaminated with pyruvate to form alanine, which can be transported to the liver for gluconeogenesis.

The gastrointestinal tract is a major site of glutamine metabolism. The gut extracts 20 to 30% of circulating glutamine in each pass. In the gut, glutamine is deaminated to form ammonia and glutamate, which can then be converted to alpha-keto-glutarate and enter the Krebs cycle. As in the kidney, alanine also can be formed in the intestine and shuttled to the liver. Glutamine seems to be particularly important for the support of intestinal mucosal integrity, since low concentrations of glutamine have been correlated with intestinal dysfunction. In fact, diminished glutamine levels have been proposed to impair the gut mucosal barrier and facilitate bacterial translocation in critically ill patients.

A logical question to be posed is why protein catabolism is accelerated in sepsis and MOF. At least some teleologic reasons seem to exist (Figure 8–4). The amino acids released into plasma from muscle proteolysis can be used for new protein synthesis, as oxidative fuels, or as a substrate for gluconeogenesis. Only about 20% of muscle protein that is broken down is used for energy generation, whereas the remainder is shuttled to the liver where accelerated gluconeogenesis occurs. The obligate need of certain tissues for glucose has been

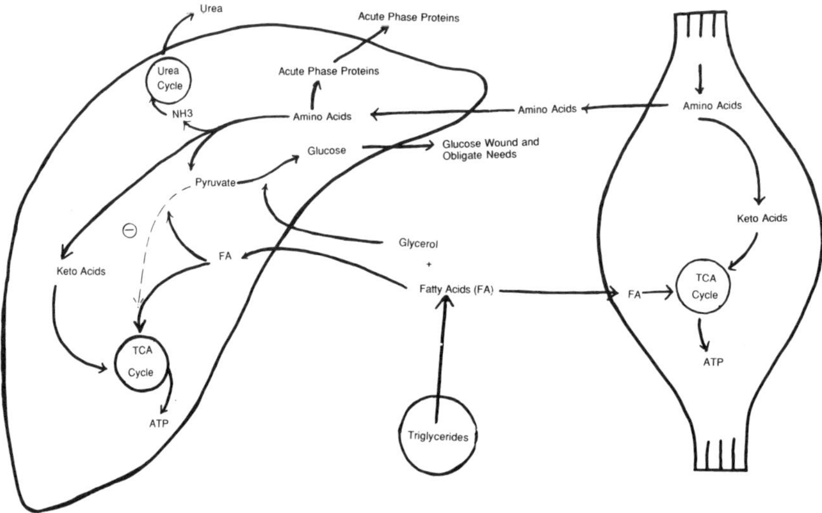

Figure 8–4.   Protein is catabolized to amino acid by muscle. Some of these amino acids are transaminated or deaminated to alpha-keto acids and used for energy production. Other amino acids are exported to the liver where they are used in acute-phase protein synthesis and glucose generation after deamination. The amino groups released are converted to urea and excreted. Other carbon skeletons may enter the TCA cycle and be used for energy generation. In catabolic states, triglyceride is broken down and used increasingly for energy generation. Both fat and protein spare glucose for obligate tissue needs. The fatty acid metabolism inhibits pyruvate dehydrogenase favoring gluconeogenesis.

previously mentioned. Hepatic glycogen stores in the liver and muscle are rapidly depleted in a catabolic setting. Thereafter, triglycerides and other nonglucose sources of energy must be used to meet energy needs. The only alternatives are protein or lipids (fatty acids or ketone bodies derived from lipid catabolism). With the exception of glycerol derived from the breakdown of triglycerides, lipid carbon is not appreciably used in the synthesis of new glucose. Since glycerol contributes only about 10% of the carbon skeleton of triglycerides, this leaves protein as the major source of carbon skeletons that can be used in the synthesis of new glucose needed to satisfy peripheral energy requirements.

A second reason for increased amino acid release from muscle is to meet the requirement for new protein synthesis by the liver, bone marrow, and wound. Although total hepatic protein synthesis is decreased after injury, specific acute-phase proteins are synthesized in increased quantities after sepsis and injury.[11–14] These proteins may confer a survival advantage after injury by supporting immune function, coagulation, and antiprotease activity. Marked elevations in C-reactive protein (CRP) in particular have been noted and CRP has been demonstrated to play a role in bacterial opsonization, complement activation, and phagocytosis.[11,15,16] Fibrinogen is elevated early after injury. The benefits for normal hemostasis are clear. Increased hepatic synthesis of several antiproteases such as alpha$_2$-macroglobulin and alpha$_1$-antitrypsin may protect against the systemic effects of proteases released from inflammatory foci. Ceruloplasmin and alpha$_2$-macroglobulin have superoxide scavenging properties. However, as sepsis progresses to MOF, acute-phase protein synthesis is altered. CRP and alpha$_1$-antitrypsin synthesis is maintained even late in sepsis, whereas other acute-phase proteins are synthesized to a lesser extent.[13] The significance of this observation is not clear. However, it is clear that, in the absence of adequate protein intake, endogenous amino acid supplied mainly by skeletal muscle proteolysis must be available for the liver to synthesize these acute-phase proteins.

Regulation of Proteolysis

The control of proteolysis is a point of great interest. It might be expected that if exogenous glucose were supplied at adequate levels to meet the obligate glucose demands of the tissues that proteolysis might be inhibited. This does not appear to be the case, since in sepsis administration of excess glucose fails to suppress protein catabolism in a way similar to that which occurs in starvation-induced proteolysis.[17–20] Ketones ordinarily inhibit proteolysis under conditions of starvation. However, since hepatic ketogenesis fails during sepsis and MOF, ketones may not be available in sufficient concentrations to suppress proteolysis.

The counterregulatory hormones such as catecholamines, glucagon, and cortisol that are elevated after injury and infection have been proposed as the cause of the accelerated proteolysis. This concept is supported by a review of the metabolic actions of glucagon and cortisol. Glucagon promotes gluconeogenesis, amino acid uptake, ureagenesis, and protein catabolism.[21,22] Cortisol enhances extrahepatic protein catabolism and promotes hepatic utilization of mobilized amino acids for gluconeogenesis and glycogenolysis. However, mixtures of these hormones in concentrations similar to those seen in sepsis have failed to elicit marked elevations in urinary nitrogen excretion in several studies.[23–28] In contrast, others have demonstrated moderate increases in urinary nitrogen when levels of cortisol, epinephrine, and glucagon were administered in concentrations similar to those in injured patients.[29] Failure to reproduce the septic response, as measured by nitrogen excretion, with administration of hormone mixtures suggests that other factors, perhaps macrophage products, are involved in addition to the catabolic hormones.

Release of macrophage products, including IL-1 or an active fragment of IL-1 (proteolysis-inducing factor (PIF)), have been implicated as a mechanism for initiating septic proteolysis.[30–35] In addition, generalized macrophage activation with monokine release has been proposed as one of the mechanisms of the MOF syndrome.[4] Nonetheless, the role of IL-1 in muscle proteolysis is unclear, since some investigators but not others have found that the in vitro administration of IL-1 increases amino acid release from skeletal muscle. Furthermore, proteolysis was not induced by the in vivo systemic administration of IL-1 and prostaglandin E$_2$ (PGE$_2$) in a dog model.[35] Regardless of the mechanism, it would seem logical to propose that the same factors that increase muscle catabolism may be linked to enhanced hepatic deamination, amino acid oxidation, urea synthesis, and acute-phase protein synthesis.

The significance of increased protein catabolism can be appreciated by its clinical effects. Marked skeletal muscle wasting is associated with depressed respiratory muscle and diaphragmatic function and the subsequent increased risk of atelectasis and pneumonia. Protein depletion is associated with immunosuppression and the development of septic complications. Altered amino acid metabolism with progressive hepatic failure and decreased clearance of aromatic amino acids may be associated with the development of encephalopathy and the synthesis of false neurotransmitters, which may in turn exacerbate the hyperdynamic septic state. For example, in late sepsis octopamine, an abnormal byproduct of tyrosine metabolism, is elevated to concentrations similar to those seen in hepatic failure.[36,37] Elevated octopamine levels may represent diversion of tyrosine away from dopamine and catecholamine synthesis.[38] Since octopamine has very little vasoconstrictive effect, its elevation may competitively inhibit the vasoconstrictive effects of the catecholamines, resulting in vasodilation and decreased total peripheral vascular resistance.

Lipid Metabolism

Lipid metabolism and administration is a controversial subject in the septic, traumatized patient. Authors have advocated the use of both low and high rates of lipid infusions as an energy substrate in order to minimize protein catabolism. Therefore, to help put this controversy into perspective, lipid metabolism during normal and abnormal states will be reviewed.

Lipid and ketone bodies normally can be used as energy substrates in most tissues and therefore may substitute for glucose. Under normal circumstances, fatty acids are mobilized from deposits of adipose tissue in response to elevated levels of cortisol, catecholamines, and glucagon or depressed levels of insulin (Fig. 8–5). The mobilized free fatty acids (FFA) are transported in the circulation bound primarily to albumin. Once the FFA have entered the cell, they are complexed to coenzyme A (CoA) in the cytosol to form fatty acyl CoA. Fatty acyl CoA is shuttled into the mitochondria via a carnitine-dependent mechanism. Lipid oxidation and energy generation occur in the mitrochondria. As more fat is catabolized, intramitochondrial levels of tricarboxylic acid (TCA) cycle intermediates, particularly citrate, become elevated. The citrate is ultimately converted to malonyl CoA. In the cytosol, malonyl CoA inhibits the carnitine-dependent mechanism responsible for promoting the entry of fatty acids into the mitochondria. This feedback inhibition of fatty acid mitochondrial entry prevents further fatty acid oxidation. As the fatty acid concentration in the cytosol increases, fatty acids are used for triglyceride synthesis. Elevated fatty acid concentrations also favor the synthesis of ketone bodies, which may be exported to other tissues where they serve as an energy source (Fig. 8–5). The FFA generated ketone bodies can be used by many tissues to meet their energy needs at a time when glucose availability is diminished.

Starvation results in enhanced fatty acid mobilization and ketone synthesis due to elevated plasma fatty acid concentrations and increased glucagon to insulin ratios.[39] Ketotic states result in depressed levels of malonyl CoA. As fatty acids are converted to ketones, less fatty acid enters the TCA cycle as acetyl CoA and less malonyl CoA is formed, thereby allowing fatty acids to continue to be used in ketone synthesis.

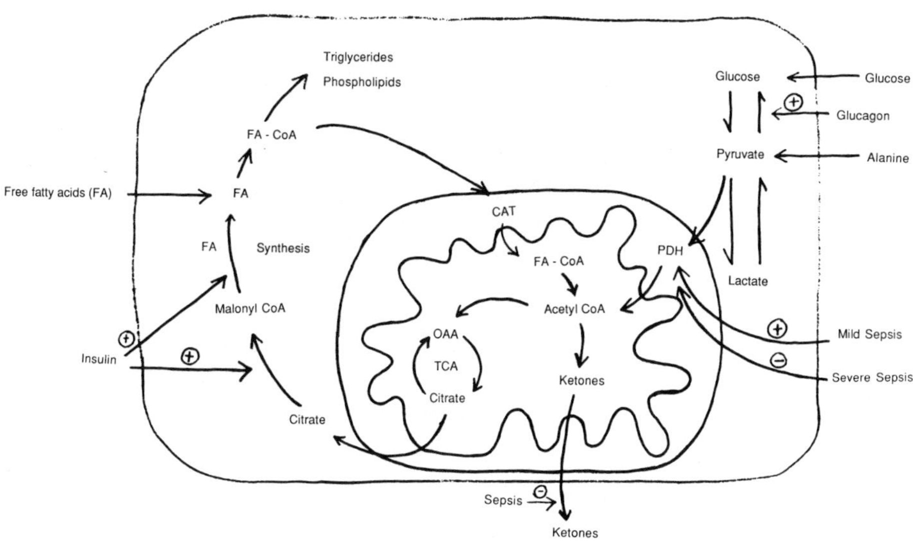

Figure 8–5. Elevated plasma triglyceride concentrations in sepsis lead to increased intracellular fatty acid (FA) concentrations. These FA may enter the mitochondria in a reaction requiring carnitine acyl transferase (CAT). Once in the mitochondria and after conversion to acetyl CoA, they can enter the tricarboxylic acid (TCA) cycle for energy generation or be used for ketogenesis. Sepsis inhibits ketogenesis and favors entry of FA carbon into the TCA cycle. As FAs enter the TCA cycle in increasing amounts, citrate concentrations increase and citrate is exported to the cytosol and converted to malonyl CoA. Elevated cytosolic malonyl CoA concentrations inhibit CAT. This inhibits entry of FA into the mitochondria and favors the use of malonyl CoA for fat synthesis, a late finding in sepsis and MOF. Worsening sepsis inhibits PDH activity and acetyl CoA generation favoring new glucose synthesis as opposed to glucose oxidation.

Lipid metabolism is altered in traumatized patients with sepsis. Endogenous lipids appear to act as a major fuel source in traumatized patients with sepsis.[40–42] Marked elevations in triglycerides and increased turnover rates for FFA have been noted.[20,43,44] Elevated FFA and glycerol production is thought to result from increased lipolysis due to elevated levels of circulating catecholamines, cortisol, and a high glucagon to insulin ratio. The FFA generated are used either for oxidation, ketone formation, or resynthesis of triglycerides in the liver.

Plasma ketone concentrations in sepsis are lower than expected given the hormonal environment. Furthermore, ketone synthesis by isolated liver preparations from septic animals is depressed compared with normal liver preparations. This failure of ketone synthesis may be related to an inhibition of carnitine acyl transferase, since this enzyme is competitively inhibited by elevated malonyl CoA levels. Thus, the net result of these processes is the inhibition of mitochondrial fat entry, which results in diminished ketone synthesis. Insulin concentrations are normal or mildly elevated in sepsis and may stimulate malonyl CoA formation, thereby inhibiting ketogenesis[45,46] (Fig. 8–3). Impairment in triglyceride removal may exist due to depression in lipoprotein lipase activity in muscle and fat of septic animals.[47,48]

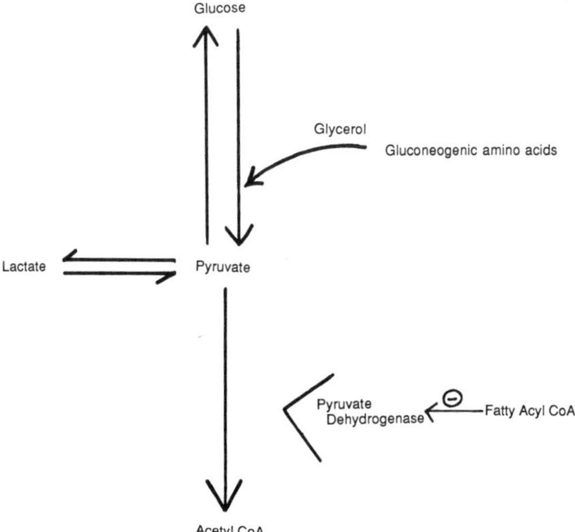

Figure 8–6.   Inhibition of pyruvate dehydrogenase by long chain fatty acyl CoA results in accumulation of pyruvate, lactate, and gluconeogenic precursors. Conversion of pyruvate to acetyl CoA is inhibited. Accumulation of pyruvate, lactate, glycerol, and amino acids favors gluconeogenesis. Elevated plasma triglyceride concentrations seen in sepsis result in increased fatty acyl CoA concentrations that inhibit pyruvate dehydrogenase.

Despite enhanced lipolysis, FFA levels are normal and triglycerides are markedly elevated. Intracellular fatty acyl CoA levels are also elevated with enhanced production of ketone bodies (acetoacetate and β-hydroxybutyrate) but not as high as expected. Since plasma ketone levels do not increase proportionately to muscle needs in sepsis,[42–44,49–52] skeletal muscle must rely increasingly on other fuels for energy.[7,18] Therefore elevated levels of fatty acyl CoA have several implications in sepsis and organ failure. For example, long chain fatty acyl CoA has been noted to reduce glucose oxidation by its inhibitory effects on pyruvate dehydrogenase (PDH) activity, which is the enzyme catalyzing the conversion of pyruvate to acetyl CoA (Fig. 8–6). Thus, as fatty acyl CoA levels increase, acetyl CoA production from pyruvate decreases. Pyruvate is then inhibited from entering the TCA cycle through PDH. This results in the accumulation of pyruvate and favors gluconeogenesis by mass action. Thus, glucose production for export to glucose-dependent tissues is enhanced due to fatty acyl CoA inhibition of PDH. Increased fatty acyl CoA concentrations should therefore enhance mitochondrial fat oxidation, glucose synthesis, and impair glucose oxidation by the TCA cycle.

Since the plasma concentration of triglycerides is increased in sepsis, FFA enters the cells and are converted in the cytosol to fatty acyl CoA, which then enters the mitochondria. If fatty acid entry into the mitochondria is great, TCA cycle intermediates will increase in concentration. Citrate (a TCA intermediate) leaves the mitochondria and enters the cytosol where it inhibits phosphofructokinase, thus sparing glycolysis and favoring gluconeogenesis. In addition citrate is converted to malonyl CoA. Malonyl CoA levels increase and lipid synthesis is favored due to inhibition of the carnitine-dependent mechanism for entry of fatty acyl CoA into the mitochondria.

The role of exogenous lipid in support of patients with sepsis is still unfolding. At a given level of caloric support, the respiratory quotient (RQ) is lower in patients with than without sepsis, suggesting that lipid may be the favored fuel over carbohydrate.[41,42,53] This lower RQ is consistent with impaired glucose oxidation and increased gluconeogenesis related to PDH inhibition in the patient with sepsis, resulting in greater reliance on lipid as an energy source.

These findings appear to fit a pattern when considered in the setting of sepsis. Most patients with sepsis are starving. They have an absolute requirement for glucose that can only briefly be met by endogenous glycogen. It cannot be met by lipid but can be achieved by the breakdown of protein. Skeletal muscle protein is therefore degraded and the resulting amino acids are shuttled to the liver. Unhindered entry of glucose carbon into the TCA cycle would significantly decrease the ability of the liver to generate glucose to meet peripheral energy needs. Thus, pyruvate (whether from glucose or alanine) is relatively inhibited from entering the TCA cycle by the inhibition of PDH activity (by high fatty acyl CoA levels). This favors glucose synthesis. Because glucose oxidation is impaired, the energy for hepatic gluconeogenesis comes from the oxidation of lipids, which are plentiful in the circulation after trauma or sepsis. Therefore lipids function as an energy source for the synthesis of glucose (and other cellular synthetic processes), while at the same time they inhibit the entry of gluconeogenic precursors into the TCA cycle. The elevated circulating lipid concentrations may also explain why the development of fatty liver is so often associated with sepsis. At high fatty acid concentrations, entry of the fatty acids into the mitochondria is inhibited by elevated malonyl CoA levels and therefore fat synthesis with subsequent hepatic storage is favored.

Carbohydrate Metabolism

Glucose entry into cells (principally skeletal muscle and fat) and its postentry metabolism is facilitated by insulin. Once in the cytosol, glucose enters the glycolytic pathway with the generation of pyruvate and subsequently acetyl CoA. The acetyl CoA may then enter the TCA cycle for energy generation or be used in fat synthesis after conversion to malonyl CoA. In the normal (postabsorptive) state, plasma insulin concentrations are elevated and glucose entry into cells is favored, resulting in glucose oxidation and glycogen synthesis. During periods of starvation, insulin concentrations are low, which allows the mobilization and utilization of fat and ketone bodies for energy.

Hyperglycemia is commonly encountered in sepsis. This occurs despite the fact that glucose uptake by the cells is increased[17,20,43,54–57] and glucose utilization and alanine and pyruvate production are increased. The increased glucose uptake by skeletal muscle is not accompanied by an increase in glucose oxidation. Compounds such as alanine and pyruvate return to the liver where they are converted into glucose for use by glucose-dependent tissues. Glucose-dependent tissues (glucose is an essential substrate) include the central and peripheral nervous system, leukocytes, red blood cells, bone marrow, renal medulla, and healing wounds. In general, these tissues are not dependent on insulin for intracellular glucose transport. The reticuloendothelial system also can be a major site of glucose utilization during sepsis.

Why hyperglycemia? It is thought that glucose oxidatior. revolves around the activity of the enzyme PDH (Fig. 8–6). In sepsis, PDH activity seems to decline, thereby diminishing the rate at which pyruvate derived from glucose can enter the TCA cycle. This inhibition results in increased concentrations of pyruvate, alanine, lactate, and other carbon skeletons that provide the substrate for gluconeogenesis. As the levels of these compounds increase, the subsequent inhibition of PDH favors the synthesis of glucose by the liver. Alanine from muscle may account for up to 75% of the increase in pyruvate levels. Thus, glucose oxidation is impaired while lactate, pyruvate, and alanine output are elevated.[58,59]

The PDH activity of different tissues is variably affected in sepsis.[60,61] Hepatic PDH activity progressively declines as sepsis worsens. Skeletal muscle PDH is more sensitive to septic inhibition, and PDH activity declines almost independent of the severity of sepsis (maximal inhibition with mild sepsis). Thus, a decline in skeletal muscle PDH activity has been suggested to be an early metabolic response to sepsis. This decrease in muscle PDH activity leads to decreased intracellular pyruvate oxidation and the release of pyruvate and lactate from the cells. These substrates are then shuttled to the liver for gluconeogenesis. The inhibition of PDH activity is thought to be one of the major causes of the hyperglycemia of sepsis and the relative "insulin resistance" that is seen. The insulin resistance is a postreceptor phenomenon occurring mainly in skeletal muscle at the level of PDH. Thus, despite the ability of glucose to enter the cell, glucose oxidation is incomplete and hepatic gluconeogenesis is augmented through an increase in the delivery of gluconeogenic precursors. In contrast to PDH activity, the sensitivity of the insulin receptor appears to remain normal in sepsis. The decline in PDH activity may also contribute to the elevated plasma lactate concentrations and the lactic acidosis of sepsis.[1,62]

Other factors besides altered PDH activity contribute to the hyperglycemia of sepsis. Elevated plasma catecholamine concentrations favor gluconeogenesis and inhibit glucose release, whereas cortisol inhibits peripheral glucose use. Plasma glucagon concentrations are markedly elevated while plasma insulin concentrations minimally change, resulting in an altered glucagon to insulin ratio. The increase in the glucagon to insulin ratio during sepsis is the reverse of what normally occurs during the postabsorptive state.[1,27,63] Additionally, the elevated glucagon concentration appears to be responsible for much of the increased hepatic glucose production seen in sepsis.

Therefore sepsis is characterized by continued fatty acid oxidation even in the presence of high glucose concentrations. The hyperglycemia in some respects correlates with outcome, since patients with sepsis whose glucose tolerance tests remain near normal have a 10% mortality rate, in contrast to the 60% mortality rate documented in patients who develop abnormal glucose tolerance tests.[64]

Several important points can be made from this discussion of substrate metabolism in sepsis:

1. Peripheral glucose demands are great and glucose synthesis is favored over glucose oxidation.
2. Protein breakdown provides pyruvate, lactate, and amino acids as substrates for hepatic gluconeogenesis.
3. Enhanced amino acid release from muscle provides substrate for new protein synthesis in the liver, bone marrow, and wound, thereby sparing glucose for use by cells with absolute glucose requirements.
4. Fat is increasingly relied on as the major source of energy production for the cell.

Role of Cytokines in Intermediary Metabolism

Within the last several years, investigators have proposed that the macrophage-monocyte cell line may be responsible for a number of the sequelae of infection and the development of septic syndromes[4,5] that may proceed to MOF. Septic syndromes have been noted in patients with severe trauma both in the presence and absence of documented infection. Bacterial products, such as endotoxin, plus other as yet unknown stimuli have been proposed to lead to systemic macrophage activation with the resultant synthesis and secretion of a number of different monokines. These monokines may have endocrine, paracrine, or autocrine effects. Endotoxin has been experimentally documented to produce a septic picture and death when injected intravenously.[65,66] Since endotoxin is a rather harmless compound when exposed directly to most body tissues, its deleterious effects appear to occur to some extent through secondary mediators liberated by activated macrophages. Endotoxin is capable of rapidly activating macrophages (splenic macrophages, hepatic Kupffer cells, pulmonary alveolar macrophages, renal mesangial cells) and stimulating them to synthesize and release monokines such as tumor necrosis factor (TNF), IL-1, platelet activating factor (PAF), and beta$_2$-interferon (IL-6). Infusions of TNF and PAF are able to reproduce the clinical picture of sepsis and several of these monokines have been documented to influence carbohydrate, lipid, protein, and trace element metabolism, as illustrated in Figure 8–7. For example, protein synthesis from cultured hepatocytes has been shown to be markedly diminished by factors released from macrophages activated by endotoxin, muramyl dipeptide, gentamicin-killed *Escherichia coli* or phorbol mystrate.[67–75] It has been postulated that this mediator-induced failure of protein synthesis by the liver may be a correlate of the hepatic dysfunction of sepsis and MOF.

Although total hepatic protein synthesis may decline, the synthesis of specific acute-phase proteins by the hepatocyte is markedly increased during sepsis and after trauma. There appears to be a reprioritization of hepatic protein synthesis away from the carrier proteins, such as albumin, and toward the acute-phase proteins. As mentioned earlier, these acute-phase proteins include fibrinogen,

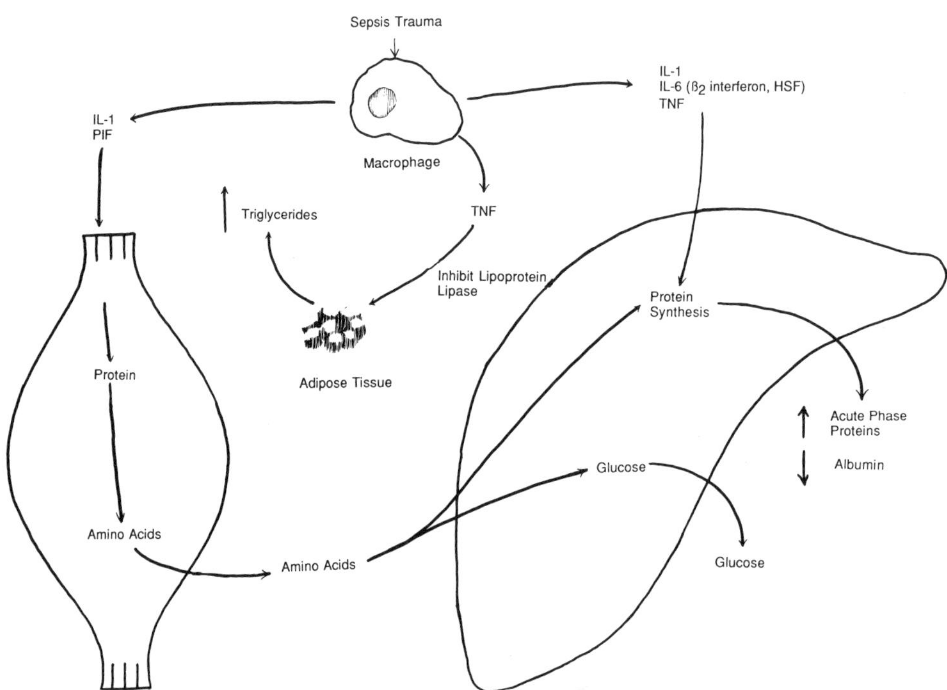

Figure 8–7. Sepsis and trauma activate macrophages with release of cytokines. IL-1, IL-6, and TNF affect hepatic acute-phase protein synthesis with increased synthesis of antiproteases, fibrinogen, and antioxidants, whereas albumin synthesis is depressed. IL-1 or PIF, or both, may enhance skeletal muscle proteolysis with amino acid release. Amino acids are extracted by the liver and used for new protein synthesis and glucose formation. TNF inhibits lipoprotein lipase, resulting in hyper-triglyceridemia.

alpha$_2$-macroglobulin, alpha$_1$-antitrypsin, ceruloplasmin, and CRP. The mechanism regulating the synthesis of these proteins appears to involve Kupffer cell and hepatocyte interactions. Kupffer cells (hepatic macrophages) in the liver are activated in some manner in vivo. This activation may occur through factors reaching the liver through the systemic or portal circulation. Translocation of bacteria across an abnormal gut mucosal barrier has been proposed as a possible activating mechanism for hepatic macrophages.[76–83] However, it would seem unlikely that the gut's permeability is altered immediately after trauma at a time when acute-phase protein synthesis is elevated. This would imply that there are other mediators, possibly derived from traumatized tissue, that are released systemically and travel to the liver and stimulate hepatocyte acute-phase protein synthesis.

Activated Kupffer cells appear to stimulate hepatocytes to produce the acute-phase proteins through the action of beta$_2$-interferon (hepatocyte stimulating factor) or IL-6.[84] Some endocrine-macrophage interaction must exist, since cortisol is required for the synthesis of acute-phase proteins to occur. Elevations in glucocorticoids in the postinjury period thus appear to facilitate hepatic acutephase protein synthesis. Other macrophage-derived factors also have been demonstrated to affect hepatic protein synthesis. Both TNF and IL-1 increase synthesis of the third component of complement (C3), whereas suppressing albumin synthesis (the so-called reprioritization of hepatic protein synthesis).[85–90] Because albumin synthesis accounts for a large percentage of hepatic protein synthesis, diminution of albumin synthesis may make amino acids more available for acute-phase protein synthesis.

Lipid metabolism is profoundly affected by sepsis and MOF. Hypertriglyceridemia is often encountered. Several mechanisms have been postulated to account for this. Catecholamines, cortisol, and glucagon all favor lipolysis and hypertriglyceridemia. Monokines also appear to play a significant role in the development of hypertriglyceridemia, since endotoxin given to experimental animals leads to marked elevation in plasma triglyceride levels. Furthermore, endotoxin-resistant animals do not develop hypertriglyceridemia when challenged with endotoxin. Endotoxin causes macrophages to release TNF, which seems to be the agent responsible for the hypertriglyceridemia. TNF may exert its effects through inhibition of lipoprotein lipase, the enzyme on the capillary cell membrane that is responsible for clearing triglycerides. Interestingly, pretreatment of animals with glucocorticoids totally suppresses the effects of endotoxin and TNF release.[91–96]

IL-1 is a peptide released by macrophages that can also have marked effects on intermediary metabolism.[97] Specifically, IL-1 can accelerate the basal metabolic rate and increase oxygen consumption. It also stimulates the liver to accumulate amino acids as well as zinc and iron from plasma pools. Interestingly, it also stimulates the pancreatic islets to release insulin and glucagon. Another proposed effect of IL-1 is to enhance skeletal muscle proteolysis and augment release of skeletal muscle amino acids.

Although other monokines have been studied, TNF, IL-1, and beta$_2$-interferon seem to exert the most profound effects on intermediary metabolism. One can look at this pattern of hormone and monokine release and propose a mechanism to explain some of the changes in metabolism that are seen after trauma and during MOF. In a traumatized patient, inflammation occurs in wounded tissue. The wound initially accumulates neutrophils followed several days later by monocytes and lymphocytes. It would seem logical that the wound is responsible for releasing a factor or factors that may act as hormones. These wound products could lead to macrophage activation in various organs (hepatic, pulmonary, renal) plus the reticulendothelial system and thereby directly affect the metabolism of other tissues, such as skeletal muscle. In sepsis, tissue macrophages in the liver, kidney, and lung, as well as the reticuloendothelial system, could be further activated by microorganisms or their products to produce monokines leading to the paracrine effects already described.

It is known that IL-1 or its putative breakdown product PIF (proteolysis inducing factor) augments skeletal muscle catabolism and release of amino acids. These amino acids then travel to the liver or gut where their extraction is enhanced by elevated glucagon and cortisol levels. Glucagon release is also enhanced by stimulation of the pancreatic islets by IL-1. Hepatic macrophages are activated and secrete beta$_2$-interferon, IL-1, and TNF, which stimulate the synthesis of acute-phase proteins in the presence of cortisol.

Release of TNF leads to a hypertriglyceridemia. The triglycerides may be used for energy generation at a time when glucose oxidation is inhibited.

Carbohydrate metabolism may be affected in several ways. As stated, IL-1 augments insulin and particularly glucagon release from the pancreatic islets. It also stimulates skeletal muscle amino acid release and thereby provides the liver with substrate for gluconeogenesis.

Integrated View of Metabolism in Sepsis and Multiple Organ Failure

Metabolic pathways and substrate utilization in the normal state are complicated and may become even more so in sepsis and trauma. Therefore certain concepts may be clearer when a clinical example is examined.

Consider a multiple trauma patient 10 days after injury who had a femur fracture and hepatic trauma requiring laparotomy. This patient, who is taking nothing by mouth, has developed fever, tachycardia, and mild hypotension; a picture consistent with sepsis. Given this scenario, how can carbohydrate, lipid, and protein metabolism be integrated into an understandable and sensible picture of metabolic alterations?

At this point, the patient has two problems, starvation and a markedly increased metabolic demand. The metabolic problem in patients with sepsis appears to be mitochondrial in origin and is a progressive deficit in energy availability for cellular processes with a decrease in oxygen consumption as sepsis worsens.[1,98] The glucose requirements of his fracture, wounds, and inflammatory cells are great at a time when his glycogen stores are depleted. His fat reserves are normal but fatty acids (except glycerol) cannot be utilized for glucose synthesis. Therefore protein from skeletal muscle is catabolized with the release of amino acids (particularly alanine), lactate, and pyruvate. Some of these amino acids (primarily BCAA) are used for muscle energy generation after transamination to form alanine or glutamine. The pyruvate, lactate, and alanine from muscle are also used by the liver for the synthesis of acute-phase proteins. These muscle-derived amino acids also will be used in protein synthesis for hematopoiesis and wound healing. Thus, muscle protein degradation provides substrate for needed gluconeogenesis and acute-phase protein synthesis. Fatty acids fuel this process while simultaneously decreasing glucose oxidation and shunting substrate into gluconeogenesis. The hormonal response with elevated plasma catecholamine, glucagon, and cortisol concentrations stimulates fat mobilization and further facilitates new glucose formation from amino acids. In addition, epinepherine inhibits insulin release from the pancreatic islets. Cortisol and glucagon both stimulate amino acid mobilization from muscle plus hepatic amino acid uptake, resulting in protein and glucose synthesis. The net result is recruitment of muscle amino acids to the liver, wound, and bone marrow for new protein synthesis. Although the monokine response is poorly defined, it would seem logical that monokines produced from macrophages in areas of tissue inflammation, injury, or infection might escape the confines of the wound and have systemic effects, acting in essence as hormones. This so-called "wound factor" could further modulate systemic changes. The monokines that seem to have the greatest metabolic effects are IL-1, TNF, and beta$_2$-interferon, all of which are primarily macrophage products.

In vitro, IL-1 or its breakdown product PIF stimulates skeletal muscle proteolysis with amino acid release in a fashion similar to that seen in sepsis. IL-1 also alters hepatic protein synthesis. Synthesis of the third component of complement is increased while albumin synthesis is markedly diminished. This would allow amino acids that are normally used for albumin synthesis to be used for protein synthesis in other more urgent areas.

TNF also plays several roles. In the liver, it inhibits albumin synthesis and augments C3 synthesis while having little effect on other acute-phase proteins. It also has a significant effect on lipid metabolism through inhibition of lipoprotein lipase and thus may in part be responsible for the hypertriglyceridemia of infection.

Beta$_2$-interferon has recently been noted to play a significant role in hepatic acute-phase protein synthesis. It is able to induce the entire spectrum of acutephase protein synthesis as well as inhibit albumin synthesis by the liver. IL-1 may modulate acute-phase protein synthesis through beta$_2$-interferon, since it has been shown to stimulate release of beta$_2$-interferon by macrophages.

As sepsis worsens and organ failure develops, liver function often deteriorates. As liver dysfunction develops, amino acid clearance, particularly the aromatic amino acids becomes impaired and the plasma concentration of these amino acids increases. This failure of hepatic amino acid clearance may have several deleterious effects. The aromatic amino acids may be metabolized to false neurotransmitters, which then may compete with catecholamines for binding sites on sympathetic nerve terminals. This may lead to vasodilation and hypotension. However, the rapidity with which septic vasodilation develops suggests that some other rapidly acting mechanism must be involved. The elevated plasma AAA concentration probably also predisposes to the development of septic encephalopathy. Aromatic amino acids compete with other neutral amino acids (mainly BCAA) for transport across the blood-brain barrier through a neutral amino acid carrier. Once in the brain, the AAA are postulated to be converted to an abnormal neurotransmitter and an encephalopathic picture may be produced. As hepatic function worsens, acute-phase protein synthesis and the synthesis of coagulation proteins are depressed.

Glucose metabolism is maintained until very late in the course of hepatic failure when hypoglycemia replaces hyperglycemia as the major abnormality of glucose metabolism. The development of fatty liver is a common finding. The etiology of fatty liver may be related to abnormalities of hepatic lipid metabolism and oxidation, that is, as fat is used for energy generation, intramitochondrial citrate and then cytosolic malonyl CoA levels are elevated. The elevated malonyl CoA levels inhibit the carnitine shuttle mechanism that allows fatty acids to enter the mitochondria. This results in the accumulation of fatty acyl CoA in the cytosol and favors lipogenesis and the development of a fatty liver. Depression of intracellular carnitine activity in sepsis may also play a role in the failure of fat to enter the mitochondria.

Much of the synopsis given of the changes in metabolism that occurs in sepsis and MOF is controversial and much more work is required before a consensus can be reached. Nonetheless, this overview may provide a useful framework with which to think about the metabolic changes that occur in sepsis and during MOF. There is no doubt that, as our understanding of septic metabolism improves, the scheme presented in this chapter will be modified.

References

1. Siegel JH, Cerra FB, Coleman B, et al. Physiological and metabolic correlations in human sepsis. Surgery 1979; 86:163.
2. Gans R, Bockhorst P, Nuytinck K, et al. Multiple organ failure: generalized auto destructive inflammation. Arch Surg 1985; 120:1109–1115.
3. Meakins J, Wicklund B, Forse R, et al. The surgical intensive care unit: current concepts in infection. Surg Clin North Am 1980; 60:117–137.
4. Border JR. The gut origin septic states in blunt multiple trauma 1SS-40 in the ICU. Ann Surg 1987; 206:427–448.
5. Carrico JC, et al. Multilple organ failure syndrome. Arch Surg 1985; 121:196–308.
6. Williamson DH, Farrell R, Kerr A, et al. Muscle-protein catabolism after injury in man as measured by urinary excretion of 3-methylhistidine. Clin Sci Mol Med 1977; 52:527.
7. Clowes GHA, O'Donnell TF, Blockburn GL. Energy metabolism and proteolysis in traumatized septic man. Surg Clin North Am 1976; 56:1169.
8. Cerra FB, Siegel JH, Coleman B, Border J, McMenany RP. Septic autocannibalism: a failure of exogenous nutritional support. Ann Surg 1980; 192:570.
9. Pittiruti M, Siegel JH, Sganga G, et al. Increased dependence on leucine in post traumatic sepsis: leucine/tyrosine clearance ration as indicator of hepatic impairment in septic multiple organ failure syndrome. Surgery 1985; 98:378.
10. Pearl R, Clowes GHA, Hirsch EF, et al. Prognosis and survival as determined by visceral amino acid clearance in severe trauma. J Trauma 1985; 25:777.
11. Koj A. Acute phase reactants: their synthesis, turnover and biologic significance. In Allison AC, ed: Structure and function of plasma proteins. New York: Plenum Press, 1974; 73.
12. Loda M, Clowes GHA, Dinarello CA, et al. Induction of hepatic protein synthesis by a peptide in blood plasma of patients with sepsis and trauma. Surgery 1984; 96:204.
13. Sganga G, Siegel JH, Brown G, et al. Reprioritization of hepatic plasma protein release in trauma and sepsis. Arch Surg 1985; 120:187.
14. Wannemacher RW, Pekarek RS, Thompson WL, et al. A protein from polymorphonuclear leukocytes (LEM) which effects the rate of hepatic amino acid transport and synthesis of acute phase globulins. Endocrinology 1975; 96:651.
15. Solomkin JS, Jenkins MK, Nelson RD, et al. Neutrophil dysfunction in sepsis. II. Evidence for the role of complement activation products in cellular deactivation. Surgery 1981; 90:391.
16. Solomkin JS, Simmons RL. Cellular and subcellular mediators of acute inflammation. Surg Clin North Am 1983; 63:225.
17. Border JR, Chenier R, McMenamy RH, et al. Multiple systems organ failure: muscle fuel deficit with visceral protein malnutrition. Surg Clin North Am 1976; 56:1147.
18. Siegel JH, Vary TL. Sepsis, abnormal metabolic control, and the multiple organ failure syndrome. In: Siegel JH, ed: Trauma, emergency surgery and critical care. New York: Livingston Churchill, 1987: 466.
19. Long CL, Kinney JM, Geiger JW. Non suppressibility of gluconeogenesis by glucose in septic patients. Metabolism 1976; 25:193.
20. Shaw JHF, Klein FS, Wolfe RR. Assessment of alanine, urea and glucose interrelationships in normal subjects and patients with sepsis with stable isotopes tracers. Surgery 1985; 97:557.
21. Exton JH, Park CR. The role of cyclic AMP in control of liver metabolism. Adv Enzyme Regul 1968; 6:391.
22. Krebs HA, Lund P, Stubbs M. Interrelations between gluconeogenesis and urea synthesis. In: Hanson RW, Mehlman MA, eds: Gluconeogenesis: its regulation in mammalian species. New York: John Wiley & Sons, 1976: 269.
23. Cherrington AD, Assimacopoulos FD, Harper SC, Corbin JD, Park CR, Exton JH. Studies on the alpha-adrenergic activation of hepatic glucose output. J Biol Chem 1976; 251:209.

24. Clutter WE, Bier DF, Shah SD, Cryer PE. Epinephrine plasma metabolic clearance rates and physiologic thresholds for metabolic and hemodynamic actions in man. J Clin Invest 1980; 66:94.
25. Frayn KN, Little RA, Maycock PF, Stoner HB. The relationship of plasma catecholamines to acute metabolic and hormonal responses to injury in man. Circ Shock 1985; 16:229.
26. Fearon DT, Ruddy S, Schur PH, et al. Activation of the properdin pathway in complement in patients with gram-negative bacteremia. N Engl J Med 1975; 292:937.
27. Liddell MJ, Daniel AM, MacLean LD, et al. The role of stress hormones in the catabolic metabolism of shock. Surg Gynecol Obstet 1979; 149:822.
28. Walters JM, Bessey PQ, Dinarella CA, et al. Both inflammatory and endocrine mediators stimulate host responses to sepsis. Arch Surg 1986; 121:179.
29. Bessey PQ, Watters JM, Aoki TT, Wilmore DW. Combined hormonal infusion stimulates the metabolic response to injury. Ann Surg 1984; 200:264–281.
30. Baracos V, Rodemann HP, Dinarello CA, Goldberg AL. Stimulation of muscle protein degradation and prostaglandin E_2 release by leukocyte pyrogen (interleukin-1). N Engl J Med 1983; 308:553.
31. Beisel WR, Sobocinski PZ. Endogenous mediators of fever-evaluated metabolic and hormonal responses. In Lipton JM ed: Fever. New York: Raven Press, 1980: 39.
32. Clowes GHA, George BG, Ryan NT. Induction of accelerated proteolysis and amino acid release from skeletal muscle by a potent non-protein factor in the plasma of septic patients. In McConn R, ed: Role of chemical mediators in the pathophysiology of acute illness and injury. New York: Raven Press, 1982: 327.
33. Clowes GHA, Hirsch E, George BC, et al. Survival from sepsis: the significance of altered protein metabolism regulated by proteolysis inducing factor, the circulating cleavage product of interleukin-1. Ann Surg 1985; 202:446.
34. Dinarello CA: Interleukin-1. Rev Infect Dis 1984; 6:51.
35. Clowes GHA, George BC, Villee CA, Saravis CA. Muscle proteolysis induced by a circulating peptide in patients with sepsis or trauma. N Engl J Med 1983; 308:545.
36. Altura M. Pharmacologic effects of alphamethyl-dopa, alpha methylnorepinephrine and octopamine on rat arteriolar, arterial and terminal vascular smooth muscle. Circ Res 1975; 36(Suppl):233.
37. Siegel JH, Giovannini I, Coleman B, et al. Pathologic synergistic modulation of the cardiovascular, respiratory and metabolic response to injury by cirrhosis and/or sepsis: a manifestation of common metabolic defect? Arch Surg 1982; 117:225.
38. Fisher JE, Horse WD, Kopin IJ. Beta hydroxylated sympathomimetic amines as false neurotransmitters. Br J Pharmacol 1965; 24:477.
39. McGarry JD, Foster D. Regulation of hepatic fatty acid oxidation and ketone body production. Annu Rev Biochem 1980; 49:395.
40. Carpenter GA, Askanazi J, Elwyn DH. Effects of hypercaloric glucose infusion on lipid metabolism in injury and sepsis. J Trauma 1979; 19:649.
41. Nanni G, Siegel JH, Coleman B, et al. Increased lipid fuel dependence in the critically-ill septic patient. J Trauma 1984; 24:14.
42. Stoner HB, Little RA, Frayn KN, et al. The effects of sepsis on the oxidation of carbohydrate and fat. Br J Surg 1983; 70:32.
43. Shaw JHF, Wolfe RR. Energy and substrate kinetics and oxidation during ketone infusion in septic dogs. Circ Shock 1984; 14:63.
44. Wolfe RR, Jahoor F, Peters E, et al. Substrate cycling in severely burned patients. (Abstr.) Circ Shock 1986; 18:359.
45. Brownsey RW, Edgell NJ, Hopkirk T, Denton RM. Studies on insulin stimulated phosphorylation of acetyl-CoA carboxylase, ATP citrate lyase and other proteins in rat epididymal adipose tissue. Biochem J 1984; 218:733–743.
46. Witters LA, Tipper JP, Bacon GW. Stimulation of site-specific phosphorylation of acetylcoenzyme A carboxylase by insulin and epinephrine. J Biol Chem 1983; 258:5643.
47. Pekala PH, Kawakami M, Angus CW, et al. Selective inhibition of synthesis of enzymes for de novo fatty acid biosynthesis by an endotoxin-induced mediator from exudate cells. Proc Natl Acad Sci USA 1983; 80:2743.
48. Scholl Ra, Lang CH, Bagby GJ. Hypertriglyceridemia and its relation to tissue lipoprotein lipase activity in endotoxemic, Escherichia coli bacteremia and polymicrobial septic rats. J Surg Res 1984; 37:394.
49. Neufeld HA, Pace JG, White L. Effect of bacterial infections on ketone concentrations in rat liver and blood and on free fatty acids concentrations in rat blood. Metabolism 1976; 25:837.
50. Pace JG. Fatty acid metabolism and ketogenesis during a streptococcus pneumonia injection in

the rat. Dissertation: Graduate School of Arts and Sciences, George Washington University, Washington, D.C., 1980: 1.

51. Wannemacher RW, Pace JG, Beall FA, et al. Role of the liver in regulation of ketone body production during sepsis. J Clin Invest 1979: 64:1565.

52. Wilmore DW, Goodwin CW, Aulick LH, et al. Effect of injury and infection on visceral metabolism and circulation. Ann Surg 1980; 192:491.

53. Wolfe RR, O'Donnell TF, Stone MD, et al. Investigation of factors determining the optimal glucose infusion rate of total parenteral nutrition. Metabolism 1980; 29:892.

54. Black PR, Brooks DC, Bessey PQ, et al. Mechanisms of insulin resistance following injury. Ann Surg 1982; 196:420.

55. Lang CH, Bugby GJ, Spitzer JJ. Carbohydrate dynamics in hypermetabolic septic rat. Metabolism 1984; 33:959.

56. Long CL, Kinney JM, Geirger JW. Nonsuppressibility of gluconeogenesis by glucose in septic patients. Metabolism 1976; 25:193.

57. Wilmore DW, Aulick LH, Masin AP Jr, Pruitt BA. Influence of burn wound on local and systemic response to injury. Ann Surg 1977; 186:444.

58. Hagg SA, Taylor SI, Ruderman NB. Glucose metabolism in perfused skeletal muscle. Biochem J 1976; 158:203.

59. Randle PJ, Garland PB, Hales CN, et al. Interactions of metabolism and the physiological role of insulin. Rec Prog Horm Res 1966; 22:1.

60. Vary TC, Siegel JH, Nakatani T, et al: Regulation of glucose metabolism by altered pyruvate dehydrogenase activity in sepsis. JPEN 1986; 10:351–355.

61. Vary TC, Siegel JH, Nakatani T, et al. Effect of sepsis on activity of pyruvate dehydrogenase complex in skeletal muscle and liver. Am. J. Physiol 1986; 250:E634.

62. Vary TC, Siegel JH, Tall BE, Morris JG. Altered glucose regulation in sepsis revealed by partial reversal of PDH inhibition by dichloracetate. Circ Shock 1986; 18:372. (Abstr.)

63. Marchuk JB, Finley RJ, Groves AC, et al. Catabolic hormones and substrate patterns in septic patients. J Surg Res 1977; 23:177.

64. Dahn M, Bouwnard, Kirkpatrick JR. The sepsis-glucose intolerance riddle: a hormonal explanation. Surgery 1979; 86:423.

65. Frank FE. Action of toxic doses of the polysaccharide from Serratia marcescens (Bacillus prodigiousus) on the dog and guinea pig. J Natl Cancer Inst 1944; 5:185–193.

66. Nishijima H, Weil MH, Shubin H, Cavinilles J. Hemodynamic and metabolic studies on shock associated with gram negative bacteremia. Medicine (Baltimore) 1973: 287–294.

67. West MA, Keller GA, Hyland BJ, Cerra FB, Simmons RL. Further characterization of Kupffer cell/macrophage-mediated alterations in hepatocyte protein synthesis. Surgery 1986; 100:416–422.

68. Keller GA, West MA, Harty JT, Wilkes LA, Cerra FB, Simmons RL. Modulation of hepatocyte protein synthesis by endotoxin activated Kupffer cells III: Evidence for the role of a monokine similar but not identical with interleukin-1. Ann Surg 1985; 201:436–442.

69. Keller GA, West MA, Cerra FB, Simmons RL. Macrophage mediated modulation of hepatic function in multiple-system failure. J Surg Res 1985; 39:555–563.

70. West MA, Keller GA, Hyland BJ, Cerra FB, Simmon RL. Hepatocyte function in sepsis. Surgery 1985; 98:388–394.

71. Keller GA, West MA, Harty JT, Cerra FB, Simmons RL. Modulation of hepatic protein synthesis during co-culture with macrophage rich peritoneal cells in vitro. Arch Surg 1985; 120:180–186.

72. Keller GA, West MA, Cerra FB, Simmons RL. Multiple systems organ failure: modulation of hepatocyte protein synthesis by endotoxin activated Kupffer cells. Ann Surg 1984; 201:87–95.

73. Keller GA, West MA, Cerra FB, Simmons RL. Macrophage mediated modulation of hepatocyte protein synthesis-effect of dexamethasone. Arch Surg 1986; 121:1199–1205.

74. Keller GA, West MA, Wilkes LA, Cerra FB, Simmons RL. Modulation of hepatocyte protein synthesis by endotoxin-activated Kupffer cells, II: mediation by soluble transferable factors. Ann Surg 1984; 201:429–435.

75. West MA, Keller GA, Cerra FB, Simmons RL. Killed E. coli stimulates macrophage mediated alterations in hepatocellular function in vitro culture: a mechanism of altered liver function in sepsis. Infect Immun 1985; 49:563–570.

76. Sori A, Rush B, Lysz T, et al. The gut as a source of sepsis after hemorrhagic shock. Am J Surg 1988; 155:187–192.

77. Maejima K, Deitch E, Berg R. Bacterial translocation from the gastrointestinal tracts of rats receiving thermal injury. Infect Immun 1984; 43:6–10.

78. Maejima K, Deitch E, Berg R. Promotion by burn stress of the translocation of bacteria from the gastrointestinal tract of mice. Arch Surg 1984; 119:166–172.

79. Deitch E, Maejima K, Berg R. Effect of oral antibiotics and bacterial overgrowth on the translocation of the gastrointestinal tract microflora in burned rats. J Trauma 1985; 25:385–392.

80. Berg R. Inhibition of E. coli translocation from the gastrointestinal tract by normal flora in gnotobiotic or antibiotic decontaminated mice. Infect Immun 1980; 29:1073–1081.
81. Baker J, Deitch E, Li M, et al. Hemorrhagic shock induces bacterial translocation from the gut. J Trauma 1988; 28:896.
82. Deitch E, Berg R, Specian R. Endotoxin promotes bacterial translocation from the gut. Arch Surg 1987; 122:185–190.
83. Deitch E, Berg R. Endotoxin but not malnutrition promotes bacterial translocation of the gut flora in burned mice. J Trauma 1987; 27:161–166.
84. Gauldie J, Richards C, Hamish D, Lansdorp P, Baumann H. Interferon B_2/B cell stimulatory factor type 2 shares identify with monocyte derived hepatocyte-estimulating factor and regulates the major acute phase protein response in liver cells. Proc Nat Acad Sci 1987; 84:7251–7255.
85. Darlington GJ, Wilson DR, Lachman LB. Monocyte conditioned medium, interleukin-1, and tumor necrosis factor stimulate the acute response in human hepatoma cells in vitro. J Cell Biol 1986; 103:787–793.
86. Koj A, Gauldie J, Regoeczl E, Sander DN, Sweeney GD. The acute phase response of cultured rat hepatocytes. Biochem J 1984; 224:505–514.
87. Andus T, Gross V, Tran Thic T, Schreiber G, Nagashima M, Heinnah P. The biosynthesis of acute phase proteins in primary cultures of rat hepatocytes. Eur J Biochem 1983; 133:561–571.
88. Kushner I. The phenomenon of the acute phase response. Ann NY Acad Sci 1982; 38:39–48.
89. Satoski K, Ishibashi I, Kazuhero H, Isuchiya Y, Sakaki Y, Okubu H, Niho Y. Kupffer cell stimulation of alpha-2 macroglobulin synthesis in rat hepatocytes and the role of glucocorticolds. Cell Struct Funct 1987; 12:35–42.
90. Perlmutter DH, Dinarello CA, Punsel PI, Culter HR. Cachectin/tumor necrosis factor regulates hepatic acute phase gene expression. J Clin Invest 1986; 78:1349–1354.
91. Beutler B, Cerami A. Cachectin. More than a tumor necrosis factor. N Engl J Med 1987; 316:379–385.
92. Dinarello CA, Mier JW. Lymphokines. N Engl J Med 1987; 317:940–945.
93. Beutler B, Cerami A. Cachectin (tumor necrosis factor): a macrophage hormone governing cellular metabolism and inflammatory response. Endocr Rev 1988; 9:57–66.
94. Tracey K, Lowry S, Fahey TJ, Albert JD, Fong Y, Herse D, Beutler B, Mangove K, Clavano S, Wei H, Cerami A, Shires GT. Cachectin/tumor necrosis factor induces lethal shock and stress hormones responses in the dog. Surg Gynecol Obstet 1987; 164:415–422.
95. Mannel DN. Biological aspects of tumor necrosis factor. Immunobiology 1986; 172:283–290.
96. Tracey KJ, Beutler B, Lowry SF, Merryweather J, Wolpe S, Milsark IW, Albert JD, Shires GT, Cerami A. Shock and tissue injury induced by recombinant human cachectin. Science 1986; 234:470–474.
97. Dinarello CA. Interleukin-1 and the pathogenesis of the acute phase response. N Engl J Med 1984; 311:413.
98. Siegel JH, Cerra FB, Peters D, et al. The physiologic recovery trajectory as the organizing principle for the quantification of hormonometabolic adaptation to surgical stress and severe sepsis. Adv Shock Res 1979; 2:177.

9

Nutritional Support in Critical Illness

Palmer Q. Bessey

> *Chirurgery is a skillful manipulation of the hands strengthened by diet and pharmacie.*
>
> —Ambroise Pare, ca. 1540

All of us eat in order to live. Nutrition provides not only the energy necessary for essential physiologic processes, such as membrane function and muscular contraction, but also the building blocks for growth and the synthesis of lean tissue. Since the critically ill patient requires increased amounts of both energy and substrate to support the increased physiologic demands of the illness and to repair damaged tissue, nutrition is an essential component of the care of all critically ill patients.

In the past, nutrition for critically ill patients was limited not only by restricted spontaneous intake, but also by the frequent inability to use the gastrointestinal tract because of ileus, fistula, hemorrhage, or other enteric diseases. This problem was largely solved by the development of intravenous nutrition, which overcame the limitations of enteral feeding. Thus, starvation can now be avoided in virtually all patients. The development of intravenous nutrition also sparked a renewal of clinical, scientific, and commercial interest in the nutritional support of patients, resulting in the development of a variety of new techniques and products.

In this chapter, I will first present a general approach to the nutritional support of patients. Then I will review how this general nutritional support scheme should be modified in patients with failure of specific organ systems. Finally, I

126

will discuss areas of active investigation and possible future developments in the field of nutrition.

Goals of Nutritional Care

Nutritional support is best designed with clear therapeutic goals in mind.[1] These goals generally fall into one of two categories. The first goal is an extension of the time-honored maxim: Do no further harm. For example, it is important to prevent nutritionally related factors or therapy from further complicating the patient's illness. These would include not only prevention of starvation and specific vitamin or nutrient deficiencies, but also avoidance of potential complications of nutritional support, such as pulmonary aspiration or diarrhea from enteral feedings, pneumothorax from total parenteral nutrition (TPN) line placement, or any of a variety of metabolic complications from inappropriate nutrient administration. Operationally, this goal can be defined as one of nutritional maintenance. Sufficient nutrients should be provided to meet the patient's nutritional requirements in the safest manner possible. This implies that the clinician has some way to judge what those requirements might be, to document what level of nutritional support is actually being provided, and to evaluate whether or not that support is effective in achieving nutritional maintenance.

The second general category of goals for optimal nutritional support includes attempts to alter the course of the patient's disease by nutritional manipulation. A simple example of this is weight gain, which occurs when the patient receives nutrition in excess of his requirements. Weight gain is a common goal for patients recovering from a critical illness and occurs as they regain muscle strength and stamina. For nutritional support to be most effective in restoring muscle mass and strength, overfeeding should be combined with a progressive exercise program. However, during the acute phases of critical illness and organ failure, this goal cannot be achieved because the patients may be inactive, sedated, or paralyzed. Furthermore, attempts at overfeeding may result in a variety of metabolic complications, including hyperosmolar states, liver dysfunction, and respiratory insufficiency. In fact, in some circumstances, overfeeding may exacerbate the severity of the patient's critical illness and alter metabolic requirements. Thus, there are potential side effects as well as benefits associated with aggressive nutritional support regimens.

When? The Timing of Nutritional Support

Although prolonged starvation can lead to death even in the absence of critical illness, transient periods of food deprivation occur commonly and are usually well tolerated. Since nutritional support techniques carry their own risks, occasionally complicate other aspects of acute care, and are costly, exogenous nutritional support may not be necessary in patients who can resume adequate, spontaneous oral intake shortly after the onset of the illness. In contrast, in patients who may have prolonged periods of starvation, the risks of further nutrient deprivation must be balanced against the risks and benefits of nutritional support.

From classic studies on human starvation,[2] loss of roughly one third of the total muscle mass or about 40% of body weight appears to be lethal. In adults who were initially healthy, it takes approximately 2 months for this degree of tissue erosion and weight loss to occur. Critically ill patients usually demonstrate increased heat production and nitrogen loss. Thus, nutritional requirements to achieve balance, that is, nutritional maintenance, are also increased. In this setting, erosion of muscle mass in the absence of adequate nutrition occurs more rapidly than in the case of starved healthy subjects.

At the other end of the spectrum, loss of 10% of the body weight in healthy subjects does not appear to impair work performance[3] and therefore may not be of clinical significance. However, in a classic study of patients undergoing gastric surgery,[4] mortality increased significantly when preoperative weight loss exceeded 20% of premorbid body weight. Other studies have documented an increased incidence of infectious complications and impaired immunologic function in patients who have lost 10 to 20% of their body weight.[5]

Based on these and other studies, it has been recommended that the goal of nutritional support during the entire course of a critical illness, including the recovery period, should be to limit weight loss to no more than 10% of the premorbid weight (ideal body weight).[5] Thus, in operational terms, limiting weight loss to less than 10% of the patient's premorbid weight is the goal of nutritional maintenance. To accomplish this goal, nutritional support should be initiated early enough in the patient's clinical course to restrict net weight loss to this amount (10%) or less.

Unfortunately, the use of daily weights to monitor nutritional status and to determine the need for additional nutritional support during a critical illness is not reliable. Changes in body weight may actually be misleading, since they more likely reflect changes in body water than changes in lean tissue mass. Therefore the effect of critical illness on lean body mass cannot be reliably determined by changes in body weight until the body fluid compartments have returned toward normal, which usually does not occur until late in recovery, often after hospital discharge.

Thus, the decision when to institute nutritional support is based primarily on an appreciation of the metabolic consequences of the patient's acute, critical illness. For example, routine nutritional support is not necessary in most patients undergoing elective surgery, since the metabolic consequences of most elective operations are slight and patients recovering from such procedures would not lose 10% of their preoperative body mass unless dietary intake is limited for 10 days or more. On the contrary, patients with a major body burn, multiple trauma, sepsis, or organ failure have markedly increased metabolic demands, and these patients could lose 10% of their premorbid body mass in as little as 5 or 6 days. Thus, for a patient in this latter group, nutritional support must be instituted much earlier in the course of disease than for the average elective surgical patient in order to achieve the goal of nutritional maintenance.

The presence of preexisting nutritional deficiencies should lead the clinician to consider nutritional support early in a patient's hospital course. Furthermore, nutritional support might be instituted almost "prophylactically," if it seemed unlikely that the patient would consume sufficient nutrients to meet nutritional needs in a reasonable period of time, either because of an expected inability to eat or because of expected increases in nutrient requirements. In fact, studies have documented that nutritional support improved outcome when instituted in the very early postoperative period in patients with abdominal trauma[6] or a variety of other acute surgical conditions.[7]

Patients with critical illness typically have increased nutritional requirements for nutritional maintenance. They should have nutritional support instituted as early in the course of the disease as practicable. Usually, this would be after hemodynamic stability and adequate oxygen delivery were secured—within 48 to 96 hours following injury or onset of critical illness. The quantity of nutrients should be increased so that full requirements are met within 5 to 7 days after the onset of critical illness.

How Much? Nutrition Assessment

The determination of a patient's nutritional requirements is the result of a process known as nutritional assessment. For the patient who is not critically ill, this may involve a variety of anthropometric measurements and laboratory tests.[8,9] These may help to define the patient's nutritional status, determine the presence or absence of malnutrition, and thus support a decision for or against nutritional support. However, for the critically ill patient, not only are these adjunctive determinations less important, but they are often unreliable. Because of the metabolic consequences of the patient's critical illness, malnutrition will surely develop unless nutritional support is begun early. Should the patient have been undernourished prior to the development of critical illness, the need for early nutritional support is more urgent.

Estimating Nutritional Requirements

Nutritional assessment of the critically ill patient initially consists of making an estimate of energy requirements. One way of estimating caloric needs involves the use of previously determined nomograms or empirically derived formulas. Several sets of standards for determining basal metabolic rate (BMR) or energy expenditure are available. These were determined from normal, healthy persons and reflect variations due to age, sex, and body size. The best known of these are the Harris-Benedict equations for men and women.[10]

Men:

$$\text{BMR (kcal/d)} = 66 + [13.7 \times \text{weight (kg)}] + [5 \times \text{height (cm)}] - [6.8 \times \text{age (yr)}]$$

Women:

$$\text{BMR (kcal/d)} = 665 + [9.6 \times \text{weight (kg)}] + [1.7 \times \text{height (cm)}] - [4.7 + \text{age (yr)}]$$

Table 9–1   Standard Basal Metabolic Rates*

Age (Years)	METABOLIC RATES (kcal/m²·hr)	
	Men	Women
1	53.0	53.0
5	49.3	48.4
10	44.0	42.5
15	41.8	37.9
20	38.6	35.3
25	37.5	35.2
30	36.8	35.1
35	36.5	35.0
40	36.3	34.9
45	36.2	34.5
50	35.8	33.9
55	35.4	33.3
60	34.9	32.7
65	34.4	32.2
70	33.8	31.7
75	33.2	31.3
80	33.0	30.9

*Adapted from Fleisch.[11]

Table 9–2   Effect of Stress on Basal Metabolic Rate*

STRESS	STRESS FACTOR†
Starvation	0.8–1.0
Elective Operation	1.0–1.1
Peritonitis, pneumonia, or major infectious disease	1.05–1.25
Long bone fracture	1.15–1.30
Multiple trauma, severe infection, head injury	1.3–1.55
Severe trauma, sepsis, + respiratory failure	1.5–1.7
Burns (body surface area)	
10%	1.25
20%	1.50
30%	1.70
40%	1.85
>50%	2.0

*Adapted from Bessey PQ. Parental nutrition and trauma. In: Rombeau JL, Caldwell MD (eds): *Parenteral Nutrition.* Philadelphia, WB Saunders Co., 1986; p. 473.

†Stress factor is used as a multiplier and reflects the increase in predicted metabolic rate due to critical illness.

The standards of Fleisch[11] are also commonly used (Table 9–1). These estimates of resting metabolic activity must be adjusted for the metabolic severity of the illness by multiplying them by a stress factor (Table 9–2). A final adjustment for the effects of feeding and activity is often made by multiplying by 1.2 or 1.25.

Table 9–3　Formulas for Estimating Daily Total Energy Requirements in Critically Ill Patients

BURN PATIENTS
Curreri[16]
Requirements = [25 × Weight (kg)] + [40 × % BSA burn]
(kcal/day)

McLaurin, Mason, et al.[17]
BMR (kcal/m²/hr)* = 54.33782 − 1.19961 × (age)(yrs) + 0.02548 × (age)² − 0.00018 (age)³
Requirements = BMR (kcal/m²/hr) × [2.33764 − 1.33764 EXP (−0.0286 × % BSA burn)] × BSA (m²) × 24 (hr/day) × 1.25
(kcal/day)

HOSPITALIZED PATIENTS
Ireton-Jones[18]
Requirements = 629 − [11 × Age (yrs)] + [25 × Weight (kg)] − [609 × Obesity†]
(kcal/day)

MECHANICALLY VENTILATED PATIENTS
Ireton-Jones[18]
Requirements = 1925 − [10 × Age (yrs)] + [5 × Weight (kg)] + [128 × Sex‡]
(kcal/day) + [292 × Trauma†] + [851 × Burn†]

Swinamer[19]
Requirements = [941 × BSA (m²)] − [6.3 × Age (yrs)] + [24.2 × Resp. Rate]
(kcal/day) + [804 × Tidal Volume (1)] + [104 × Temp. (°C)] − 4231

---

*This value should be reduced 7 to 10% for women.
†Present = 1, Absent = 0.
‡Male = 1, Female = 0.

This approach to nutritional assessment is simple, inexpensive, and generally applicable to all patients. However, it may not adequately reflect individual patient variation, since the basic formulas are based on data obtained several decades ago and therefore estimates vary according to the clinician's experience and bias. In fact, recent studies of contemporary patient populations, in which metabolic rates were determined by indirect calorimetry, suggest that estimates of energy expenditure based on the just mentioned approaches are too high.[12] This is of concern because overfeeding of the critically ill patient can lead to ventilatory[13] and hepatic[14] dysfunction and can aggravate the patient's metabolic responses.[15] However, the potential error of derived estimates of nutritional requirements can be minimized by using the patient's ideal rather than actual body weight in calculating basal caloric needs. In this way, the calculated nutritional values should more closely reflect the mass of metabolically active tissue (lean body mass) rather than the fat mass or extra body water. Additionally, the stress factor should be estimated conservatively (Table 9–2). In my experience, estimates of energy expenditure using these approaches have agreed closely with measured values in a variety of critically ill patients. Other investigators have derived empiric formulas for estimating energy expenditure in various populations of critically ill patients (Table 9–3).[16-19] These contemporary formulas derived from studies of critically ill patients have the same limitations as described for the Harris-Benedict equations.

Metabolic rate or energy expenditure can also be determined by indirect calorimetry (measurement of oxygen consumption and carbon dioxide production) at the bedside using one of several commercially available, portable metabolic carts. This method is routinely used for nutritional assessment and follow-up at many institutions,[20] since an estimate of energy needs based on indirect calorimetry is thought to be a more reliable, objective assessment of a patient's energy requirements than those obtained using standard equations. However, there are potential errors inherent in this approach also. The techniques of indirect calorimetry are not standardized and there may be variation due to the particular instrumentation utilized. Furthermore, these measurements are made over a finite period of time and extrapolated to 24 hours. Current instruments utilize either an open or closed system design, each of which has its own advantages and limitations. For example, open circuit instruments appear to be superior in patients spontaneously breathing room air, whereas closed circuit techniques are better for ventilated patients requiring high inspired oxygen concentrations.[21] An air leak anywhere in the system, (from the mouthpiece, mask, chest tube, or from around the tracheal cuff) is a major source of error in both design systems. In addition, there are a variety of patient and environmental factors that may affect the result of indirect calorimetry. These include such factors as patient comfort, anxiety, drugs, noise, activity, light, or temperature. This is especially true when 24-hour caloric needs are based on a measurement made over as short a time span as 15 minutes. To minimize these potentially confounding influences, instruments have been designed to interface with mechanical ventilators and to display the patient's integrated, 24-hour, measured energy expenditure. Since these instruments are moderately expensive to purchase and to operate, some centers have justified this expense by documenting a reduction in overfeeding and thus a savings in cost of TPN. However, no controlled studies are available to determine whether or not there is a difference in outcome between nutritional support based on empiric estimates of energy expenditure or that based on routine indirect calorimetry.

Nutritional Monitoring

Clearly, there are potential errors associated with both approaches to the initial determination of a patient's energy requirements. In addition, nutritional needs may change during the patient's hospital course. For example, energy requirements frequently increase with the development of complications or during the recovery period when the level of activity increases. Thus, nutritional assessment should be done repeatedly during a patient's course and should include some determination of the efficacy of the patient's nutritional support regimen. Nutritional support is therefore similar to most other supportive therapies for critically ill patients (for example, intravenous fluids, ventilator support, catecholamines, antibiotics) in that an initial level of support or dose is instituted and then its efficacy is determined by measuring appropriate physiologic or biochemical parameters (such as urine output, blood gases, cardiac output, antibiotic concentrations). Based on these parameters, therapy may be modified.

The most practical and widely used parameter to monitor nutritional support is nitrogen balance. A positive nitrogen balance is associated with a net whole body accretion of nitrogen. This occurs when protein synthesis exceeds protein breakdown, such as during normal growth. In contrast, negative nitrogen balance is associated with net whole body loss of nitrogen. This occurs when protein synthesis is less than protein breakdown, such as during starvation. Nitrogen equilibrium (nitrogen balance equals 0) is seen when synthesis and breakdown are matched and there is no net change in lean tissue mass. Nitrogen equilibrium is the nutritional status of most normal adults. Critically ill patients typically have a marked increase in protein breakdown and nitrogen loss, which is clinically apparent as negative nitrogen balance and muscle wasting. The achievement of positive nitrogen balance or at least nitrogen equilibrium is therefore a major objective of nutritional support. A positive nitrogen balance or nitrogen equilibrium is thought to be associated with preservation of lean body tissue mass and with clinical recovery. Thus, nutritional support is usually adjusted to try to match nitrogen loss with nitrogen intake. However, this approach is not always possible, especially in the early phases of a critical illness when muscle wasting from disuse may contribute significantly to total nitrogen loss.

Unfortunately, the measurement of total body nitrogen loss is imprecise. Nitrogen is lost mainly in the urine, but it is also lost in stool and other gastrointestinal fluids, as well as in the skin, sweat, hair, nails, wound exudate, and blood. Since it is not practical to quantitate the nitrogen lost by each of these routes, the determination of nitrogen loss is usually based on measurement of urinary nitrogen excretion. Classically, the total nitrogen content of a 24-hour urine collection is measured. However, the measurement of total nitrogen is not a standard assay in most clinical laboratories. Therefore, urinary nitrogen content is based on measurements of urea nitrogen. Urea is the major nitrogenous component of urinary nitrogen, and measurement of urea nitrogen is universally available. Commonly used laboratory assays for urea nitrogen also measure the nitrogen contained in ammonia. When determined by this method, urea nitrogen has been found to represent 80% of total urinary nitrogen excretion in critically ill patients receiving maintenance nutritional support.[22] The nitrogen lost from the gastrointestinal tract, through skin desquamation, and in sweat is usually estimated to be 2 g/day in adults. However, nitrogen loss by these routes may be increased in the presence of diarrhea, excessive wound exudate, or blood loss. Thus, nitrogen loss can be estimated using the following formula:

$$\text{Nitrogen loss (g)} = [\text{urinary urea nitrogen (g)}/0.8] + 2$$

Accurate records of nutritional intake are essential, not only for determination of nitrogen intake, but also to evaluate the efficacy of the patient's nutritional support. These records are commonly maintained by the clinical dietician and include the patient's total caloric intake, plus the amounts of carbohydrate, fat, and protein or amino acids the patient received. Nitrogen comprises approximately 16% of protein or amino acid solutions by weight. Thus:

$$\text{Nitrogen intake (g)} = \text{protein or amino acid intake (g)}/6.25$$

and:

$$\text{Nitrogen balance} = \text{nitrogen intake} - \text{nitrogen loss}$$

The determination of the balance of nitrogen intake and loss is at best a crude reflection of whole body protein metabolic processes. It may be influenced by renal function, by changes in total body water, as well as by the concentrations of urea and other circulating nitrogenous compounds. Furthermore, if the nutritional records are inaccurate, or if errors are made in the collection of timed urine samples, the calculated nitrogen balance will not accurately reflect true nitrogen balance. However, other nutritional parameters are no more reliable. As already mentioned, changes in body weight in the critically ill patient are usually due to changes in body water. As patients recover, they typically mobilize and excrete a portion of their expanded extracellular fluid.[23] Thus, weight loss in the setting of net sodium and water loss may be associated with recovery and not necessarily reflect inadequate nutritional support. Similarly, the concentrations of albumin and other serum proteins are influenced by changes in body water. Thus, although the levels of some of the serum proteins, such as albumin, are typically reduced during critical illness and return toward normal as the patient recovers, they are not specific indicators of the adequacy of nutritional support.

Nitrogen balance may be improved by increasing either nitrogen intake or total caloric intake, or both. In this regard, indirect calorimetry may be helpful in determining the adequacy of energy intake. However, in critically ill patients positive nitrogen balance or nitrogen equilibrium may not always be attainable, especially if the patient is immobilized. Since large calorie and nitrogen loads may entail additional metabolic risks, nitrogen balance values must be viewed in context with other parameters and the patient's overall course. Helpful information may be obtained by measuring other substances excreted in the urine. The actual specimen collection is often the most difficult part of a balance study. Once the sample is obtained, chemical analyses are simple and cheap. Measurement of creatinine excretion will allow an assessment of renal function (creatinine clearance). Furthermore, since creatinine excretion is fairly constant, an abrupt reduction in creatinine excretion without a change in serum creatinine concentration might indicate an inaccurate collection. Measurement of sodium excretion can be helpful in assessing extracellular fluid changes, whereas potassium excretion may help guide appropriate potassium replacement.

What? The Components of Nutritional Support

The major components of any nutritional support regimen are protein and amino acids plus carbohydrates and fats. Protein and amino acids contain nitrogen and thus provide the building blocks for protein synthesis and wound healing, whereas the oxidation of carbohydrates and fats provides energy to support the body's metabolic machinery. Not all fats are metabolized for energy. Some specific types of lipid are essential for the synthesis of specialized lipid compounds, such as the prostaglandins. In addition, electrolytes, vitamins, and trace minerals are required for proper enzyme function and cellular activity.

Nitrogen Substrate: Protein and Amino Acids

In fasting normal subjects the oxidation of protein accounts for approximately 15% of the metabolic rate under basal conditions.[24] Therefore it has been assumed that 15% of nutritional support should be with nitrogen-containing substrate. In patients the BMR is typically increased, but the proportion due to protein oxidation is roughly the same.[25] Many standard nutritional support regimens therefore provide about 15% of total calories as protein or amino acids. However, recent studies suggest that providing proportionally greater amounts of protein or amino acids than is oxidized may be beneficial in critically ill patients.[26,27] This concept of increased nitrogen needs is supported by experiments documenting that when an infusion of cortisol, glucagon, and epinephrine was given to normal humans to simulate the metabolic alterations of critical illness, the efficiency of nitrogen retention was blunted. To achieve nitrogen equilibrium in this model, nitrogen substrate would have had to comprise approximately 20% of the administered calories.[28]

Thus, in planning a nutritional support regimen for a critically ill patient, at least 15 to 20% of the estimated total energy requirements should be provided as protein or amino acids. The higher proportion is used for patients with markedly increased energy requirements. Older patients or patients who were nutritionally depleted prior to their acute illness may also benefit from a higher than standard proportion of nitrogen substrate.[29] The limiting factor in the administration of nitrogen is renal function and urea clearance. High nitrogen loads will lead to increased urea production and elevated concentrations of blood urea nitrogen (BUN). BUN levels up to 40 or 50 mg/dl appear to be well tolerated.

There are several approaches to determining nitrogen needs in critically ill patients, all of which are roughly equivalent. One may calculate the amount of nitrogen substrate based on the patient's weight. Critically ill patients usually require 1.5 to 2.5 g of protein (amino acid) per kilogram of ideal body weight.[30] The higher value is used for the severe illnesses. Alternatively, the relationship between nitrogen and energy may be determined by the ratio of nonprotein calories to nitrogen. Normal persons can be maintained with a nonprotein calorie to nitrogen ratio of 150:1 or higher. Critically ill patients appear to benefit from lower ratios in the range of 125:1 to 100:1. This statement is equivalent to saying that they benefit from a nutrition support regimen in which a higher than normal proportion of total calories is provided as nitrogen substrate (protein or amino acids). These two approaches lead to similar support regimens.

For example, consider an 18-year-old man, weighing 80 kg (body surface area equals 2 m^2), who sustains a 20% body surface area burn. Following the techniques already outlined, his energy requirements would be based on a 50% increase in his BMR of 40 kcal/m^2/hr and thus would be estimated at 3456 kcal/day. If his nutrition support regimen contained 3500 kcal, 20% (700 kcal) of which was provided by protein, he would receive 175 g of protein (28 g of nitrogen) and 2800 nonprotein calories. This would be equivalent to 2.2 g protein/kg body weight and a nonprotein calorie to nitrogen ratio of 100:1. It is critical to remember that both nitrogen substrate (protein and amino acids) and energy (calories) are required for nutritional maintenance or positive nitrogen balance.

High caloric diets without sufficient nitrogen are inadequate to achieve nitrogen equilibrium. Conversely, diets that contain large quantities of protein or amino acids but are hypocaloric will also be inadequate. In the latter case, nitrogen substrate will be used for energy instead of protein synthesis and will have a similar effect on net nitrogen balance as a calorically equivalent amount of glucose.[31]

Energy Substrate: Carbohydrate and Fat

Although carbohydrate and fat are the principal body fuels, certain tissues, including the central nervous system, renal medulla, and hematopoietic cells, utilize glucose almost exclusively. Not only is glucose inexpensive, it is effective in promoting net nitrogen retention, in part by stimulating the release of insulin. Normal subjects can assimilate large quantities of glucose and can seemingly utilize glucose to meet all of their energy requirements. The successful use of glucose and amino acid solutions for intravenous feeding over the past 20 years in the United States is a testament to this fact. However, this experience has also demonstrated that certain lipids, such as the polyunsaturated fatty acids, are essential nutrients. These essential fats are required not only for energy but as precursors for certain endogenous lipid compounds, such as the prostaglandins. In the absence of these unsaturated fatty acids, a characteristic essential fatty acid deficiency syndrome will develop in time.[32] Thus, even though nutrition support consists mainly of glucose and amino acid solutions, some lipid intake must be provided to prevent essential fatty acid deficiency. The lipid requirements are often met by infusion of a lipid emulsion high in linoleic and linolenic acids.

Critically ill patients also utilize increased amounts of glucose. The patient's wound, or mass of inflammatory cells, primarily consumes glucose as a respiratory fuel.[33,34] This additional need is matched by increased endogenous glucose production by the liver. Thus, there is an increase in the mass flow of glucose through the glucose distribution space (extracellular fluid compartment roughly 20% body weight). This increased glucose flow is a typical response to injury, infection, and other critical illness and is proportional to the severity of illness.[35] Glucose flow returns toward normal as convalescence proceeds. It may increase still further if complications or infections develop, but with multisystem organ failure glucose production may also fail.[36] In normal subjects, glucose administration readily suppresses endogenous glucose production. However, this is not the case for critically ill patients. Shaw et al.[37] determined the effect of glucose infusion on glycogenolysis and gluconeogenesis in critically ill patients with sepsis. They found that the basal rate of glucose production was elevated above control values and that an infusion of exogenous glucose at a moderately low rate, which would have suppressed glucose production in normal persons, decreased hepatic glycogenolysis but did not affect either gluconeogenesis from alanine or urea production. Significantly higher glucose infusion rates were required before urea production decreased and glucose oxidation increased.

Despite the increased flow and basal rate of glucose uptake, critically ill patients are typically hyperglycemic, especially when exogenous glucose is administered. Terms such as "traumatic diabetes" and "diabetes of injury," which have been utilized in the past, suggest an insulin deficiency state as an explanation of why these patients are hyperglycemic. This concept is appealing because it would also explain why protein breakdown is increased in these patients. However, a true insulin deficiency state does not appear to be present, since the insulin response to exogenous glucose in critically ill patients appears unimpaired.[38] Black and coworkers[39] examined this question by maintaining a fixed hyperglycemic state with an infusion of glucose (hyperglycemic glucose clamp study) in injured patients and in age-matched controls. In response to fixed hyperglycemia, glucose disposal continually increased in the control subjects and was associated with a steady increase in serum insulin concentration. In contrast, patients convalescing normally from moderately severe injury demonstrated a decreased rate of glucose disposal in response to fixed hyperglycemia. In the patients, insulin concentrations increased and were actually greater in the patients than in the normal control subjects. Whereas there was a very close association between glucose disposal and insulin concentration in normal subjects, there was no association between these two parameters in the injured patients. Thus, glucose disposal was limited in the injured subjects (6 to 7 mg/ kg/min) even in the presence of an increasing insulin level.

To quantitate further the efficacy of insulin in injured subjects, Black and associates[39] performed euglycemic insulin clamp studies on a similar group of injured subjects. In this technique, a primed, constant infusion of insulin maintains fixed hyperinsulinemia when glucose concentrations are clamped at normal values by altering the rate of glucose infusion. Under these conditions, the rate of glucose infusion reflects glucose disposal and indicates whole body responsiveness to insulin. Black et al. achieved similar levels of hyperinsulinemia and euglycemia in both patients and control subjects. At all insulin doses and insulin concentrations achieved, glucose disposal was lower in the patients than in the control subjects. These studies provided quantitative evidence of insulin resistance in critically ill patients. Based on the relationship between insulin dose and glucose disposal, it appeared that this decrease in whole body insulin responsiveness was the result of a postreceptor defect. Brooks and his coworkers[40] measured glucose uptake across the forearm of injured patients during insulin clamp studies. Forearm glucose uptake was reduced in patients compared with control subjects, indicating that peripheral tissue, primarily skeletal muscle, was a major site of post-traumatic insulin resistance.

This finding that injured subjects were more limited than healthy volunteers in the maximum amount of glucose they could utilize effectively is similar to observations made in several other studies that utilized different methodologies and involved different types of critically ill patients.[41–43] Collectively, the data suggest that this maximum rate of glucose disposal is inversely related to the severity of injury (Table 9–4). Whereas normal patients or subjects following elective operation may be able to utilize glucose to meet all of their nonprotein calorie needs, patients with severe injuries or other critical illness can only utilize enough glucose to meet approximately 50% of their total caloric requirements. Despite hyperglycemia, critically ill patients will continue to depend on fat oxidation to meet a significant proportion of their energy needs. Thus, in the

Table 9–4　Maximum Glucose Oxidation or Disposal

Patients	DISPOSAL RATES		
	mg/kg·min	*g/kg·d*	*kcal/d (70kg)*
Post-operative (44)	7	10.1	2400
Moderate Injury (42)	6	8.6	2050
Severe Burn (45)	5	7.2	1710

nutritional support of critically ill patients, a mixed fuel system consisting of both carbohydrate and fat is commonly utilized.[44,45] Glucose or other carbohydrates typically provide between 50 and 70% of the total calories. The difference between estimated total energy intake and the sum of carbohydrate and protein (amino acid) calories is provided by fat. Most commonly utilized enteral nutrition products provide nutrients in approximately these proportions. Intravenous feedings may also provide a similar nutrient mix.

Electrolytes, Vitamins, and Trace Minerals

Nutritional support must occasionally be modified to maintain serum electrolyte concentrations within normal ranges. Enteral nutritional products usually contain sufficient electrolytes so that further supplementation is not necessary. Patients maintained solely on enteral nutrition may require extra water to maintain normal extracellular fluid tonicity. Furthermore, the sodium and potassium contents of some products may cause problems in patients with cardiac or renal failure.

Since potassium and magnesium are principally intracellular cations, their serum concentrations may not reflect total body stores. In fact, it is common for patients to have low normal or normal serum potassium or magnesium levels, in the presence of large total body deficits of these cations. Not only are the losses of these cations increased in hypercatabolic patients, but their increased levels of incorporation into the intracellular matrix further increases daily requirements. Thus, potassium and magnesium should be provided in generous amounts (100 to 150 mEq of potassium and 30 mEq of magnesium per day) to maintain serum concentrations in the mid to high normal range. Metabolic acid-base status must be carefully monitored in patients receiving nutritional support, especially those receiving intravenous feedings. Since metabolic acidosis or alkalosis is associated with hyperchloremia or hypochloremia, respectively, it is frequently necessary to adjust the amount of chloride administered in order to prevent these abnormalities. Sodium and potassium can be provided either as acetate or chloride salts. Thus, in the hyperchloremic patient, sodium or potassium should be provided as acetate salts. The acetate anion is converted by the liver into bicarbonate, and this will alkalinize the extracellular fluid. Under normal conditions, approximately two thirds of the anions accompanying sodium and potassium should be provided as chloride and the remainder as acetate.

Vitamins and trace minerals are also essential and important components of nutritional support. Although the exact requirements for vitamins and trace minerals in the critically ill patient have not been defined, it appears that in most patients a daily dose of a mixed vitamin preparation and a mineral preparation will prevent the development of deficiency states. However, because of the importance of some of these substances in supporting the physiologic processes necessary for recovery from critical illness, extra quantities are frequently administered. These substances include vitamin A (necessary for growth, reproduction and immunity); vitamin C (collagen formation and wound healing); zinc (wound healing and nitrogen retention); and selenium (antioxidant properties).

Where? The Route of Nutrient Administration

Key decisions in planning the nutritional care of critically ill patients covered so far include when to begin support, how much to give, and what constitutes an appropriate nutrient mix. It is also important to select the route by which nutritional support will be administered. One must consider whether the patient's nutritional goals can be met with spontaneous oral feedings, or will supplemental enteral feedings, TPN, or a combination of approaches be necessary.

Ideally, patients should meet their nutritional needs through the spontaneous intake of food. This is an appropriate long-term goal for most patients. However, for critically ill patients, there often is a period of time when it is not possible to meet nutritional needs purely through the spontaneous oral intake of nutrients. For those patients who cannot or will not eat sufficient amounts of nutrients to meet their needs, nutritional support should be delivered into the gastrointestinal tract as long as it is functional. Even in the presence of an ileus or gastric paresis, nutritional balance can be maintained by the provision of an elemental diet via a tube placed in the small bowel.[6] Unfortunately, the use of enteral feeding in critically ill patients is often limited by the development of diarrhea. This often is the result of diet-induced alterations in the normal ecology of the bacterial flora as well as the absence of certain complex polysaccharides in the enteral formula, such as pectin. In addition, because of the hypermotility, nutrient absorption is probably limited.

Intravenous feedings have the advantages that they can be administered to virtually any patient and they deliver essential nutrients directly to the systemic circulation. However, intravenous feedings are associated with more metabolic complications than enteral feedings. Additionally, intravenous feedings have unique risks that are associated with the central vein catheters that are required for nutrient delivery, and this is the most expensive form of nutritional support. Furthermore, even though intravenous feedings can be used to support patients who do not have a functioning gastrointestinal tract, they may not provide optimal nourishment for gut recovery, a topic discussed later.

As patients recover from their critical illness and gastrointestinal function returns, enteral nutrition should be instituted and intravenous feedings tapered off. Patients should be encouraged to eat as soon and as much as they are able. In reassessing nutritional requirements, it would be expected that the patient's heightened nutritional requirements would return toward basal values as the patient recovers. However, patients at this point frequently still require increased levels of nutritional support, since they are beginning to replete the lean tissue mass that was lost during the catabolic period of their illness. Additionally, their level of physical activity typically increases as they recover. From a practical point of view, the optimal amount of energy and nitrogen may change little over the course of a patient's convalescence. However, there are some patients who have a long delayed recovery. These patients are often quite debilitated and may require prolonged ventilatory support. Their ability to replete lean tissue and to exercise are limited. In these cases, reduction of the amount of nutritional support may be appropriate to prevent the complications of over-feeding (ventilator dependence and hepatic dysfunction).

Nutrition Support and Organ System Failure

Although many critically ill patients will recover after a period of stabilization, others will develop or present with organ system failure. Adequate nutritional support is particularly important in those high-risk patients to avoid the development of any further metabolic complications. Although appropriate nitrogen and calorie intake must be maintained, the presence of organ system failure may make this goal more difficult to achieve.

Cardiopulmonary Failure

Cardiopulmonary failure poses a serious threat to the patient and may frustrate attempts at nutritional support. Unless tissue oxygen delivery is sufficient to maintain the oxidative processes required for the effective utilization of administered nutrients, wound healing and recovery may not occur. Thus, the maintenance of satisfactory tissue perfusion and oxygen delivery is a primary objective of critical care. The nutritional care of the patient with cardiac failure may be affected by the need for volume restriction. However, since concentrated nutrient mixtures for both enteral and parenteral feedings are available, fluid intake can usually be maintained within an acceptable limit. In addition to nutrients, patients also may receive a large volume of fluids in association with regularly scheduled medications, as well as the administration of blood and blood products. Therefore efforts should generally be made to restrict the intake of fluid from all sources. In many patients, diuretics will be required to maintain the intravascular volume at an acceptable level in the presence of large fluid loads. Reducing the amount of nutritional support in an attempt to limit fluid intake may not be a wise trade-off, since this approach could lead to poor wound healing, impaired host immunity, and other nutritionally related complications that might frustrate recovery.

Respiratory insufficiency and the need for ventilatory support is common in critically ill patients. If ventilatory support is prolonged, pulmonary infections usually develop. Adequate nutritional support is important in maintaining host defenses against pulmonary infections and in promoting recovery from ventilatory insufficiency. However, nutritional support, especially when provided in excess of needs, may contribute to ventilatory failure. Excess carbohydrate intake promotes lipogenesis, which leads to an increase in carbon dioxide production and, hence, to an increase in the minute ventilation required to maintain normal end-tidal carbon dioxide.[13] Provision of hypercaloric glucose-based feedings in critically ill patients not only increases carbon dioxide production, but also increases oxygen consumption and therefore adds to the stress of critical illness.[15] The use of both carbohydrate and fat to provide nonprotein caloric needs and the avoidance of overfeeding minimizes this potential complication of nutritional support.

Renal Failure

Urea and other nitrogenous compounds, as well as potassium, magnesium, phosphate, organic acids, sodium, and water all are excreted by the kidneys. When renal failure develops, the excretion of any or all of these substances is impaired and characteristic syndromes associated with excess amounts and concentrations of these substances may complicate patient care. The planning and provision of nutrition support to patients with renal failure is complex, since the administered nutrients may exacerbate uremia, hypervolemia, and electrolyte and acid-base disorders.

Patients with chronic, stable renal failure may be maintained on low protein diets supplemented by essential amino acids.[46,47] This strategy can assist in the control of uremia and associated symptoms. In contrast, when acute renal failure develops in a critically ill, hypermetabolic patient who continues to have high rates of net protein breakdown, nutritional support with a diet containing normal or increased amount of nitrogen must be provided in an attempt to limit erosion of the lean body mass. In planning nutritional support for the critically ill patient with renal failure, initial energy needs are estimated as previously described. Assessing protein or amino acid needs is somewhat more difficult than assessing energy needs, since excessive protein administration will exacerbate urea formation and uremia, whereas inadequate protein intake will not maintain nitrogen equilibrium.

Because of the renal impairment, there may be significant accumulation of urea in these patients. This accumulation of nitrogen as urea must be accounted for when estimating nitrogen balance. Since urea is distributed throughout the total body water, change in total body urea can be determined from the following formula:

$$\Delta \text{ body urea (g of N/24 hr)} = \Delta \text{BUN (g/dl)} \times 0.6 \times \text{weight (kg)}$$

Nitrogen balance can then be calculated as:

$$\text{N balance (g/day)} = \text{N intake (g/day)} - [\text{N loss (g/day)} + \Delta \text{ body urea}$$

(g of N/24 hr)]

In critically ill patients with renal failure, moderately large quantities of protein must often be given, which contributes to increased urea formation. Hence hypercatabolic patients receiving adequate nutrition support may require frequent hemodialysis, as often as every day. An alternative technique to hemodialysis is continuous arteriovenous hemofiltration (CAVH). In this technique, an arteriovenous connection is established and a hemofilter is placed in the circuit. Arterial blood pressure provides the driving force. An ultrafiltrate is formed that consists of plasma, water, and nonprotein-bound small and middleweight solutes. The ultrafiltrate formed is then drained into a collection bag. Since the total filtration rate may amount to as much as 15 L/day, the filtrate must be replaced, at least in part, with an electrolyte solution in order to prevent hypovolemia from developing. Depending on the total volume of filtrate and on the degree of hypercatabolism and rate of urea formation, CAVH may be able to maintain the BUN in an acceptable range and thereby reduce or eliminate the need for hemodialysis. Thus, since each liter of filtrate formed usually contains high concentrations of urea, a significant amount of urea will be lost through CAVH. For example, if a patient's BUN is 100 mg/dl and 10 L of filtrate is formed with CAVH in a day, then the patient has lost 10 g of urea nitrogen. Bartlett and associates[48] instituted aggressive nutritional support in patients with renal failure and found that CAVH simplified the provision of nutritional support and allowed the patients to be maintained in a positive caloric balance. In this study, the patients supported with nutrition and CAVH appeared to have an improved outcome compared with comparable patients managed with conventional dialysis techniques.

Hepatic Failure

The liver participates extensively in the metabolic response to critical illness. It is the site of glucose synthesis, which proceeds at an accelerated rate in order to support the patient's increased energy needs as well as to provide fuel for the healing wound. In addition to glucose production, the liver must synthesize acute-phase proteins and metabolize exogenously administered drugs and endogenously produced compounds, such as aromatic amino acids and ammonia. Failure of the liver to metabolize these endogenously produced compounds is thought to contribute toward the development of encephalopathy in patients with hepatic failure. To counteract this trend, amino acid formulations for intravenous feedings have been developed, which are high in branched chain amino acids (BCAA) and low in the aromatic amino acids. Studies comparing the effect of nutritional support with these modified amino acid solutions versus dextrose alone or dextrose in combination with oral antibiotics seem to show an improvement in encephalopathy with these special amino acid solutions.[49] However, this advantage is reduced when patients treated with specialized amino acid formulations are compared with patients who receive isonitrogenous and isocaloric feedings.[50] Thus, although some investigators recommend the use of amino acid solutions that are high in BCAA and low in aromatic amino acids in patients with hepatic failure to prevent or reduce encephalopathy, the optimal form of nutritional support for patients with hepatic insufficiency remains controversial.

Future Directions

The approach to nutritional support outlined herein is applicable to all patients. It should result in nutritional support that is as safe and as effective as current technology and understanding of metabolic events allow. There are other effective and safe approaches to the nutritional support of hospitalized patients that differ in some details from the one presented here. No matter which approach is followed, as long as careful attention is paid to the patient's metabolic needs, the complications of malnutrition in the classic sense (inadequate calorie or nitrogen intake) can be avoided in almost all patients. However, despite the availability and use of nutritional support techniques, patients still die with multiple organ system failure and sepsis, apparently related to metabolic exhaustion. Developments along the lines to be discussed may permit improved metabolic and nutritional support in the future.

Altering Responses to Critical Illness

The metabolic responses to critical illness appear to have survival value. For example, young patients are able to mount more intense hypermetabolic responses than elderly persons and have higher survival rates. However, when uncontrolled and prolonged, these metabolic responses are debilitating and may be associated with organ failure and death. Therefore development of therapeutic strategies that reduce the deleterious but not the beneficial aspects of the hypermetabolic response would be of major clinical importance. Since the counterregulatory hormones (epinephrine, glucagon, cortisol) seem to play an important role in mediating many of these hypermetabolic events,[51] several investigators have attempted to modify this neuroendocrine response by adrenergic blockade or regional anesthesia. These manuevers were associated with an improvement in postoperative nitrogen balance and decreased muscle protein breakdown.[52–54] Additionally, in a recent report, the continuous administration or propranolol to burned children reduced cardiac work without adversely affecting mortality, postburn course, or would healing.[55] This technique might eventually benefit elderly critically ill patients with limited cardiovascular reserves.

Endotoxin is a potent stimulus of systemic inflammatory and metabolic responses,[56] and critically ill patients may be exposed to endotoxin from absorption through their wounds or gut, or from the processing of bacteria. Endotoxin appears to exert its effects through the systemic release of tumor necrosis factor (TNF),[57] which in turn leads to a hypermetabolic state that involves the cyclooxygenase pathway. Another cytokine, interleukin-2 (IL-2) which is released from activated lymphocytes, may induce systemic responses that are similar to those caused by endotoxin and TNF.[58] These responses also appear to be mediated in part by cyclooxygenase pathways. However, IL-2 appears to work in concert with gamma-interferon rather than TNF. Thus, studies are needed to determine whether cyclooxygenase inhibitors such as aspirin, indomethacin, acetaminophen, and ibuprofen will attenuate the systemic symptoms and endocrine responses induced by endotoxin and IL-2 without altering beneficial secondary cytokine elaboration or leukocyte proliferation.[59] Although these agents are commonly used clinically on an intermittent dosage schedule to treat patients with high fevers, it is not known whether or not continuous administration of these drugs would significantly reduce the intensity of host systemic responses during critical illness without adversely affecting immunologic function.

Disease or Tissue-Specific Nutrients: Nutritional Pharmacology

The advent of intravenous nutrition techniques has enabled the clinician to assume precise control over nutrient intake. Many investigators have tried to determine nutrient requirements in different disease states and then to design disease-specific nutrition support regimens. Several amino acid formulas are now commercially available as a result of these investigations. There is one for hepatic failure, which is low in the aromatic amino acids and high in BCAA, and another formula, developed for use in renal failure, contains almost exclusively essential amino acids. Use of a renal failure formula is based on an improved survival in patients treated with parenteral nutritional formulas containing essential amino acids.[60] However, more recent data suggest that a renal failure formula has no benefit over amino acid formulas that provide roughly equivalent amounts of essential and nonessential amino acids.[61]

Amino acid solutions enriched with the BCAA leucine, isoleucine, and valine have been developed specifically for hypermetabolic, critically ill patients. The BCAA and their alpha-keto and analogues are thought to be important regulators of skeletal muscle protein metabolism.[62] Therefore it has been proposed that extra quantities of BCAA might attenuate net protein catabolism.[63] Whether or not BCAA are clinically beneficial is not clear, although several clinical studies have been published that support this hypothesis.[64-66] However, other studies are not supportive.[64,65] For example, when intracellular muscle amino acids were measured following injury, BCAA concentrations were greater than normal[67] and they increased still further with infection. Additionally, a clinical study by Bower and colleagues,[68] in surgical patients with sepsis studied over a 10-day period, found only marginal differences in nitrogen balance and a trend toward improved cumulative balance with the BCAA mixture. However, there appeared to be no direct effect on skeletal muscle catabolism and there was no difference in clinical outcome. Thus, although BCAA-enriched solutions can be administered safely to critically ill patients, the biologic benefits reported to date have been small and transitory and no consistent effect on clinical outcome has been demonstrated.

Based on an appreciation that different tissues or organs within the body may have different nutrient requirements, especially during periods of stress or disease, therapeutic nutritional strategies may be developed that are specific for individual tissues or organs. For example, the gastrointestinal tract, once considered to be passive and quiescent during critical illness, may actually play a major role in perpetuating and amplifying the systemic responses to trauma or stress.[69] Since the gastrointestinal tract may serve as a portal of entry for bacteria or their toxins, selective nutritional support of the gut may be important in minimizing the debilitating effects of many disease states. Gut mucosal barrier integrity is maintained in part by luminal bulk and by specific nutrients, such as short chain fatty acids and glutamine. Critically ill patients are typically placed on nasogastric suction and bowel rest, which deprives them of bulk and short chain fatty acids derived from the bacterial fermentation of orally administered polysaccharides. Currently available amino acid solutions do not contain glutamine, because its relative instability in solution would limit the shelf life of the amino acid solutions. Thus, current standard intravenous nutritional therapy effectively starves the gut and thereby may facilitate erosion of the gut mucosal barrier. Further support for the importance of glutamine as an intestinal nutrient comes from animal studies where it was shown that the addition of glutamine to parenteral nutrition formulations, in place of other nonessential amino acids, increased mucosal cellularity of the jejunum, ileum, and colon.[70] In other studies, the addition of glutamine to standard nutrient solutions ameliorated both the toxic effects of methotrexate on the gastrointestinal tract and improved nitrogen balance.[71] Although glutamine is a nonessential amino acid, it is quantitatively the most abundant free intracellular amino acid in skeletal muscle. A variety of studies have suggested that intracellular glutamine concentration may regulate skeletal muscle protein metabolism.[72,73] A decrease in intracellular glutamine concentration is a common response to critical illness. Therefore the addition of glutamine or a stable compound that could be metabolized to glutamine in vivo might not only preserve gastrointestinal integrity, but also reduce net skeletal muscle protein breakdown by maintaining intracellular glutamine concentrations.

Other nutritional manipulations may alter cellular function advantageously. Alexander and coworkers[74] included fish oil as the lipid source in nutritional support of a standard animal burn model. Fish oil is rich in eicosapentaenoic acid which is one of the omega-3 series of lipids. Safflower oil, which is composed chiefly of linoleic acid (an omega-6 series lipid), was used in the control group. The animals receiving the fish oil diets had improved survival and immunologic function. It was proposed that these improvements were related to differences in the prostaglandins and related compounds induced by the differences in precursor fatty acids. In other studies, the amino acid arginine has been found to have a variety of beneficial effects, including improved nitrogen retention, rates of wound healing, and thymotropic activity.[75]

Growth Factors

Another strategy for improving the metabolic support of critically ill patients involves the use of growth factors. Currently, the goal of nutritional therapy is to support the hypermetabolic responses to critical illness by increased nutrient delivery. Yet, this approach of increased feeding may intensify hypermetabolic responses, since rates of synthesis are increased to match the rates of catabolic processes. This is akin to accelerating to top speed in the hopes that this will increase your chances of reaching your destination before the car falls apart. Certain anabolic hormones, such as insulin and growth hormone, or growth factors, such as epidermal growth factor, may be able selectively to promote anabolism without intensifying the hypermetabolic process. Although insulin concentrations are generally increased in critically ill patients receiving nutritional support, additional insulin administration may be beneficial. Inculet and associates[76] reported a clinical study in which they achieved improved nitrogen utilization in postoperative patients receiving TPN by the addition of exogenous insulin. Furthermore, the apparent mild beneficial effects of TPN enriched with BCAAs may be related to increased insulin elaboration induced by this formulation rather than the BCAAs themselves.[68]

Growth hormone is another anabolic hormone that is normally increased following injury and other critical illness. Several years ago, exogenous growth hormone from animal sources was administered to burn patients and led to an increase in nitrogen balance.[77] However, these investigations were not pursued because of the toxicity of the growth hormone preparation. Recently, since recombinant human growth hormone has become available, Manson and Wilmore[78] tested its anabolic effects in intravenously fed normal volunteers. The diets provided an adequate amount of nitrogen but only half of the subjects' estimated caloric requirements. Subjects who received daily doses of growth hormone achieved positive nitrogen balance compared with the control subjects who remained in negative balance. In a recent clinical study Jiang and coworkers[79] preserved lean body mass and function in patients given hypocaloric intravenous feedings and growth hormone following elective gastrectomy or colectomy. Other investigations testing growth hormone in a variety of critically ill patients are currently underway. Preliminary results indicate that growth hormone administration may promote positive nitrogen balance and increase wound healing in these patients as well. If this strategy is shown to be effective, it may accelerate recovery time and obviate the need for hypercaloric feedings with their attendant risks and complications.

Finally, a wide variety of growth factors have been identified that appear to be important in the proliferation of many different cell types. These substances are the focus of several different lines of investigation, which ultimately may lead to clinically useful therapy.

References

1. MacBurney MM, Wilmore DW. Rational decision-making in nutritional care. Surg Clin North Am 1981; 31:571–582.
2. Levenson SM, Seifter E. Starvation: metabolic and physiologic responses. In Fischer JE (ed). Surgical nutrition. Boston: Little, Brown, 1983: 423–478.
3. Daws TA, Consolazio CF, Hilty SL, et al. Evaluation of cardiopulmonary function and work performance in man during caloric restriction. J Appl Physiol 1972; 33: 211–217.
4. Studley HO. Percentage of weight loss: a basic indicator of surgical risk in patients with chronic peptic ulcer. JAMA 1936; 106: 458–460.
5. Wilmore DW, Kinney JM. Panel report on nutritional support of patients with trauma or infection. Am J Clin Nutr 1981; 34: 1213–1222.

6. Moore EE, Jones TN. Benefits of immediate jejunostomy feeding after major abdominal trauma—a prospective, randomized study. J Trauma 1986; 26: 874–881.
7. Askanazi J, Hensle TW, Starker PM, et al. Effect of immediate postoperative nutritional support on length of hospitalization. Ann Surg 1986; 203: 236–239.
8. Buzby GP, Mullen JL. Nutritional assessment. In Rombeau JL, Caldwell MD (eds). Enteral and tube feeding. Philadelphia: WB Saunders, 1984: 127–147.
9. Blackburn GL, Bistrian BR, Maimi BS, et al. Nutritional and metabolic assessment of the hospitalized patient. JPEN 1977; 1: 11–22.
10. Harris JA, Benedict FG. Biometric studies of basal metabolism in man. Publication no. 279. Washington, DC: The Carnegie Institute of Washington, 1919.
11. Fleisch A. Le metabolisme basal standard et sa determination au moyen du "Metabocalculator." Helv Med Acta 1951; 18: 23–44.
12. Turner WW Jr, Ireton CS, Hunt SL, Baxter CR. Predicting energy expenditures in burned patients. J Trauma 1985; 25: 11–16.
13. Askanazi J, Elwyn DH, Silverberg PA, et al. Respiratory distress secondary to a high carbohydrate load: a case report. Surgery 1980; 87: 596–598.
14. Sheldon GF, Peterson SR, Sanders R. Hepatic dysfunction during hyperalimentation. Arch Surg 1978; 113: 504–508.
15. Askanazi J, Carpentier YA, Elwyn DH, et al. Influence of total parenteral nutrition on fuel utilization in injury and sepsis. Ann Surg 1980; 191: 40–46.
16. Curreri PW, Richmond MJ, et al. Dietary requirements of patients with major burns. J Am Diet Assoc 1974; 65: 415–417.
17. McLauren NK, Mason AD Jr, Goodwin CW, et al. Estimating energy requirements of burned patients: a comparative study. In US Army Institute of Surgical Research annual progress report FY 1983, San Antonio, TX: Fort Sam Houston, 1983: 278–290.
18. Ireton-Jones CS, Turner WW Jr. The energy equations: formulae for estimating energy expenditures in hospitalized patients. JPEN 1989; 13: 20S.
19. Swinamer DL, Grale M, Hamilton SM, Roberts P, Kim EG. A predictive equation for assessing energy expenditures in mechanically ventilated critically ill patients. JPEN 1989; 13: 19S.
20. Feurer IN, Mullen JL. Bedside measurement of resting energy expenditure and respiratory quotient via indirect calorimetry. Nutr Clin Prac 1986; 1: 43–49.
21. Branson D, Hurst JD, Davis K, Bower R. Comparison of open circuit and closed circuit methods for measuring oxygen consumption. JPEN 1989; 13: 195.
22. Bessey PQ, Dickenson MR. Estimates of total urinary nitrogen based on urea nitrogen determination. In preparation.
23. Elwyn DH, Bryan-Brown CW, Shoemaker WC. Nutritional aspects of body water dislocations in postoperative and depleted patients. Ann Surg 1975; 182: 76–85.
24. Benedict FJ. A study of prolonged fasting. Publication no. 203, Washington, DC: Carnegie Institute of Washington, 1915; pp 402–403.
25. Duke JH, Jorgensen SB, Broell JR, et al. Contribution of protein to caloric expenditure following injury. Surgery 1970; 68: 168–174.
26. Alexander JW, MacMillan BG, Stinnett JD, Ogle CK, Bozian RC, Fischer JF, Dukes JB, Morris MJ, Krummel R. Beneficial effects of aggressive protein feeding in severely burned children. Ann Surg 1980; 192: 505–517.
27. Border JR, Hassett J, LaDura J, Seibel R, Steinberg S, Mills B, Losi P, Border D. The gut origin septic states in blunt multiple trauma (ISS = 40) in the ICU. Ann Surg 1987; 206: 427–448.
28. Bessey PQ. Nutrition support of the critically ill: how much nitrogen? Surg Forum 1988; 39: 41–44.
29. Heimburger DC, Young VR, Bistrian BR, Ettinger WH, Lipschitz DA, Rudman D. The role of protein in nutrition, with particular reference to the composition and use of enteral feeding formulas. A consensus report. JPEN 1986; 10: 425–430.
30. Cerra FB. Nutritional and metabolic support. In Mattox KL, Moore EE, Feliciano DL (eds). Trauma. Norwalk, CT: Appleton & Lange, 1988; pp 869–877.
31. McDougal WS, Wilmore DW, Pruitt BA Jr. Effect of intravenous isoosmotic nutrient infusions on nitrogen balance in critically ill injured patients. Surg Gynecol Obstet 1977; 145: 408–414.
32. Wene JD, Connor WE, DenBentsen L. The development of essential fatty acid deficiency in healthy men fed fat-free diets intravenously and orally. J Clin Invest 1975; 56: 127–134.
33. Im MJC, Hoopes JE. Energy metabolism in healing skin wounds. J Surg Res 1970; 10: 459–464.
34. Im MJC, Freshwater MF, Hoopes JE. Enzyme activities in granulation tissue: energy for collagen synthesis. J Surg Res 1976; 20: 121–125.
35. Wilmore DW, Mason AD Jr, Pruitt BA Jr. Alterations in glucose kinetics following thermal injury. Surg Forum 1975; 26: 81–83.
36. Wilmore, DW, Goodwin, CW, Aulick, AH, et al. Effect of injury and infection on visceral metabolism and circulation. Ann Surg 1980; 192: 491–504.

37. Shaw JHF, Klein S, Wolfe RR. Assessment of alanine, urea, and glucose kinetics in normal volunteers and severely septic patients using stable isotopic tracers. Surgery 1985; 97: 557–567.
38. Allison SP, Hinton P, Chamberlain MJ. Intravenous glucose-tolerance, insulin, and free fatty acid levels in burned patients. Lancet 1968; 2: 1113–1116.
39. Black PR, Brooks DC, Bessey PQ, et al. Mechanisms of insulin resistance following injury. Ann Surg 1982; 196: 420–435.
40. Brooks DC, Bessey PQ, Black PR, et al. Post-traumatic insulin res stance in uninjured skeletal muscle. J Surg Res 1984; 37: 100–107.
41. Long JM, Wilmore DW, Mason AD Jr, Pruitt BA Jr. Effect of carbohydrate and fat intake on nitrogen excretion during total intravenous feeding. Ann Surg 1977; 185: 417.
42. Wolfe RR, O'Donnell TF Jr, Stone MD, et al. Investigation of factors determining optimal glucose infusion rate in total parenteral nutrition. Metabolism 1980; 29: 892–900.
43. Wolfe RR, Durkot MJ, Allsop JR, Burke JF. Glucose metabolism in severely burned patients. Metabolism 1979; 28: 1031–1039.
44. Nordenstrom J, Carpentier YA, Askanazi J, et al. Metabolic utilization of intravenous fat emulsion during total parenteral nutrition. Ann Surg 1982; 196: 221–231.
45. Goodenough RD, Wolfe RR. Effect of total parenteral nutrition on free fatty acid metabolism in burned patients. JPEN 1983; 8: 357–366.
46. Bergstrom J, Furst P, Noree LU. Treatment of chronic uremic patients with protein-poor diet and oral supply of essential amino acids. I. Nitrogen balance studies. Clin Nephrol 1975; 3: 187–194.
47. Kanpf D, Fischer HC, Kessel M. Efficiency of an unselected protein diet (25 g) with minor oral supply of essential amino acids and keto analogues compared with selective protein diet (40 g) in chronic renal failure. Am J Clin Nutr 1980; 33: 1671–1672.
48. Bartlett RH, Mault JR, Dechert RE, Palmer J, Swartz RD, Port FK. Continuous arteriovenous hemofiltration: Improved survival in surgical acute renal failure. Surgery 1986; 100: 400–405.
49. Cerra FB, Cheung NK, Fischer JE, Kaplowitz N, Schiff ER, Dienstad JL, Bower RH, Mabry CD, Leevy CM, Kiernan T. Disease-specific amino acid infusion (F080) in hepatic encephalopathy: a prospective, randomized, double-blind, controlled trial. JPEN 1985; 9: 288–295.
50. Galloway JR, Hooks, MA, Millikan WJ, Henderson JM, Towns M, Kutner MH, Warren WD. The nutritional effects of F080 versus standard intravenous hyperalimentation in malnourished cirrhotics with subclinical encephalopathy (A23). JPEN 1989; 13: 85.
51. Bessey PQ, Watters JM, Aoki TT, Wilmore DW. Combined hormonal infusion simulates the metabolic response to injury. Ann Surg 1984; 200: 264–281.
52. Tsuji H, Shirasaka C, Asoh T, Uchida I. Effects of epidural administration of local anesthetics or morphine on postoperative nitrogen loss and catabolic hormones. Br J Surg 1987; 74: 421–425.
53. Hulton N, Johnson DJ, Smith RJ, et al. Hormonal blockade modifies post-traumatic protein catabolism. J Surg Res 1985; 39: 310–315.
54. Brandt MR, Fernandes A, Mordhorst R, Kehlet H. Epidural analgesia improves postoperative nitrogen balance. B Med J 1978; 1: 1106–1108.
55. Herndon DN, Barrow RE, Rutan TC, Minifree P, Jahoor F, Wolfe RR. Effect of propranolol administration on hemodynamic and metabolic responses of burned pediatric patients. Ann Surg 1988; 208: 484–492.
56. Revhaug A, Michie HR, Manson JM, et al. Inhibition of cyclooxygenase attenuates the metabolic response to endotoxin in humans. Arch Surg 1988; 123: 162–170.
57. Michie HR, Spriggs DR, Manogue KR, et al. Tumor necrosis factor and endotoxin induce similar metabolic responses in human beings. Surgery 1988; 104: 280–286.
58. Michie HR, Manogue KR, Spriggs DR, et al. Detection of circulating tumor necrosis factor after endotoxin administration. N Engl J Med 1985; 318: 1481–1486.
59. Michie HR, Eberlein TJ, Spriggs DR, Manogue KR, Berami AJ, Wilmore DW. Interleukin-2 initiates metabolic responses associated with critical illness in humans. Ann Surg 1988; 208: 493–503.
60. Abel RM, Beck CH, Abbot WM, et al. Improved survival from acute renal failure after treatment with intravenous essential L-amino acids. N Engl J Med 1973; 288: 695–699.
61. Feinstein EI, Blumenkrantz MJ, Healy M, Koffler A, Silberman H, Massry SG, Kopple JD. Clinical and metabolic responses to parenteral nutrition in acute renal failure. Medicine (Baltimore) 1981; 60: 124–137.
62. Buse MG, Reid SS. Leucine: a possible regulator of protein turnover in muscle. J Clin Invest 1975; 56: 1250–1261.
63. Freund H, Yoshimura N, Lunetta L, et al. Infusion of branched chain amino acids in decreasing muscle catabolism *in vivo*. Surgery 1978; 83: 611–618.
64. Freund H, Hoover HC Jr, Atamian S, et al. Infusion of branched chain amino acids in post-operative patients: anticatabolic properties. Ann Surg 1979; 190: 18–23.

65. Cerra FB, Mazuski J, Chute E, et al. Branched chains support postoperative protein synthesis. Surgery 1982; 92: 192–199.
66. Cerra FB, Mazuski J, Chute E, et al. Branched chain metabolic support: a prospective randomized, double-blind trial in surgical stress. Ann Surg 1984; 199: 286–291.
67. Askanazi J, Carpientier YA, Michelson B, et al. Muscle and plasma amino acids following injury: influence of inter-current infection. Ann Surg 1980; 192: 78–85.
68. Bower RH, Muggia-Sullam M, Vallgren S, et al. Branched chain amino acid-enriched solutions in the septic patient: a randomized, prospective trial. Ann Surg 1986; 203: 13–20.
69. Wilmore DW, Smith RJ, O'Dwyer ST, Jacobs DO, Ziegler TR, Wang X-D. The gut: a central organ after surgical stress. Surgery 1988; 104: 917–923.
70. Hwang TL, O'Dwyer ST, Smith RJ, Wilmore DW. Preservation of the small bowel mucosa using glutamine enriched parenteral nutrition. Surg Forum 1986; 37: 56–58.
71. O'Dwyer ST, Smith RJ, Scott T, Wilmore DW. Glutamine enriched nutrition decreases intestinal injury and increases nitrogen retention. Br J Surg 1987; 74: 1162.
72. Rennie MJ, Hundal HS, Babij P, MacLennan P, Taylor PM, Watt PW. Characteristics of a glutamine carrier in skeletal muscle have important consequences for nitrogen loss in injury, infection and chronic disease. Lancet 1986; 2: 1008.
73. Johnson DJ, Jiang ZM, Colpoys M, Kapadia CR, Smith RJ, Wilmore DW. Branched chain amino acid uptake and muscle free amino acid concentrations predict postoperative muscle nitrogen balance. Ann Surg 1986; 204: 513.
74. Alexander JW, Saito H, Ogle CK, et al. The importance of lipid type in the diet after burn surgery. Ann Surg 1986; 204: 1–8.
75. Barbul A. Arginine biochemistry, physiology, and therapeutic implications. JPEN 1986; 10: 227.
76. Inculet RI, Finley RJ, Duff JH, Pace R, Rose C, Groves AC, Woolf LI. Insulin decreases muscle protein loss after operative trauma in man. Surgery 1986; 99: 752–758.
77. Wilmore DW, Moylan JA Jr, Bristow BF, Mason AD Jr, Pruitt BA Jr. Anabolic effects of growth hormone and high caloric feedings following thermal injury. Surg Gynecol Obstet 1974; 138: 875–884.
78. Manson JM, Wilmore DW. Positive nitrogen balance with human growth hormone and hypocaloric intravenous feeding. Surgery 1986; 100: 188–197.
79. Jiang Z-M, He G-Z, Zhang S-Y, Wang X-R, Yang N-F, Zhu Y, Wilmore DW. Low dose growth hormone and hypocaloric nutrition attenuate the protein catabolic response following major operation. Ann Surg 1989; 210: 513–525.

10

Role of Infection and the Use of Antimicrobial Agents During Multiple System Organ Failure

David L. Dunn

Pathophysiologic Basis of Infection in Relation to Multiple System Organ Failure

We reside in a state of equilibrium with our resident microbial flora. Overt perturbation of this equilibrium occurs when host defenses are disrupted and microbial invasion takes place. In this setting, severe clinical infection and attendant potentially lethal sequelae, such as bacteremia, shock, and multiple system organ failure (MSOF), may occur, providing perhaps the strongest line of evidence of the important role of infection as an etiology of MSOF.[1–11] Interestingly, nearly one third of patients who develop MSOF do not ever have an infectious source identified.[3,6,12–15] The suspicion exists, however, that many cases of MSOF that occur without clinical infection ever discovered may have a similar underlying etiology related to the host inflammatory response.

150

**Table 10–1   Microorganisms Isolated
During Episodes of Gram-Negative
Bacterial Sepsis**

Frequent	*Less Frequent*
Escherichia coli	*Proteus* sp.
Klebsiella sp.	*Providencia* sp.
Enterobacter sp.	*Bacteroides* sp.
Serratia sp.	*Aeromonas* sp.
Pseudomonas aeruginosa	*Citrobacter* sp.
	Acinetobacter sp.

The manner in which infection causes failure of organs separated spatially from the infected site has intrigued investigators for years. Although initially it seemed that blood-borne bacteria or bacterial toxins were responsible, it would appear that more complex interactions probably take place. The triggering and amplification of numerous components of several host mediator systems play an important role, and increasing evidence has accumulated that indicates that MSOF may occur subsequent to such an overexuberant host response. Neither bacteria, bacterial toxins, nor host-mediated events alone can account for all the alterations that occur in host physiology, and thus some composite effect may be responsible. In particular, several groups of investigators have developed experimental models and made clinical observations that make it clear that cellular mediators are released in response to a variety of stimuli, including bacterial products, and that excessive mediator secretion causes target organ damage and failure.[6,16–22] Precise translation of this information to the clinical setting and demonstration of similar pathogenetic mechanisms has been difficult, and a unified sequence of events leading to MSOF has proved to be elusive.

One of the best studied types of infection that often precedes MSOF is that due to gram-negative enteric bacilli. Gram-negative bacterial organisms frequently produce nosocomial infections, which are associated with a significant increase in morbidity and mortality rates. Although respiratory, urinary, and surgical wound infections are common, the highest lethality occurs in patients with gram-negative infections who develop bacteremia due to a large number of serotypically distinct microorganisms (Table 10–1). Lethality of gram-negative bacteremia is significant (10 to 20%) even in previously healthy persons and may exceed 30% in patients with compromised host defenses. A large number of factors predispose persons to gram-negative sepsis. These include underlying disease processes that may lead to varying degrees of global host immunosuppression (surgical procedures, diabetes mellitus, renal or cardiac failure, iatrogenic immunosuppression occurring in transplant patients, or patients undergoing chemotherapy), perturbations in local host defenses (surgical wound, intubation), and alterations in host microflora (inanition, concurrent or prior antimicrobial therapy).[23–29]

Gram-negative bacterial sepsis is frequently accompanied by a wide range of physiologic disturbances, which may include systemic acidosis, arterial hypoxemia, disordered substrate and oxygen utilization, abnormal metabolism, hyperkalemia, hyperglycemia, decreased systemic vascular resistance, elevated cardiac output, and hypotension.[30,31] Activation of the complement and coagulation cascades occurs and has been associated with leukopenia due to polymorphonuclear leukocyte aggregation, macrophage stimulation, and thrombocytopenia.[32–34] Release of cellular products, such as superoxide radicals, lysosomal enzymes, prostaglandins, and monokines, which in excess damage host tissues, appears to follow the initial activation steps.[6,16,35] This portion of the host response, which normally acts to contain and localize infection, may injure the host during systemic infection, leading to the high mortality events of septic shock and MSOF. Isolated pulmonary failure (adult respiratory distress syndrome) is common following systemic sepsis, and gut, hepatic, and renal failure may occur subsequently.[20,36] Many studies have clearly correlated an increase in mortality with an increased number of organs failing during MSOF.[6–8,10,11,13,37]

The diagnosis of systemic sepsis is frequently suspected when the previously mentioned physiologic alterations occur after a known or suspected source of infection is identified, but the diagnosis is truly confirmed only after blood cultures become positive for a specific microorganism. Identification of the presence of gram-negative endotoxin (lipopolysaccharide [LPS]) is problematic at best because available assays such as the limulus lysate test are subject to a great deal of variation.[38] Antibody detection tests for LPS, gram-positive or fungal cell wall components have been examined experimentally and clinically, but most suffer from lack of specificity and are not routinely available.[39] During the time in which a diagnosis of infection is being established, clinical deterioration frequently occurs and therapy must be instituted prior to the availability of confirmatory cultural data.

An abundance of information exists regarding the mechanisms by which gram-negative bacteria interact with mammalian host defenses, and how this may cause organ injury and lethality. The gram-negative cell wall consists of two separate inner and outer membrane bilayers separated by a periplasmic space (Fig. 10–1). The outer membrane contains proteins, lipoproteins, and LPS.[40–42] Administration of isolated LPS to animals reproduces many of the adverse effects on the host that occur during gram-negative bacterial sepsis and MSOF.[43] For this reason, this compound has been intensively examined in an attempt to determine how it exerts its effects on the mammalian host.

LPS consists of repeating O-antigen polysaccharide subunits linked to a polysaccharide core region, which, in turn, is attached to membrane-bound lipid A. The O-antigen polysaccharide subunits are unique for each organism, and thus largely responsible for the wide serotypic diversity seen among strains of even a particular gram-negative bacterial species. The core region of LPS demonstrates a significant degree of structural conservation among genera of gram-negative bacteria and consists of a short series of saccharide residues. The innermost portion of core LPS consists of two to three saccharide residues in most gram-negative bacteria and is thought to be the most highly conserved portion of this region. Lipid A is embedded within the outer membrane and consists of diglucosamine residues associated with nonhydroxylated fatty acids of 12–16 car-

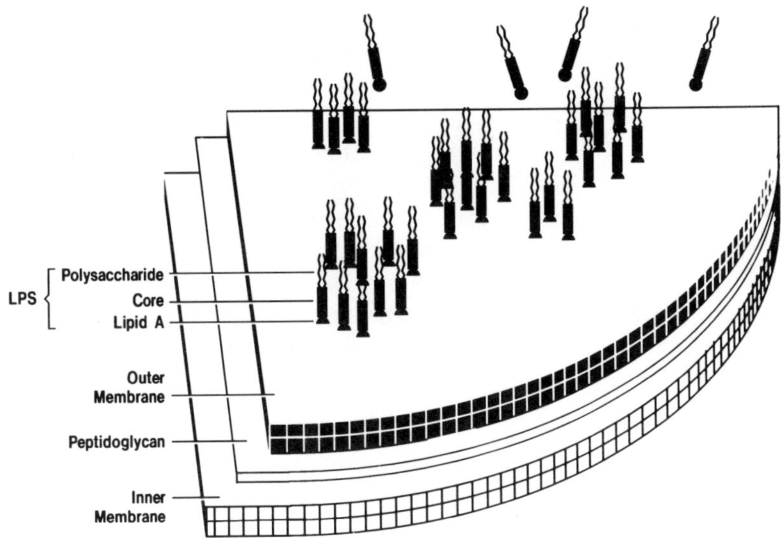

Figure 10–1.   Structure of the gram-negative bacterial cell wall.

bon atom chain length.[44-47] Although relatively insoluble in aqueous solutions, injection of isolated lipid A produces toxicity in a variety of animal models, leading to the hypothesis that the hydrophilic O-antigen solubilizes LPS in the mammalian host milieu, whereas lipid A interacts with lipid components of the host cell membrane.

Immunologic responses to LPS include nonspecific polyclonal B cell proliferation, tolerance to a subsequent LPS or bacterial challenge, as well as production of antibody directed against various portions of the LPS molecule following repeated challenge with either LPS or intact bacteria.[48,49] Physiologic responses similar to those seen during gram-negative bacterial sepsis occur during LPS administration (vide supra) and include hypotension, hypoxemia, acidosis, bacterial translocation across the gut, complement and coagulation cascade activation, white blood cell and platelet margination, and death.[50,51]

It has become increasingly clear that the lethal sequelae that occur during gram-negative bacterial sepsis may be a result of the interaction of LPS with various components of the host immune system. LPS triggers macrophages to release a variety of monokines, including tumor necrosis factor (TNF) and interleukin-1 (IL-1).[52-56] Direct injection of TNF has been shown experimentally to reproduce many of the toxic effects of LPS on the mammalian host. Macrophages isolated from inbred strains of mice that are LPS resistant (C3H/HeJ) do not produce TNF in response to LPS, whereas those from an LPS responder strain (C3H/HeN) exhibit high levels of TNF secretion.[52,53,57] LPS may elicit TNF secretion after the lipid A portion of the LPS molecule imbeds itself within the lipid bilayer of the mammalian cell membrane, triggering a signal for TNF production. Apart from such mediator effects, however, LPS itself may also exert direct toxicity on mammalian cells.[58] LPS-induced toxicity is most probably related to both effects.

Examples of animal models that have been used to mimic clinical gram-negative sepsis include those in which bacterial proliferation occurs and presumed LPS toxicity takes place due to release during bacterial growth or after antibiotic-induced lysis, or in which isolated LPS is administered intravenously, often in combination with a lethality-enhancing substance, such as actinomycin D or galactosamine. No one model completely reproduces the host alterations seen during clinical gram-negative sepsis, and quantitation of LPS release during bacterial growth and after bacteriolysis is extremely difficult. Although the injection of LPS does not exactly reproduce all of the effects of gram-negative bacillary sepsis, the accumulated evidence supports a major role of LPS as the compound responsible for many alterations in host physiology as well as host lethality.

Microbiology and Antimicrobial Therapy of Infection During Multiple System Organ Failure

One of the most difficult therapeutic decisions that the surgeon caring for a patient with rapidly progressive MSOF must make is whether or not to institute therapy with antimicrobial agents. Accumulating evidence suggests that, although many patients with MSOF may initially have an underlying septic source, those initially nonseptic patients frequently may acquire a nosocomial infection while being treated for various aspects of MSOF. The dilemma thus centers around attempts to determine whether or not the patient has a source of infection, and at what point does the evidence provide enough support of this diagnosis, so that it would be imprudent to withhold antimicrobial therapy.

The first step in solving this problem revolves around performing several diagnostic maneuvers in an attempt to obtain concrete microbiologic information (Fig. 10–2). Blood, urine, and sputum should be cultured for potential bacterial pathogens as well as fungi and viruses. A carefully directed diagnostic evaluation based on the patient's current status as well as the past medical history and antecedent illness that led to hospitalization will then further direct evaluation and therapy. For example, routine studies such as the chest and sinus radiographs in a patient who has undergone prolonged intubation for the purpose of mechanical ventilation may identify diffuse pneumonitis, a discrete infiltrate, or sinusitis. Subsequent bronchoscopy or sinus aspiration can then be performed to obtain specific site cultures. Catheter sepsis, surgical wound, and urinary tract infections must also be considered. Although relatively low-frequency events, necrotizing soft tissue infections, tetanus, and toxic shock syndrome may occur in or about the surgical wound, are associated with few if any of the classic signs of wound infection (for example, erythema, pain, fluctuance, drainage) but are frequently associated with signs of septic shock, MSOF, and high lethality.[59–63] A high index of suspicion based on unusual but classic signs allows the surgeon to establish the diagnosis and appropriately treat the infection (Table 10–2). The use of frozen sections of potentially infected tissue to determine the extent of debridement for necrotizing soft tissue infection has also been

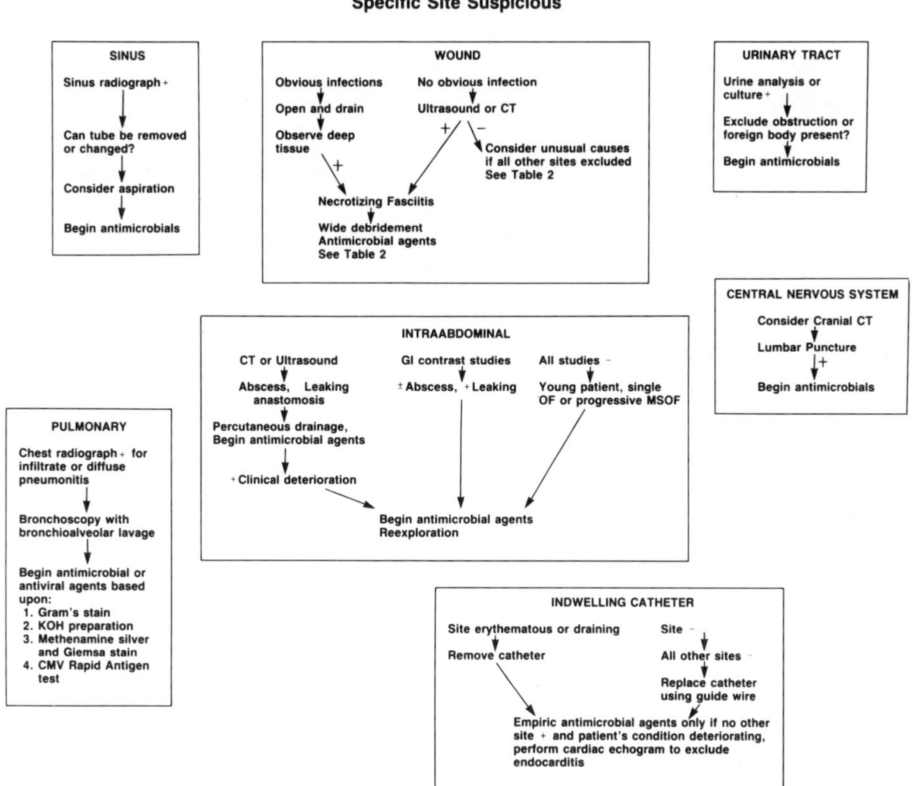

Figure 10–2.   Microbiologic evaluation for suspected sepsis during MSOF.

advocated, but is controversial.[62] Many surgeons debride well beyond the border of infection that is grossly visible at the time of surgery, and rely on planned reexploration to a greater degree.

Patients who have undergone exploratory laparotomy and bowel resection or who have abdominal signs and symptoms obviously should be evaluated for a potential intra-abdominal source of sepsis. An initial flat plate and upright or decubitus roentgenogram of the abdomen may be helpful, but often an ultrasound or a computed tomographic scan of the abdomen should be performed in order to exclude the presence of biliary tract disease or an intra-abdominal abscess. Concomitant administration of gastrointestinal and intravenous contrast (the latter only if renal function is normal) generally enhance the quality of the study, but are not mandatory. Examination of the gastrointestinal tract using water-soluble contrast to ensure that a leaking anastomosis or a perforated viscus is not present may be required. Intra-abdominal fluid collections may be readily diagnosed (more than 85% accuracy) and safely sampled, using a small needle, and may be drained via a percutaneously placed catheter should purulent material be aspirated, or if the initial Gram's stain or potassium hydroxide preparation is positive.[64,65]

Table 10–2   Unusual Soft Tissue Infections Associated with MSOF

Infection	Offending Organisms	Signs	Treatment
Necrotizing soft tissue	Polymicrobial: gram-positive anaerobic cocci, gram-negative aerobic bacilli, gram-positive aerobic cocci, Clostridia sp. (all frequent)	Violacious or bronze skin; blebs; crepitus; thin, grayish drainage	Open wound: computed tomography scan to determine extent of disease. Extensive surgical debridement. Penicillin plus vancomycin plus aminoglycoside plus antianaerobic agent
Tetanus	*Clostridium tetani*	Trismus; opisthotonos; minimal or no wound erythema or drainage	Open wound: tetanus hyperimmune globulin, tetanus toxoid, penicillin
Toxic shock syndrome	Toxic shock syndrome toxin-1-producing *Staphylococcus aureus*	Minimal or no wound erythema or drainage; diffuse epidermal desquamation	Open wound: vancomycin

The presence of a leaking anastomosis or a perforated viscus invariably mandates laparotomy, the rare exception being a delayed, anastomotic dehiscence that is contained and converted into a controlled fistula by percutaneous drainage in a patient who would be subjected to undue morbidity by reexploration. The surgical clinician cannot be lulled into a false sense of security after percutaneous drainage has been performed, and laparotomy must be reconsidered should the patient's condition deteriorate. Cultures can be obtained at the time of percutaneous aspiration or laparotomy and will serve to direct therapy better, perhaps through alterations in the initial empiric antimicrobial regimen. Several investigators have advocated the use of open peritoneal lavage (minilaparotomy) in the setting of suspected intra-abdominal sepsis in which extensive diagnostic tests have failed to document any other source. This is certainly less traumatic for the patient than a formal laparotomy and may serve to establish an intra-abdominal source of sepsis.[66–69] The value of empiric laparotomy during MSOF is controversial, and some investigators have advocated performing this procedure only when clinical signs and symptoms or diagnostic studies have indicated the presence of a potential intra-abdominal source of infection, or in younger patients without a defined intra-abdominal source of infection but with single organ failure or worsening MSOF.[4,5,65,70–75]

Once a potential source of sepsis has been established, every attempt should be made to obtain appropriate specimens from that site for aerobic bacterial, fungal, and viral cultural analysis. Anaerobic cultures of suspected sites of infection should be performed, but areas of the body such as the oropharynx where anaerobes are frequent saprophytes are not often helpful. Gram's stain and potassium hydroxide preparations of body fluid may be useful, serving to

Table 10–3   Organisms Frequently Present in the Gastrointestinal Microflora of Humans*

Site	CFU	Predominant Microorganisms	Examples
Oropharynx		Aerobic: gram-positive cocci	*Staphylococcus aureus, Staphylococcus epidermidis*
		Anaerobic: gram-negative bacilli	Lactobacilli
			Branhamella catarrhalis
		gram-negative cocci, gram-positive cocci	nonhemolytic streptococci
Stomach	$<10^2$	—	—
Upper small intestine	$<10^5$	Facultative: gram-positive cocci, gram-positive bacilli	*Streptococcus fecalis* Lactobacilli
Lower small intestine and colon	10^{11}–10^{12}	Anaerobic: gram-negative bacilli gram-positive bacilli	*Bacteroides fragilis* Lactobacilli, Eubacterium sp.
		Gram-positive cocci	*Peptostreptococcus sp.,* Peptococcus sp.
		Facultative: Gram-positive cocci, Gram-negative bacilli	*Streptococcus fecalis* *Escherichia coli*, Klebsiella sp., Enterobacter sp.
		Yeast	*Candida albicans* and Candida sp.

*From Sommers.[76] Reprinted with permission.

direct initial empiric antimicrobial therapy. Quantitative cultures may be justified in some cases in which aerosensitive or fastidious organisms are involved, and serve to delineate better the degree of infection.

In many cases the patient continues to follow a clinical course compatible with severe sepsis without any source of infection being identified, and a decision must be made whether or not to begin antimicrobial therapy on an empiric basis. At present, there is little definitive information to help the surgical clinician in this regard. No randomized trials have been performed in patients with MSOF, since these patients represent an exceedingly diverse group in terms of underlying disease processes, extent and etiology of MSOF, as well as the pathogens identified. Several lines of reasoning exist, however, which serve to guide initial therapy. Primarily, it has become increasingly apparent that the initial inoculum frequently arises from the indigenous microflora of the host, although environmental sources also exert a significant impact. For the practicing surgeon, the gastrointestinal microflora are thus of frequent concern. Although the oropharynx contains both aerobic and anaerobic microorganisms, the normal stomach and upper small intestine contain few microbes. The lower small intestine and colon, however, contain large numbers of aerobes and anaerobic forms.[76] The latter organisms predominate both in overall diversity and numerical predominance (Table 10–3). Although both types of microorganisms may provide the initial inoculum should perforation of a viscus occur, the anaerobes appear to provide a significant barrier that prevents aerobic gram-negative bacilli from achieving numerical predominance and invading the host, even when no perforation has occurred.

The initial pathogens that predominate during the incipient stages of intra-abdominal infection are facultative gram-negative aerobes such as *Escherichia coli*,

Table 10–4 Comparison of Microorganisms Frequently Encountered During the Initial and Subsequent Stages of Infection Associated with MSOF in Surgical Patients[*†‡]

Initial	*Subsequent*
Escherichia coli	*Staphylococcus epidermidis*
Bacteroides fragilis and Bacteroides sp.	*Candida albicans* and Candida sp.
Enterobacter sp.	*Pseudomonas aeruginosa*
Klebsiella sp.	
Streptococcus fecalis and Streptococcus sp.	
Eubacteria sp.	
Canadida albicans and Candida sp.	

[*]Organisms are listed in order of decreasing frequency.
[†]Secondary bacterial peritonitis was present initially in majority of patients.
[‡]See Marshall et al.,[8] Swenson et al.,[77,79] Stone and Hester,[78] Dunn and Simmons,[80] Brook,[81] and Rotstein et al.[82]

anaerobes such as *Bacteroides fragilis,* and aerobic and anaerobic gram-positive cocci.[77–81] During repeated episodes of intra-abdominal soilage, patients more frequently develop infections due to gram-positive cocci, such as *Staphylococcus epidermidis,* enterococcus, gram-negative organisms, such as *Pseudomonas aeruginosa,* and fungi (primarily Candida sp.).[8,82] Although it seems reasonable to treat gram-positive sepsis with appropriate agents (such as vancomycin), a clear impact on patient mortality has not been demonstrated. These organisms are typically outside the initial spectrum of antimicrobial treatment, and under normal circumstances may be of low pathogenicity. In the patient with MSOF with global immunosuppression due to sepsis, treatment of obviously aggressive single site or multiple site infections, or bacteremia seems rational.[82–88] A comparison of the organisms encountered during initial and persistent intra-abdominal sepsis is shown in Table 10–4. The suspicion exists that these low pathogenicity organisms are, in fact, selected out by the initial prophylactic or treatment antimicrobial regimens.[89]

The treatment of gram-negative bacteremia with antimicrobial agents is well established, and a number of studies have demonstrated a salutary effect when appropriate treatment is begun early in the course of disease. Evidence also exists that empiric antimicrobial therapy directed against gram-negative aerobes may have a salutary effect in febrile, neutropenic patients with hematologic malignancies.[90–93] Other studies, however, have demonstrated that gram-positive microorganisms are also important nosocomial pathogens in this latter group of patients.[94] Both gram-negative and gram-positive facultative aerobes play an important role in the development of nosocomial infections in the surgical intensive care unit, and anaerobic microorganisms are common components of both intra-abdominal and soft tissue infections.[88] For that reason, empiric antimicrobial therapy is often directed against both these two former types of pathogens, and against the latter if a non-nosocomial source is concomitantly suspected.

Controversial issues regarding the use of empiric antimicrobial therapy in this setting concern the use of multiple agent regimens in which each agent is specifically targeted against a specific class of pathogens, versus the use of more broad-spectrum agents (second and third generation cephalosporins, carboxypenicillins, acylampicillins, penicillins plus beta-lactamase inhibitors, monobactams, carbapenems) which may suffer slightly from a lack of individual pathogen specificity, but overall are directed against several groups of pathogens. These broad-spectrum agents are being used more and more commonly as empiric therapy, particularly because they often avoid many of the toxic effects, such as nephrotoxicity, that are present with combined modality regimens. Other broad-spectrum classes of agents remain virtually untested in surgical patients with severe sepsis (such as amdinocillin, spectinomycin analogs such as trospectomycin, and quinolones). Careful selection among all these agents is required based on known spectra of activity.

Several studies have demonstrated single-agent therapy to be equivalent to an aminoglycoside plus an antianaerobic agent (clindamycin or metronidazole) for the treatment of peritoneal contamination due to gangrenous appendicitis or penetrating gastrointestinal injury, as long as the spectrum of activity includes aerobes and anaerobes.[95–106] Extended spectrum agents should not be used for prophylaxis, not when less expensive, more routine agents can be directed against a specific pathogen. They are often ideal for treatment of the patient with MSOF with several pathogenic organisms present, or with a nosocomial infection due to a resistant organism that is within the spectrum of activity of a particular extended spectrum agent and not other antimicrobials (Tables 10–5 and 10–6).

The importance of obtaining initial cultures and sensitivity results prior to embarking on a course of empiric antimicrobial therapy cannot be overemphasized. Once significant pathogens are identified, and their resistance patterns are known, appropriate changes in the initial empiric antimicrobial regimen can be instituted. It should be noted, however, that radical changes in the initial antimicrobial regimen in the setting of obvious clinical improvement may not be warranted. Care must also be taken to select antimicrobial agents based on known activity patterns in a given institution.

A variety of factors influence the action of antimicrobial agents during infection in the mammalian host. Once a specific pathogen is identified, minimal inhibitory concentrations (MIC) may be performed and compared with either measured or known achievable serum levels for a particular antimicrobial agent. It should be noted that the MIC dilution method is performed with a single isolated organism, which is inoculated during log phase into Mueller-Hinton broth containing varying amounts of an antibiotic. After an 18- to 24-hour period, the tube that exhibits no growth is then chosen, and the reciprocal of this dilution is termed the MIC. Determination of serum bactericidal levels may be of use in some cases and involves obtaining the patient's own antibiotic-containing serum to determine inhibitory concentrations against a specific pathogen or series of pathogens. Although this test suffers from many of the aforementioned drawbacks, it may be especially helpful in patients who are being treated with several antimicrobial agents. In general, antimicrobial agents that achieve in excess of

**Table 10–5   Activity of Antimicrobial Agents Used
for Empiric Treatment of Sepsis During MSOF**

Gram-positive cocci
  Vancomycin
  First generation cephalosporin
  Carbapenems
  Ampicillin and acylampicillins (primarily enterococcus)
  Penicillin derivative plus beta-lactamase inhibitor

Gram-negative bacilli
  Second or third generation cephalosporin with or without aminoglycoside
  Carboxypenicillins or acylampicillins with or without aminoglycoside
  Carbapenems
  Monobactams
  Penicillin derivative plus beta-lactamase inhibitor with or without aminoglycoside

Anaerobic gram-negative bacilli
  Clindamycin
  Metronidazole
  Selected second and third generation cephalosporins
  Carbapenems
  Penicillin derivative plus beta-lactamase inhibitor

Fungi
  Amphotericin B
  5-Fluorocytosine
  Ketoconazole and other imidazoles

a four- to eightfold increase over the MIC during the peak serum level have
been demonstrated to be efficacious in experimental animal models of infection
as well as clinical studies.[107–113]

Confounding factors that do not allow direct extrapolation of this microbiologic
information to a specific surgical patient include evidence that: (1) many surgical

**Table 10–6   Potential Antimicrobial Regimens Used for Empiric Treatment of
Polymicrobial Bacterial Infections Occurring During MSOF**

Suspect gram-negative bacilli (facultative plus anaerobic)
  Aminoglycoside plus antianaerobic agent
  Carbapenem
  Selected second and third generation cephalosporins with or without antianaerobic
  agent
  Monobactam plus antianaerobic agent
  Carboxypenicillin or penicillin derivative plus beta-lactamase inhibitor with or
  without antianaerobic agent

Suspect gram-negative bacilli (facultative and anaerobic) plus gram-positive organisms
  Ampicillin or acylampicillin plus aminoglycoside plus antianaerobic agent
  Vancomycin plus aminoglycoside plus antianaerobic agent
  Carbapenem

**Table 10–7 Disparate Host and Microbial Factors that
May Influence Antimicrobial Efficacy and Still Eventuate
in the Eradication of Infection**

Inoculum Size	In vitro Sensitivity	Antimicrobial Tissue Level
Low	Moderate	Adequate
Low	Exquisite	Low
High	Moderate	High
High	Exquisite	Adequate

infections are polymicrobial in nature and may involve synergistic microbial interactions; (2) the initial inoculum size is not known and may in many cases exceed the inoculum size tested in the laboratory (the unstated suspicion being that antimicrobial activity differs, depending on the size of the bacterial inoculum); and (3) the host milieu (pH, blood supply) may affect both the activity as well as penetration of antimicrobial agents. Table 10–7 lists several hypothetical examples in which alterations in host milieu, antimicrobial tissue penetration, and sensitivity determinations all could influence the eventual outcome. Despite these caveats, it is clear that every effort should be made to identify the underlying pathogens involved and to administer antimicrobial agents that effectively achieve tissue levels at the site of infection and that have appropriate efficacy against the specific pathogens identified.

The issue of the efficacy of empiric antifungal and antiviral therapy is also unresolved at present. Many patients with MSOF have a combination of bacterial, fungal, and viral pathogens cultured from various sites. Similar to the problems encountered with bacterial organisms, the first diagnostic dilemma concerns whether or not the fungal or viral organism indeed represents a pathogen. Candida sp. are the most frequent fungal pathogens isolated and are common elements of the host microflora. In general, local, apparently noninvasive candidal infections involving the integument and mucous membranes are treated with oral decontamination and topical antifungal therapy using topical agents such as nystatin.[114] Candida urinary tract infections can be treated with topical amphotericin B as a continuous bladder irrigation.

More difficult decisions concern the use of amphotericin B in patients who have fungal pathogens isolated from several sites. Solomkin et al.[115] demonstrated that those patients with three sites positive, or with peritoneal or blood cultures positive for Candida, fared better if amphotericin B therapy was started early in the course of infection. Thus, an obvious site of infection, such as pneumonitis with a positive fungal culture on bronchoscopy, positive fungal blood cultures, the presence of retinal changes compatible with Candida sepsis, or Candida present within the peritoneal cavity are generally considered indications for a limited course of amphotericin B therapy (300 to 500 mg). This issue, however, remains controversial, and the role of combination therapy with 5-fluorocytosine or therapy with imidazoles, such as miconazole and ketoconazole, remains to be established.[116–122] Infection due to other fungi (Aspergillus sp., Mucor sp., Rhizopus sp.) are less common, but may be seen as invasive infections involving a specific organ or the surgical wound in immunocompromised patients.

The contribution of viral pathogens to MSOF has not been established, although they have been identified with increasing frequency in surgical patients, and severe infection can produce MSOF.[123,124] Herpes group virus (herpes simplex virus [HSV] and cytomegalovirus [CMV]) are the most common pathogens identified and are associated with protean manifestations. Manifestations of CMV may include fever, hepatitis, pancreatitis, pneumonitis, and respiratory failure, retinitis, gastrointestinal ulceration and massive hemorrhage, unrelenting hypotension, associated gram-negative or fungal sepsis, MSOF, and death. Although HSV more frequently presents as a more limited infection of the skin and mucous membranes, infrequently lethal pneumonitis, hepatitis, encephalitis, or gastrointestinal ulceration may occur. Dual HSV and CMV are also associated with higher morbidity than CMV infection alone in renal transplant patients.[125]

Rapid diagnosis of viral pathogens can be accomplished by use of specific monoclonal antibodies directed against viral antigens. This test can be accomplished in 12 to 18 hours. Earlier diagnosis is based on identification of CMV inclusion bodies from a specific site, whereas culture reports or titer increases generally require a longer period of time. The availability and efficacy of antiviral agents such as acyclovir, ganciclovir, and CMV immune globulin with activity against HSV, HSV and CMV, and CMV, respectively, have been demonstrated in several clinical studies.[126–128]

Newer Modalities to Prevent or Treat Infection During Multiple System Organ Failure

It has become increasingly evident that the host intestinal microflora represents a potential source of those organisms that appear as nosocomial pathogens. Prolonged intubation for the purpose of mechanical ventilation is associated with initial oropharyngeal and subsequent gastric colonization with facultative gram-negative aerobic organisms, such as *E. coli, Pseudomonas aeruginosa,* and *Klebsiella pneumoniae.*[129,130] This phenomenon has also been associated with an increased incidence of gram-negative respiratory infections. These same organisms may colonize and proliferate in the distal gastrointestinal tract despite so-called colonization resistance due to anaerobic organisms. Translocation of these organisms and their derived LPS may represent a significant pathogenetic mechanism of MSOF and gram-negative sepsis when disruption of gut barrier function occurs (see Chapter 4).[131–133]

In order to reduce the quantity of aerobic gram-negative bacillary organisms present within the intestinal tract, selective gut decontamination has been attempted. This involves the use of orally administered antimicrobial agents that achieve high intraluminal antimicrobial levels directed against gram-negative aerobes and yeast, while leaving the host anaerobic intestinal microflora relatively undisrupted. Although a reduction in overall infectious episodes has been demonstrated primarily in neutropenic patients with underlying hematologic malignancies, a clear-cut impact on host mortality has not been clearly shown.[134–137] Intravenous antimicrobial agents may disrupt components of the intestinal microflora to varying degrees, and this may factor into the choice of agents during empiric therapy or treatment of a specific source of infection.[138,139]

The treatment of clinical gram-negative bacterial sepsis and shock presently consists of: (1) antimicrobial therapy directed initially against the most likely pathogens or those that are present at obvious sites of tissue infection, and subsequently against those isolates identified from blood cultures; (2) administration of intravenous fluids and hemodynamic monitoring to ensure maximal tissue perfusion; and (3) appropriate alimentation (since the host septic response is catabolic). Although mortality is reduced using these treatment modalities, it remains substantial. Aside from the previously mentioned forms of therapy, several different approaches have been tested either to bind LPS directly or to diminish the deleterious effects of LPS on the mammalian host.

Corticosteroids have been tested extensively in both experimental and clinical sepsis. Their use is particularly appealing due to the hypothesis that they may somehow stabilize lysosomal and cell membranes disrupted by LPS. Although many experimental studies have provided evidence that administration of corticosteroids may reduce septic lethality, in most cases the effect is maximized by steroid treatment prior to the septic insult. Two clinical trials examining the effect of corticosteroid administration during septic shock reached the conclusion that administration of these agents did not reduce septic lethality and may adversely influence outcome in some patients.[140,141] Other antiinflammatory agents have been tested experimentally but have not clearly been found to be efficacious in the treatment of clinical sepsis.[142]

Endogenous opioids (such as beta-endorphin) are released into the cerebral ventricles and systemic circulation in conjunction with endogenous adrenocorticotropic hormone, which promotes corticosteroid secretion during various types of stress and shock, including LPS administration.[143] Many studies have demonstrated the salutary effects of opioid antagonist administration to animals subjected to shock due to a variety of causes, including sepsis. Mortality, however, has not been affected routinely when opioid antagonists are administered without other agents.[142,144,145] Those clinical studies performed to date have not uniformly indicated a successful treatment of septic shock.[146–148] Other opioid antagonists, such as thyrotropin-releasing hormone, may prove to be more efficacious.[149]

Fibronectin, polyclonal and monoclonal antibody preparations directed against the toxic LPS molecule have been administered to patients with sepsis in an effort to enhance both bacterial clearance, bacteriolysis, and host leukocyte phagocytosis. Despite several clinical trials, administration of cryoprecipitate, which contains high levels of fibronectin, has not been clearly demonstrated to be efficacious.[150,151] Antibody directed against O-antigen is serotype specific, has been demonstrated to bind to the intact bacterial cell membrane as well as isolated LPS, and provides potent protection in animal models of gram-negative bacterial sepsis or endotoxemia.[152,153]

Antibody preparations that possess core LPS-lipid A binding specificity have more extensive activity against a variety of gram-negative pathogens but are less protective compared with type-specific antibody preparations. Selected portions of LPS or synthetic lipid A or lipid A precursors have been used in highly selective immunization schemes and for the selection of monoclonal antibodies (MAbs).[154,155] Although specificity to the inner core LPS or lipid A region appears to maximize cross-reactivity,[156-158] not all investigators have been able to demonstrate that these cross-reactive epitopes are invariably expressed on smooth LPS (composed of O-antigen as well as core LPS-lipid A) or intact smooth strain bacteria.[159,160] Western immunoblot analysis has allowed more precise definition of the binding specificity of a variety of MAbs, and the weight of evidence favors an inner core LPS-lipid A epitope as that which will maximize cross-reactivity.[156]

In most animal models, pretreatment with anticore LPS-lipid A antibody preparations serves to optimize protection, although antibody can still exert a protective effect when administered after the onset of the septic insult and can act in concert with antibiotics to reduce lethality.[161-163] The reason why cross-reactive antibody preparations are less potent is probably related both to antigen density and antibody penetration onto the outer membrane. Polymyxin B, a polypeptide antibiotic, also binds to this region but is extremely toxic when administered systemically. Administration of this drug may reduce lethality during experimental gram-negative bacteremia or endotoxemia, but toxicity has largely precluded clinical utility to date, although selective removal using extracorporeal hemofiltration may be possible.[164,165]

The presence of intrinsic anticore LPS-lipid A antibody has been shown to occur in normal persons and may affect outcome during gram-negative sepsis.[166-168] Several studies have demonstrated a reduction in mortality when anti-LPS polyclonal antiserum was administered to patients with sepsis.[169,170] Other studies, however, did not demonstrate anti-LPS antiserum efficacy when the preparation was administered as single-dose prophylaxis to neutropenic patients to prevent septic complications, or demonstrated a decrease in the incidence of septic shock, but not the number of infectious complications in surgical patients.[171,172] Clinical studies using purified cross-reactive, cross-protective monoclonal and polyclonal antibody preparations are currently underway. Experimental studies have demonstrated that treatment with antibody directed against TNF can reduce septic mortality and the use of anti-TNF antibody in clinical trials may substantiate the significance of this mediator during human sepsis.[173]

The use of agents that alter the host intestinal microflora or inhibit the host response toward LPS holds promise, but cannot yet be considered of proved efficacy. The most critical and, as yet, unanswered question is to what degree interventions directed against bacterial proliferation or host-mediator systems can reverse the progression of the septic response after the initial insult has taken place. In all probability the septic insult may take place in a series of discrete events, each of which serves to alter further and activate host defense mechanisms that either directly or through secondary mediator systems damage host tissue and cause MSOF. Interventions that prevent or initially limit the septic insult will probably be the most potent. These interventions may consist of the prophylactic administration of antimicrobial agents or antibody preparations prior to surgical procedures that are associated with a high incidence of infectious complications, early empiric antimicrobial therapy for bacteremia, and perhaps selective gut decontamination. Subsequent, but similar, interventions may serve to decrease the frequency and intensity of the ongoing septic insult. These modalities in combination with newer agents directed specifically against LPS as well as certain host mediator systems may serve to limit morbidity and mortality during MSOF.

Acknowledgment.   I thank Anita Wallace, B.A., for her help in preparing this manuscript.

References

1. Norton L, Moore G, Eiseman B. Liver failure in the postoperative patient; the role of sepsis and immunologic deficiency. Surgery 1975;78:6–13.
2. Baue AE. Multiple, progressive, or sequential systems failure. Arch Surg 1975;110:779–781.
3. Eiseman B, Beart R, Norton L. Multiple organ failure. Surg Gynecol Obstet 1977;144:323–326.
4. Polk HC, Shields CL. Remote organ failure: a valid sign of occult intra-abdominal infection. Surgery 1977;81:310–313.
5. Norton LW. Does drainage of intraabdominal pus reverse multiple organ failure? Am J Surg 1985;149:347–350.
6. Fry DE. Multiple system organ failure. Surg Clin North Am 1988;68:107–122.
7. Fry DE, Pearlstein L, Fulton RL, Polk HC. Multiple system organ failure: the role of uncontrolled infection. Arch Surg 1980;115:136–140.
8. Marshall JC, Christou NV, Horn R, Meakins JL. The microbiology of multiple organ failure: the proximal gastrointestinal tract as an occult reservoir of pathogens. Arch Surg 1988;123:309–315.
9. Bohnen J, Boulanger M, Meakins JL, McLean APH. Prognosis in generalized peritonitis; relation to cause and risk factors. Arch Surg 1983;118:285–290.
10. Fry DE, Garrison RN, Heitsch RC, Calhoun K, Polk HC. Determinants of death in patients with intraabdominal abscess. Surgery 1980;88:517–523.
11. Pine RW, Wertz MJ, Lennard ES, Dellinger EP, Carrico CJ, Minshew BH. Determinants of organ malfunction or death in patients with intra-abdominal sepsis: a discriminant analysis. Arch Surg 1983;118:242–249.
12. Meakins JL, Wicklund B, Forse RA, McLean APH. The surgical intensive care unit: current concepts in infection. Surg Clin North Am 1980;60:117–132.
13. Faist E, Baue AE, Dittmer H, Herberer G. Multiple organ failure in polytrauma patients. J Trauma 1983;23:775–787.
14. Hassett J, Cerra FB, Siegel J, Moyer E, Caruana J, Yu L, Peters D, Border J, McMenamy R. Multiple systems organ failure: mechanisms and therapy. Surg Annu 1982;14:25–72.
15. Machiedo GW, Lo Verme PJ, McGovern PJ, Blackwood JM. Patterns of mortality in a surgical intensive care unit. Surg Gynecol Obstet 1981;152:757–795.
16. Holman RG, Maier RV. Superoxide production by neutrophils in a model of adult respiratory distress syndrome. Arch Surg 1988;123:1491–1495.
17. Trunkey DD. Inflammation and trauma. Arch Surg 1988;123:1517.
18. Pruitt BA. The pathogenesis of multiple organ failure. Arch Surg 1988;123:1518.
19. Nuytinck KS, Offermans XJMW, Kubat K, Goris JA. Whole-body inflammation in trauma patients: an autopsy study. Arch Surg 1988;123:1519–1524.
20. Cerra FB, West M, Keller G, Mazuski J, Simmons RL. Hypermetabolism/organ failure: the role of the activated macrophage as a metabolic regulator. Prog Clin Biol Res 1988;264:27–42.
21. Lubbesmeyer HJ, Kimura R, Maguire JP, Irei M, Traber LD, Traber DL, Herndon DN. Pulmonary microvascular changes following fluid resuscitation in an ovine model of endotoxemia. Arch Surg 1988;123:345–350.
22. Watters JM, Bessey PQ, Dinarello CA, Wolff SM, Wilmore DW. Both inflammatory and endocrine mediators stimulate host responses to sepsis. Arch Surg 1986;121:179–190.
23. Dunn DL. Immunotherapeutic advances in the treatment of gram-negative bacterial sepsis. World J Surg 1987;11:233–240.

24. Dunn DL. Vaccines and antibody immunotherapy in surgical patients. Am J Surg 1987;153:409–416.
25. Dunn DL. Antibody immunotherapy of gram-negative bacterial sepsis. Pharmacotherapy 1987;7:S31–35.
26. Haley RW, Hooton TM, Culver DH, Stanley RC, Emori TG, Hardison CD, Quade D, Shachtman RH, Schaberg DR, Shah BV, Schatz GD. Nosocomial infections in U.S. hospitals, 1975–1976: estimated frequency by selected characteristics of patients. Am J Med 1981;70:947–959.
27. Kreger BE, Craven DE, Carling PC, McCabe WR. Gram-negative bacteremia: III. Reassessment of etiology, epidemiology and ecology in 612 patients. Am J Med 1980;68:332–343.
28. Kreger BE, Craven DE, McCabe WR. Gram-negative bacteremia: IV. Re-evaluation of clinical features and treatment in 612 patients. Am J Med 1980;68:344–355.
29. Bryan CS, Reynolds KL, Brenner ER. Analysis of 1,186 episodes of gram-negative bacteremia in non-university hospitals: the effects of antimicrobial therapy. Rev Infect Dis 1983;5:629–638.
30. Siegel JH, Cerra FB, Coleman B, Giovannini I, Shetye M, Border JR, McMenamy RH. Physiological and metabolic correlations in human sepsis. Surgery 1979;86:163–193.
31. Fry DE, Kaelin CR, Giammara BL, Rink RD. Alterations in oxygen metabolism in experimental bacteremia. Adv Shock Res 1981;6:45–54.
32. Solomkin JS, Cotta LA, Satoh PS, Hurst JM, Nelson RD. Complement activation and clearance in acute illness and injury: evidence for C5a as a cell-directed mediator of the adult respiratory distress syndrome in man. Surgery 1985;97:668–678.
33. Bengtson A, Heideman M. Anaphylatoxin formation in sepsis. Arch Surg 1988;123:645–649.
34. Schirmer WJ, Schirmer JM, Naff GB, Fry DE. Systemic complement activation produces hemodynamic changes characteristic of sepsis. Arch Surg 1988;123:316–321.
35. Border JR. Hypothesis: sepsis, multiple systems organ failure, and the macrophage (Editorial.) Arch Surg 1988;123:285–286.
36. Seidenfeld JJ, Pohl DF, Bell RC, Harris GD, Johanson WG. Incidence, site, and outcome of infections in patients with the adult respiratory distress syndrome. Am Rev Respir Dis 1984;33:242–252.
37. Knaus WA, Draper EA, Wagner DP, Zimmerman JE. Prognosis in acute organ-system failure. Ann Surg 1985;202:685–693.
38. Elin RJ, Robinson RA, Levine AS, Wolff SM. Lack of clinical usefulness of the limulus test in the diagnosis of endotoxemia. N Engl J Med 1975;293:521–524.
39. Gagliardi NC, Nolan JP, Feind DM, DeLissio M. A rapid sensitive monoclonal assay for lipid A in solution. J Immunol Methods 1986;91:243–247.
40. Inouye M. What is the outer membrane? In Inouye M (ed): Bacterial outer membranes: biogenesis and function. New York: John Wiley & Sons, 1979, pp 1–12.
41. Costerton JW, Ingram JM, Cheng KJ. Structure and function of the cell envelope of gram-negative bacteria. Bacteriol Rev 1974;38:87–110.
42. Braun J. Molecular organization of the rigid layer and the cell wall of *Escherichia coli*. J Infect Dis 1973;128:S9–S16.
43. Rietschel ETH, Schade U, Jensen J, Wollenweber HW, Luderitz O, Greisman SG. Bacterial endotoxins: chemical structure, biological activity and role in septicemia. Scand J Infect Dis 1982;31:S8–S21.
44. Luderitz O, Galanos C, Legmann V, Nurminen M, Rietschel ET, Rosenfelder G, Simon M, Westphal O. Lipid A: chemical structure and biological activity. J Infect Dis 1973;128:S17–S29.
45. Schmidt G, Fromme I, Mayer H. Immunochemical studies on core lipopolysaccharides of Enterobacteriaceae of different genera. Eur J Biochem 1970;14:357–366.
46. Luderitz O, Staub AM, Westphal O. Immunochemistry of O and R antigens of Salmonella and related Enterobacteriaceae. Bacteriol Rev 1966;30:192–255.
47. Galanos C, Luderitz O, Rietschel ET, Westphal O. Newer aspects of the chemistry and biology of bacterial lipopolysaccharide with special reference to their lipid A component. Int Rev Biochem 1977;14:239–355.
48. Wannemuehler MJ, Michalek SM, Jirillo E, Williamson SI, Hirasawa M, McGhee JR. LPS regulation of the immune response: Bacteroides endotoxin induces mitogenic, polyclonal, and antibody responses in classical LPS responsive but not C3H/HeJ mice. J Immunol 1984;133:299–305.
49. Morrison DC, Ryan JL. Bacterial endotoxins and host immune responses. Adv Immunol 1979;28:293–450.
50. Morrison DC, Ulevitch RJ. The effects of bacterial endotoxins on host mediation systems. Am J Pathol 1978;93:527–617.
51. Deitch EA, Berg R, Specian R. Endotoxin promotes the translocation of bacteria from the gut. Arch Surg 1987;122:185–190.
52. Beutler B, Cerami A. Cachectin: more than a tumor necrosis factor. N Engl J Med 1987;316:379–385.

53. Old LJ. Tumour necrosis factor: another chapter in the long history of endotoxin. Nature 1987;330:602–603.
54. Dinarello CA. Interleukin-1. Rev Infect Dis 1984;6:51–95.
55. Dinarello CA, Wolff SM. Molecular basis of fever in humans. Am J Med 1982;72:799–819.
56. Dinarello CA, Clowes GHA Jr, Gordon AH, Saravis CA, Wolff SM. Cleavage of human interleukin-1: isolation of a peptide fragment from plasma of febrile humans and activated monocytes. J Immunol 1984;133:1332–1338.
57. Tracey KJ, Beutler B, Lowry SF, Merryweather J, Wolpe S, Milsark IW, Hariri RJ, Fahey III TJ, Zentella A, Albert JD, Shires GT, Cerami A. Shock and tissue injury induced by recombinant human cachectin. Science 1986;234:470–474.
58. Mazuski JE, Platt JL, West MA, Simmons RL, Towle HC, Cerra FB. Direct effects of endotoxin on hepatocytes. Arch Surg 1988;123:340–344.
59. Landercasper J, Miller III CH, Boyer DD. Toxic shock syndrome and multiple-system organ failure after breast biopsy. Surgery 1987;102:96–98.
60. Dornan KJ, Thompson DM, Conn AR, Wittmann BK, Stiver HG, Chow AW. Toxic shock syndrome in the postoperative patient. Surg Gynecol Obstet 1982;154:65–68.
61. Miller JD. The importance of early diagnosis and surgical treatment of necrotizing fasciitis. Surg Gynecol Obstet 1983;157:197–200.
62. Stamenkovic I, Lew PD. Early recognition of potentially fatal necrotizing fasciitis; the use of frozen-section biopsy. N Engl J Med 1984;310:1689–1696.
63. Giuliano A, Lewis F Jr, Hadley K, Blaisdell FW. Bacteriology of necrotizing fasciitis. Am J Surg 1977;134:52–53.
64. Hoogewoud HM, Rubli E, Terrier F, Hassler H. The role of computerized tomography in fever septicemia and multiple system organ failure after laparotomy. Surg Gynecol Obstet 1986;162:539–543.
65. Hinsdale JG, Jaffe BM. Reoperation for intra-abdominal sepsis: indications and results in a modern critical care setting. Ann Surg 1984;191:1:31–36.
66. Hoffman J, Lanng C, Shokouh-Amiri MH. Peritoneal lavage in the diagnosis of acute peritonitis. Am J Surg 1988;155:359–360.
67. Richardson JD, Flint LM, Polk HC. Peritoneal lavage: a useful diagnostic adjunct for peritonitis. Surgery 1983;94:826–829.
68. Barbee CL, Gilsdorf RB. Diagnostic peritoneal lavage in evaluating acute abdominal pain. Ann Surg 1975;181:853–856.
69. Powell DC, Bivins BA, Bell RM. Diagnostic peritoneal lavage. Surg Gynecol Obstet 1982;155:257–264.
70. Hamilton SM. Monitoring and investigation of intra-abdominal sepsis. Can J Surg 1988;31:327–330.
71. Bunt TJ. Non-directed relaparotomy for intra-abdominal sepsis: a futile procedure. Am Surg 1986;52:294–298.
72. Ferraris VA. Exploratory laparotomy for potential abdominal sepsis in patients with multiple organ failure. Arch Surg 1983;118:1130–1133.
73. Harbrecht PJ, Garrison RN, Fry DE. Early urgent relaparostomy. Arch Surg 1984;119:369–374.
74. Pitcher WD, Musher DM. Critical importance of early diagnosis and treatment of intra-abdominal infection. Arch Surg 1982;117:328–333.
75. Sinanon M, Maier RV, Carrico CJ. Laparotomy for intra-abdominal sepsis in patients in an intensive care unit. Arch Surg 1984;119:652–658.
76. Sommers HM. Indigenous microbiota in humans. In Howard RJ, Simmons RL (eds): Surgical infectious diseases, 2nd ed. East Norwalk, CT: Appleton and Lange, 1988, pp 15–22.
77. Swenson RM, Lorber B, Michaelson TC, Spaulding EH. The bacteriology of intra-abdominal infections. Arch Surg 1974;109:398–399.
78. Stone HH, Hester TR Jr. Incisional and peritoneal infection after emergency celiotomy. Ann Surg 1973;177:669–678.
79. Lorber B, Swenson RM. The bacteriology of intra-abdominal infections. Surg Clin North Am 1975;55:1349–1354.
80. Dunn DL, Simmons RL. The role of anaerobic bacteria in intraabdominal infections. Rev Infect Dis 1984;6:S139–S146.
81. Brook I. Bacterial studies of peritoneal cavity and postoperative surgical wound drainage following perforated appendix in children. Ann Surg 1980;192:208–212.
82. Rotstein OD, Pruett TL, Simmons RL. Microbiologic features and treatment of persistent peritonitis in patients in the intensive care unit. Can J Surg 1986;29:247–250.
83. Dougherty SH, Flohr AB, Simmons RL. "Breakthrough" enterococcal bacteremia in surgical patients: 19 cases and a review of the literature. Arch Surg 1983;188:232–238.
84. Garrison RN, Fry DE, Berberich S, Polk HC. Enterococcal bacteremia: clinical implications and determinants of death. Ann Surg 1982;196:43–47.

85. Bryan CS, Reynolds KL, Brown JJ. Mortality associated with enterococcal bacteremia. Surg Gynecol Obstet 1985;160:557–562.
86. Shlaes DM, Levy J, Wolinsky E. Enterococcal bacteremia without endocarditis. Arch Intern Med 1981;141:578–581.
87. Barrall DT, Kenney PR, Slotman GJ, Burchard KW. Enterococcal bacteremia in surgical patients. Arch Surg 1985;120:57–63.
88. Ing AF, McLean AP, Meakins JL. Multiple-organism bacteremia in the surgical intensive care unit: a sign of intraperitoneal sepsis. Surgery 1981;90:779–786.
89. Moellering RC Jr. Enterococcal infections in patients treated with moxalactam. Rev Infect Dis 1982;4:S708–S711.
90. Peterson PK, McGlave P, Ramsay NKC, Rhame F, Goldman AI, Kersey J. Empirical antibacterial therapy in febrile, granulocytopenic bone marrow transplant patients. Antimicrob Agents Chemother 1984;26:136–138.
91. Verhagen C, de Pauw BE, Donnelly JP, Williams KJ, de Witte T, Janssen JTP. Ceftazidime alone for treating *Pseudomonas aeruginosa* septicaemia in neutropenic patients. J Infect 1986;13:125–131.
92. Pizzo PA, Hathorn JW, Hiemenz J, et al. A randomized trial comparing ceftazidime alone with combination antibiotic therapy in cancer patients with fever and neutropenia. N Engl J Med 1986;315:552–558.
93. The EORTC International Antimicrobial Therapy Cooperative Group. Ceftazadime combined with a short or long course of amikacin for impirical therapy of gram-negative bacteremia in cancer patients with granulocytopenia. N Engl J Med 1987;317:1692–1698.
94. Shenep JL, Hughes WT, Roberson PK, Blankenship KR, Baker DK, Meyer WH, Gigliotti F, Sixbey JW, Santana VM, Feldman S, Lott L. Vancomycin, ticarcillin, and amikacin compared with ticarcillin-clavulanate and amikacin in the empirical treatment of febrile, neutropenic children with cancer. N Engl J Med 1988;319:1053–1058.
95. Crenshaw C, Glanges E, Webber C, McReynolds DB. A prospective random study of a single agent versus combination antibiotics as therapy in penetrating injuries of the abdomen. Surg Gynecol Obstet 1983;156:289–294.
96. Nichols RL, Smith JW, Klein DB, Trunkey DD, Cooper RH, Adinolfi MF, Mills J. Risk of infection after penetrating abdominal trauma. N Engl J Med 1984;311:1065–1070.
97. Gentry LO, Feliciano DV, Lea AS, Short HD, Mattox KL, Jordan GL. Perioperative antibiotic therapy for penetrating injuries of the abdomen. Ann Surg 1984;200:561–566.
98. Rowlands BJ, Ericsson CD. Comparative studies of antibiotic therapy after penetrating abdominal trauma. Am J Surg 1984;148:791–795.
99. Fabian TC, Boldreghini SJ. Antibiotics in penetrating abdominal trauma: comparison of ticarcillin plus clavulanic acid with gentamicin plus clindamycin. Am J Med 1985;79:157–160.
100. Jones RC, Thal ER, Johnson NA, Gollihar LN. Evaluation of antibiotic therapy following penetrating abdominal trauma. Ann Surg 1985;201:576–585.
101. Nelson RM, Benitez PR, Newell MA, Wilson RF. Single-antibiotic use for penetrating abdominal trauma. Arch Surg 1986;121:153–156.
102. Hackford AW, Tally FP, Reinhold RB, Barza M, Gorbach SL. Prospective study comparing imipenem-cilastatin with clindamycin and gentamicin for the treatment of serious surgical infections. Arch Surg 1988;123:322–326.
103. Busuttil RW, Davidson RK, Fine M, Tompkins RK. Effect of prophylactic antibiotics in acute nonperforated appendicitis: a prospective, randomized, double-blind clinical study. Ann Surg 1981;194:502–509.
104. Berne TV, Yellin AW, Appleman MD, Heseltine PNR. Antibiotic management of surgically treated gangrenous or perforated appendicitis: comparison of gentamicin and clindamycin versus cefamandole versus cefoperazone. Am J Surg 1982;144:8–13.
105. Baird IM. Multicentered study of cefoperazone for treatment of intraabdominal infections and comparison of cefoperazone with cefamandole and clindamycin plus gentamicin for treatment of appendicitis and peritonitis. Rev Infect Dis 1983;5:S165–S172.
106. Heseltine PNR, Yellin AE, Appleman MD, Gill MA, Chenella FC, Berne TV, Leedom JM. Imipenem therapy for perforated and gangrenous appendicitis. Surg Gynecol Obstet 1986;162:43–48.
107. Guglielmo BJ, Rondondi LC. Comparison of antibiotic activities by using serum bactericidal activity over time. Antimicrob Agents Chemother 1988;32:1511–1514.
108. Reller LB, Stratton CW. Serum dilution test for bactericidal activity. II. Standardization and correlation with antimicrobial assays and susceptibility tests. J Infect Dis 1977;136:196–204.
109. Wolfson JS, Swartz MN. Serum bactericidal activity as a monitor of antibiotic therapy. N Engl J Med 1985;312:968–975.
110. Bryan CS, Marney SR, Alford RH, Bryant RE. Gram-negative bacillary endocarditis: interpretation of the serum bactericidal test. Am J Med 1975;58:209–215.

111. Ellner PD, Neu HC. The inhibitory quotient: a method for interpreting minimum inhibitory concentration data. JAMA 1981;246:1575–1578.
112. Klastersky J, Daneau D, Swings G, Weerts D. Antibacterial activity in serum and urine as a therapeutic guide. J Infect Dis 1974;129:187–193.
113. Washington JA II. Bactericidal tests. In Washington JA II (ed): Laboratory Procedures in Clinical Microbiology. New York: Springer-Verlag, 1981, pp 715–728.
114. Shepp DH, Klosterman A, Siegel MS, Meyers JD. Comparative trial of ketoconazole and nystatin for prevention of fungal infection in neutropenic patients treated in a protective environment. J Infect Dis 1985;152:1257–1263.
115. Solomkin JS, Flohr A, Simmons RL. Candida infections in surgical patients: dose requirements and toxicity of amphotericin B. Ann Surg 1982;195:177–185.
116. Rodrigues RJ, Wolff WI. Fungal septicemia in surgical patients. Ann Surg 1974;180:741–746.
117. Meunier-Carpentier Francoise, Kiehn TE, Armstrong D. Fungemia in the immunocompromised host: changing patterns, antigenemia, high mortality. Am J Med 1981;71:363–370.
118. Dyess DL, Garrison RN, Fry DE. *Candida* sepsis: implications of polymicrobial blood-borne infection. Arch Surg 1985;120:345–348.
119. Spebar MJ, Pruitt BA. Candidiasis in the burned patient. J Trauma 1981;21:237–239.
120. Bodey GP. Candidiasis in cancer patients. Am J Med 1984;13–19.
121. Stone HH, Kolb LK, Currie CA, Geheber CE, Cuzzell JZ. Candida sepsis: pathogenesis and principles of treatment. Ann Surg 1974;179:697–711.
122. March PK, Tally FP, Kellum J, Callow A, Gorbach SL. Candida infections in surgical patients. Ann Surg 1983;198:42–47.
123. Simmons RL, Matas AJ, Rattazzi LC, Balfour HH Jr, Howard RJ, Najarian JS. Clinical characteristics of the lethal cytomegalovirus infection following renal transplantation. Surgery 1977;82:537–545.
124. Deutschman CS, Konstantinides FN, Tsai M, Simmons RL, Cerra FB. Physiology and metabolism in isolated viral septicemia: further evidence of an organism-dependent, host-dependent response. Arch Surg 1987;122:21–25.
125. Dunn DL, Matas AJ, Fryd DS, Simmons RL, Najarian JS. Association of concurrent herpes simplex virus and cytomegalovirus with detrimental effects after renal transplantation. Arch Surg 1984;119:812–817.
126. Meyers JD, Reed EC, Shepp DH, Thornquist M, Dandliker PS, Vicary CA, Flournoy N, Kirk LE, Kersey JH, Thomas ED, Balfour HH. Acyclovir for prevention of cytomegalovirus infection and disease after allogeneic marrow transplantation. N Engl J Med 1988;318:70–75.
127. Fischel RJ, Freise CE, Bonser RS, Hertz MI, Jamieson SW, Dunn DL. Successful management of fulminant cytomegalovirus induced acute lung injury following double lung transplantation. Clin Transplant 1988;2:331–335.
128. Snydman DR, et al. Use of cytomegalovirus immune globulin to prevent cytomegalovirus disease in renal-transplant recipients. N Engl J Med 1987;317:1049–1054.
129. Atherton ST, White DJ. Stomach as source of bacteria colonising respiratory tract during artificial ventilation. Lancet 1978;2:968–969.
130. Border JR, Hassett J, LaDuca J, Seibel R, Steinberg S, Mills B, Losi P, Border D. The gut origin septic states in blunt multiple trauma (ISS = 40) in the ICU. Ann Surg 1987;206:427–448.
131. O'Dwyer ST, Michie HR, Ziegler TR, Revhaug A, Smith RJ, Wilmore DW. A single dose of endotoxin increases intestinal permeability in healthy humans. Arch Surg 1988;123:1459–1464.
132. Deitch EA, Maejima K, Berg R. Effect of oral antibiotics and bacterial overgrowth on the translocation of the GI tract microflora in burned rats. J Trauma 1985;25:385–392.
133. Maejima K, Deitch EA, Berg R. Promotion by burn stress of the translocation of bacteria from the gastrointestinal tract of mice. Arch Surg 1984;119:166–172.
134. Storring RA, McElwain TJ, Jameson B, Wiltshaw E. Oral nonabsorbed antibiotics prevent infection in acute nonlymphoblastic leukemia. Lancet 1977;32:837–840.
135. Aerdts SJA, van Dalen R, Clasener HAL, Vollaard EJ. Prophylaxis of infection by selective decontamination in mechanically ventilated patients. A preliminary report. Drugs 1988;35:97–99.
136. van Saene HKF, Stoutenbeek CP, Zandstra DF. Cefotaxime combined with selective decontamination in long term intensive care unit patients: virtual absence of emergence of resistance. Drugs 1988;35:29–34.
137. Clasener HAL, Vollaard EJ, van Saene HKF. Long-term prophylaxis of infection by selective decontamination in leukopenia and in mechanical ventilation. Rev Infect Dis 1987;9:295–328.
138. Michea-Hamzehpour M, Auckenthaler R, Kunz J, Pechere JC. Effect of a single dose of cefotaxime or ceftriaxone on human faecal flora: a double blind study. Drugs 1988;35:6–11.
139. Nord CE, Heimdahl A, Kager L, Malmborg AS. The impact of different antimicrobial agents on the normal gastrointestinal microflora of humans. Rev Infect Dis 1984;6:S270–S275.
140. Bone RC, Fisher CJ Jr, Clemmer TP, Slotman GJ, Metz CA, Balk RA, and the Methylpredni-

solone Severe Sepsis Study Group. A controlled clinical trial of high-dose methylprednisolone in the treatment of severe sepsis and septic shock. N Engl J Med 1987;317:653–658.

141. The Veterans Administration Systemic Sepsis Cooperative Study Group. Effect of high-dose glucocorticoid therapy on mortality in patients with clinical signs of systemic sepsis. N Engl J Med 1987;317:659–665.

142. Long WM, Sprung CL. Corticosteroids, nonsteroidal anti-inflammatory drugs, and naloxone in the sepsis syndrome. World J Surg 1987;11:218–225.

143. Carmody JJ. Opiate receptors: an introduction. Anaesth Intensive Care 1987;15:27–37.

144. Hinshaw LB, Beller BK, Chang ACK, Flournoy DJ, Lahti RA, Passey RB, Archer LT. Evaluation of naloxone for therapy of *Escherichia coli* shock. Arch Surg 1984;119:1410–1418.

145. Hinshaw LB, Archer LT, Beller BK, Chang ACK, Flournoy DJ, Passey RB, Long JB, Holaday JW. Evaluation of naloxone therapy for *Escherichia coli* sepsis in the baboon. Arch Surg 1988;123:700–704.

146. Rock P, Silverman H, Plump D, Kecala Z, Smith P, Michael FR, Summer W. Efficacy and safety of naloxone in septic shock. Crit Care Med 1985;13:28–33.

147. Allolio B, Fischer H, Kaulen D, Deub U, Winkelmann W. Naloxone in treatment of circulatory shock resistant to conventional therapy. Klin Wochenschr 1987;65:213–217.

148. DeMaria A, Heffernan JJ, Grindlinger GA, Craven DE, McIntosh TK, McCabe WR. Naloxone versus placebo in treatment of septic shock. Lancet 1985;1:1363–1365.

149. Teba L, Zakaria M, Dedhia HV, Schiebel F, Beamer KC. Beneficial effect of thyrotropin-releasing hormone in canine hemorrhagic shock. Circ Shock 1987;21:51–57.

150. Todd TR, Glynn MFX, Silver E, et al. A randomized trial of cryoprecipitate replacement of fibronectin deficiencies in the critically ill. Am Rev Respir Dis 1984;129:102.

151. Saba TM, Kiener JL, Holman JM Jr. Fibronectin and the critically ill patient: current status. Intensive Care Med 1986;12:350–358.

152. Dunn DL, Ewald DC, Chandan N, Cerra FB. Immunotherapy of gram-negative bacterial sepsis: a single murine monoclonal antibody provides cross-genera protection. Arch Surg 1986;121:58–62.

153. Dunn DL. Antibody immunotherapy of gram-negative bacterial sepsis in an immunosuppressed animal model. Transplantation 1988;45:424–429.

154. Brade L, Kosma P, Appelmelk BJ, Paulsen H, Brade H. Use of synthetic antigens to determine the epitope specificities of monoclonal antibodies against the 3-deoxy-D-manno-octulosonate region of bacterial lipopolysaccharide. Infect Immun 1987;55:462–466.

155. Rietschel Et, Brade L, Brandenburg K, Flad HD, de Jong-Leuveninck J, Kawahara K, Lindner B, Loppnow H, Luderitz T, Schade U, Seydel U, Sidorczyk Z, Tacken A, Zahringer U, Brade H. Chemical structure and biologic activity of bacterial and synthetic lipid A. Rev Infect Dis 1987;9:S527–S536.

156. Bogard WC, Dunn DL, Abernethy KC, Kilgarriff C, Kung PC. Isolation and characterization of murine monoclonal antibodies specific for gram-negative bacterial lipopolysaccharide: association of cross-genus reactivity with lipid A specificity. Infect Immun 1987;55:899–908.

157. Pollack M, Raubitschek AA, Larrick JW. Human monoclonal antibodies that recognize conserved epitopes in the core in the core-lipid A region of lipopolysaccharides. J Clin Invest 1987;79:1421–1430.

158. Baumgartner JD, O'Brien TX, Kirkland TN, Glauser MP, Ziegler EJ. Demonstration of cross-reactive antibodies to smooth gram-negative bacteria in antiserum to *Escherichia coli* J5. J Infect Dis 1987;156:136–143.

159. McCallus DE, Norcross NL. Antibody specific for *Escherichia coli* J5 cross-reacts to various degrees with an *Escherichia coli* clinical isolate grown for different lengths of time. Infect Immun 1987;55:1042–1046.

160. Shenep JL, Gigliotti F, Davis DS, Hildner WK. Reactivity of antibodies to core glycolipid with gram-negative bacteria. Rev Infect Dis 1987;9:S639–S643.

161. Appelmelk BJ, Verwey-Van Vught AMJJ, Maaskant JJ, Schouten WF, Thijs LG, Maclaren DM. Use of mucin and hemoglobin in experimental murine gram-negative bacteremia enhances the immunoprotective action of antibodies reactive with the lipopolysaccharide core region. Antonie Van Leeuwenhoek 1986;52:537–542.

162. Dunn DL, Bogard WC, Cerra FB. Efficacy of type-specific and cross-reactive murine monoclonal antibodies directed against endotoxin during experimental sepsis. Surgery 1985;98:283–289.

163. Dunn DL, Dunn DL, Priest BP, Condie RM. Protective capacity of polyclonal and monoclonal antibodies directed against endotoxin during experimental sepsis. Arch Surg 1988;123:1389–1393.

164. Flynn PM, Shenep JL, Stokes DC, Fairclough D, Hildner WK. Polymyxin B moderates acidosis and hypotension in established, experimental gram-negative septicemia. J Infect Dis 1987;156:706–712.

165. Hanasawa K, Tani T, Oka T, Yoshioka T, Aoki H, Endo Y, Kodama M. Selective removal of

endotoxin from the blood by extracorporeal hemoperfusion with polymyxin B immobilized fiber. Perspect Shock Res 1988;264:337–341.

166. Law BJ, Marks MI. Age-related prevalence of human serum IgG and IgM antibody to the core glycolipid of *Escherichia coli* strain J5, as measured by ELISA. J Infect Dis 1985;151:988–994.
167. Fomsgaard A, Dinesen B, Baek L. Anti-lipopolysaccharide antibodies measured by enzyme-immunoassay in Danish blood donors. Acta Pathol Microbiol Immunol Scand 1987;95:9–13.
168. Nys M, Damas P, Joassin L, Demonty J. A direct enzyme-linked immunosorbent assay (ELISA) for antibodies to enterobacterial Re core glycolipid and lipid A: results in healthy subjects and in patients infected by gram-negative bacteria. Med Microbiol Immunol (Berl) 1987;176:257–271.
169. Ziegler EJ, McCutchan JA, Fierer J, Galuser MP, Sadoff JC, Douglas H, Braude AI. Treatment of gram-negative bacteremia and shock with human antiserum to a mutant *Escherichia coli*. N Engl J Med 1982;307:1225–1230.
170. Lachman E, Pitsoe SB, Gaffin SL. Anti-lipopolysaccharide immunotherapy in management of septic shock of obstetric and gynaecological origin. Lancet 1984;1:981–983.
171. McCutchan JA, Wolf JL, Ziegler EJ, Braude AI. Ineffectiveness of single-dose human anti-serum to core glycolipid (*E. coli* J5) for prophylaxis of bacteremic, gram-negative infections in patients with prolonged neutropenia. Schweiz Med Wochenschr 1983;113S:40–45.
172. Baumgartner JD, McCutchan JA, Van Melle G, Vogt M, Luethy R, Glauser MP, Ziegler EJ, Klauber MR, Muehlen E, Chiolero R, Geroulanos S. Prevention of gram-negative shock and death in surgical patients by antibody to endotoxin core glycolipid. Lancet 1985;2:59–63.
173. Beutler B, Milsark IW, Cerami AC. Passive immunization against cachectin/tumor necrosis factor protects mice from lethal effect of endotoxin. Science 1985;229:869–871.

11

Cardiovascular Dysfunction in Multiple Organ Failure

STEVEN A. CONRAD, JEROME L. FINKELSTEIN, MICHAEL R. MADDEN, JILL BURK, AND CLEON W. GOODWIN

Early clinical studies of sepsis and extensive trauma identified the hyperdynamic cardiovascular state that frequently accompanies these conditions. It was generally thought that the cardiovascular system played a passive role and was not adversely affected because it was able to achieve a hyperdynamic state. We now know that the cardiovascular system plays a pivotal role in the pathogenesis of sepsis, the response to major trauma, and the subsequent multiple organ failure syndrome. It is both a target organ system in the systemic response to trauma and sepsis, and its failure plays a major role in the pathogenesis of multiple organ failure.

The major function of the cardiovascular system is the delivery of oxygen to peripheral tissues. Oxygen is the most flow-dependent of the substances carried by the blood, and lack of it rapidly results in cellular dysfunction. From this concept emerges the rather simplistic definition of cardiovascular failure as a

172

failure to provide sufficient delivery of oxygen to tissues. The mechanisms of this failure, however, are complex. This review will present the determinants of cardiovascular function, specifics on cardiovascular dysfunction in trauma and sepsis, and an approach to treatment of this dysfunction with the goal of prevention of multiple organ failure. It should be recognized that the clinical presentation of sepsis, the systemic responses to major trauma and operation, and the presentation of multiple organ failure syndrome (MOFS) of any etiology are essentially indistinguishable. In large part, the pathogenetic mechanisms underlying the development of the clinical picture of these three states are similar. Sepsis is by far the major cause of or contributor to MOFS. Therefore the term "MOFS" or sepsis/MOFS will be used to refer collectively to the presentations of this syndrome.

Regulation of Normal Cardiovascular Function

Regulation of the contractile function of the heart was first investigated systematically by Frank[1] and by Starling et al.[2] around the turn of the century. The concepts of Starling's Law as the major determinant of stroke output persisted unquestioned until relatively recently, when the interactions of a number of cardiac and extracardiac factors have been further characterized. We now know that ventricular preload, afterload, compliance, geometry, interventricular dependence, and neurohumoral factors interact in a rather complex fashion to determine cardiovascular function in health and disease.

Left Ventricular Function

The major determinants of stroke output include: (1) the intrinsic level of myocardial contractility; (2) end-diastolic volume, or preload; and (3) the level of tension developed during ejection, or afterload. Heart rate, in addition to stroke output, determines the minute cardiac output. These three major determinants are individually influenced by several factors (Table 11–1), each of which must be considered when evaluating cardiac function.

MYOCARDIAL CONTRACTILITY

The intrinsic contractility for a given preload and afterload is affected by a host of factors. Ischemia, electrolyte and acid-base disturbances, adrenergic state, and the presence of myocardial depressant factors can affect this intrinsic contractility. Contractility is a difficult parameter to assess. One of the best hemodynamic measurements used to assess contractility in the catheterization laboratory is the maximal instantaneous rate of change of pressure with time (dP/dt_{max}), but even this measurement is not totally independent of preload and afterload. At the bedside, one must rely on more crude measurements, such as stroke volume, stroke work, and ejection fraction, while taking into consideration the state of preload and afterload.

Table 11–1   Determinants of Myocardial Function

Myocardial contractility	Sympathetic stimulation
	Circulating catecholamines
	Heart rate (Bowditch phenomenon)
	Afterload (Anret effect)
	Calcium availability
	Myocardial ischemia/hypoxia
	Myocardial edema/inflammation
	Myocardial depressants
Preload	Venous return
	Intravascular volume
	Venous capacitance
	Intrathoracic pressure
	Ventricular compliance
	Ventricular geometry
Afterload	Arteriolar tone
	Microvascular resistance
	Adrenergic tone
	Adrenergic receptor density
	Vasoactive mediators
	Ventricular size
	Ventricular wall thickness
	Intraventricular pressure
	Valvular dysfunction

VENTRICULAR PRELOAD

Perhaps the best definition of preload is end-diastolic myocardial fiber length. Isolated muscle preparations demonstrate a relationship between fiber length and force of myocardial contraction. In the intact heart, however, preload may best be described as ventricular end-diastolic volume. An increase in end-diastolic volume, even on a beat to beat basis, results in an increased force of contraction, and hence an increased stroke volume. Pressure required to distend the ventricle is related to the end-diastolic volume by ventricular compliance. Since bedside measurement of intracardiac pressures is easier than that of ventricular volume, end-diastolic volume is inferred in the clinical setting by end-diastolic pressure. However, a number of factors can alter compliance, reducing the usefulness of pressure measurements for assessing preload. Nonetheless, it is a readily available and clinically relevant measurement.

Alterations in compliance are common in critically ill patients. Myocardial ischemia and acute or remote infarction can reduce compliance. Ventricular hypertrophy from chronic hypertension or hypertrophic cardiomyopathy also decreases compliance. Cardiomyopathies of various causes can either increase or decrease compliance.

Preload is also affected by the relationship between intravascular volume and vascular capacitance either one of which can be altered in critical illness. Pericardial disease or increases in intrathoracic pressure from positive pressure ventilation can also adversely affect preload through reduction of venous return and limitation of diastolic filling.

An interdependence exists between preload and afterload. Marked increases in afterload, especially in the presence of diminished myocardial contractility, can reduce stroke output unless preload can be increased to compensate. Significant reductions in afterload can result in a decrease in preload and subsequently stroke output.

VENTRICULAR AFTERLOAD

Afterload is more a concept than a clinical entity, and is perhaps best thought of as the amount of ventricular wall stress developed during contraction. Stroke volume is inversely related to afterload, particularly at supranormal levels of afterload and in the compromised ventricle. In the normal ventricle operating at normal preload and afterload, changes in afterload have little effect on stroke output. The physiologic response to an increase in afterload is to increase preload (end-diastolic volume), so that stroke volume remains constant in the presence of a decreased ejection fraction. Since the function of the compromised ventricle can be markedly affected by afterload, maintenance of an appropriate afterload may be crucial for optimal ventricular performance.

Right Ventricular Function

The right ventricle differs from the left in several ways that deserve special consideration. The chamber is crescent shaped and "wrapped around" the left ventricle, since the septum normally functions more as a part of the left ventricle. Because of this configuration, less fiber shortening is required for ventricular ejection. The right ventricle normally functions as a low-pressure, high-volume pump, in contrast to the high-pressure conditions of the left ventricle. In the absence of adaptation, it is not capable of generating high ejection pressures and therefore is highly susceptible to increases in afterload. Normally, the pulmonary vasculature has the capacity to accommodate increased flows without increased pulmonary artery pressures; thus the right ventricle normally does not become exposed to high afterload, even with exercise. With pathologic increases in afterload, the right ventricle is more dependent on preload than the left. The thin walls and geometry of the right ventricle also permit ventricular dilation more readily, and hence preload augmentation.

Cardiovascular Dysfunction in Sepsis/Multiple Organ Failure

The initial response to sepsis and extensive tissue injury is an increased cardiac output, decreased systemic vascular resistance, and normal or mildly decreased blood pressure. Despite the absence of clinical evidence of cardiovascular depression, abnormalities in myocardial contractility, intravascular volume, and vascular function are present. As these abnormalities progress, clinical presentation of cardiovascular failure becomes manifest.

Left Ventricular Dysfunction

Sepsis and MOFS adversely affect ventricular dysfunction through changes in preload and afterload in addition to effects on myocardial contractility.

REDUCTION IN MYOCARDIAL CONTRACTILITY

Myocardial contractility is depressed in sepsis and multiple organ failure. The mechanisms have not been fully elucidated. A circulating myocardial depressant factor or factors have been demonstrated in the serum of patients with sepsis,[3] but this finding is not universal.[4] The ventricle dilates and end-diastolic volume and ventricular compliance are increased. Ejection fraction is decreased and stroke volume decreases even in the presence of an increased preload. These alterations in ventricular performance are usually transient, reversing with recovery from sepsis and MOFS.

Myocardial ischemia may contribute to myocardial depression, but its role is not clear. Although overall myocardial blood flow and oxygen delivery is increased,[5] regional dysfunction has been identified,[6] and patchy areas of necrosis have been identified.[7]

REDUCTION IN PRELOAD

Left ventricular (LV) preload is frequently reduced in the patient with sepsis or multiple organ failure for several reasons. A reduction in circulating blood volume may result from hemorrhage or transudation of fluid into the extracellular interstitial space. A reduction in diastolic filling can result from increases in venous capacitance and decreases in venous return, reduction in right ventricular (RV) output from pulmonary hypertension,[8] and possibly alteration of LV geometry from RV overload.

Right Ventricular Dysfunction

The role of the right ventricle as an important determinant of cardiac performance has been fully appreciated only recently.[9] RV dysfunction is not easily recognized, but can contribute to poor LV performance through reduction in LV preload.

The principal causes of acute RV failure seen in multiple organ failure are depression of myocardial contractility and acute increases in afterload. Causes of depression in contractility parallel those of the left ventricle, with myocardial depressant substances and myocardial ischemia playing major roles. Increased RV afterload is probably the major cause of RV dysfunction. Increased pulmonary vascular resistance is common in MOFS, due to pulmonary vascular changes of multiple organ failure, acute respiratory distress syndrome, hypoxia-induced pulmonary vasoconstriction, vasoconstrictor drugs, and pulmonary emboli. Positive pressure ventilation is a major contributor and will be discussed in more detail later. RV volume overload also plays a role in RV dysfunction, resulting from valvular insufficiencies, septal defects, or fluid overloading during resuscitation.

Bedside Evaluation of Ventricular Function

A number of methods for assessing ventricular function are available, but those that can be performed at the bedside are somewhat limited. The availability of arterial and pulmonary artery catheterization has been a major advance in the management of cardiovascular dysfunction in the critically ill and will be discussed in more detail later. Noninvasive methods can provide additional information.

Radionuclide angiography using portable data acquisition equipment enables measurement of RV and LV ejection fractions. Combined with measurement of stroke volume from thermodilution cardiac output, ventricular volumes can be calculated. The best clinical measurements to assess ventricular contractility include ejection fraction and end-diastolic volume, and the response to therapy is easily determined.

Two-dimensional and Doppler echocardiography are very useful and quite easily performed in the critical care unit. Estimates of ventricular volumes, regional and global myocardial contractility, valvular function, and even cardiac output can be determined noninvasively. Transesophageal Doppler systems are available for continuous cardiac output measurement.

Microvascular Dysfunction

MOFS is characterized by an impairment of microcirculatory function resulting in a mismatch of oxygen supply and demand at the tissue level. Despite the development of a hyperdynamic state, oxygen utilization is reduced. The microcirculation is characterized by increased permeability, heterogenous vasoconstriction and vasodilation, and vasomotor instability. The mechanism of microcirculatory dysfunction is not clear, but endotoxin appears to play an initiating role. Activated granulocytes and monocytes also contribute. A full discussion of microvascular function and the pathogenesis of microvascular failure is given in Chapter 7.

One of the characteristics of the microvascular dysfunction of sepsis and MOFS is impaired oxygen utilization, even when systemic oxygen delivery is above normal. Normally, oxygen consumption is independent of delivery above a critical value (approximately, 330 ml$\cdot$min$^{-1}\cdot$m^{-2}). In sepsis and MOFS, the critical value can be markedly increased to values that may be unattainable. The existence of a flow dependence in the presence of even normal delivery suggests a tissue oxygen debt that is not clinically apparent.

Clinical Management

Initiation of therapy for cardiovascular support in sepsis and MOFS must be rapid and guided by cardiovascular assessment. This clinical syndrome is quite distinct from simple hemorrhagic shock, in which there is blood volume loss with minimal tissue injury. Major tissue injury and sepsis result in systemic activation of mediator systems that can affect distant organs not directly involved

Table 11–2 Major Goals of Cardiovascular Support for Prevention and Treatment of Sepsis and MOFS*

Cardiac index	>4.5 L·min^{-1}·m^{-2}
Blood volume	500 ml above normal
Oxygen delivery	>600 ml·min^{-1}·m^{-2}
Oxygen consumption	>170 ml·min^{-1}·m^{-2}
Blood pressure	Normal
Pulmonary vascular resistance	<250 dyne·s·cm^{-5}·m^{2}

*From Shoemaker.[34] Reprinted with permission.

(see Chapters 5 and 8). The cardiovascular system is not spared from these effects, as already described. This section will concentrate on management of cardiovascular dysfunction in sepsis and early multiple organ failure.

Goals of Management

There is growing evidence to support the concept that the more rapid and complete the initial resuscitation of the cardiopulmonary system, the greater the chance of prevention of multiple organ failure and subsequent survival. The ability to maintain a hyperdynamic state is associated with a greater survival in sepsis than is development of a hypodynamic state.[10] In these patients, reduced peripheral oxygen transport, myocardial performance, and blood volume were associated with diminished survival. Based on present knowledge of the cardiovascular and microvascular abnormalities in sepsis and major trauma, one should attempt to achieve an elevated cardiac output, oxygen transport, and peripheral oxygen utilization as a means to improve survival and prevent multiple organ failure.

Shoemaker et al.[11] evaluated a protocol in critically ill surgical patients aimed at achieving hyperdynamic cardiac function and supranormal oxygen delivery and consumption. The major goals of this protocol are listed in Table 11–2. The protocol group had a mortality of 12.5% compared with 35% in the control group. The incidence of postoperative sepsis was reduced from 44 to 11%. This study demonstrates that aggressive adherence to a treatment protocol aimed at maximizing oxygen delivery and consumption may have significant impact on patient outcome.

Role of Hemodynamic Monitoring

The goals just discussed of improving oxygen transport and utilization mandate a means of objectively monitoring hemodynamic status and response to therapy. The combination of thermodilution of the pulmonary artery and systemic arterial catheters allows assessment of hemodynamics as well as oxygen transport and utilization variables.

Arterial catheterization permits monitoring of the pressure waveform and direct measurement of the mean systemic blood pressure. It also permits sampling of blood for measurement of arterial saturation. The pulmonary artery

Table 11–3   Calculation of Derived Hemodynamic Variables

Variable	Units	Formula*
Cardiac index (CI)	$L \cdot min^{-1} \cdot m^{-2}$	CO / BSA
Stroke index (SI)	$ml \cdot beat^{-1} \cdot m^{-2}$	CI / HR
Systemic vascular resistance (SVRI)	$dyne \cdot s \cdot cm^{-5} \cdot m^2$	$(MAP - RAP)/CI \cdot 80$
Pulmonary vascular resistance index (PVRI)	$dyne \cdot s \cdot cm^{-5} \cdot m^2$	$(MPAP - PAWP)/CI \cdot 80$
Left ventricular stroke work index (LVSWI)	$g \cdot m \cdot m^{-2}$	$SI \cdot (MSAP - PAWP) \cdot 0.0136$
Right ventricular stroke work index (RVSWI)	$g \cdot m \cdot m^{-2}$	$SI \cdot (MPAP - RAP) \cdot 0.0136$
Arterial oxygen content (CaO_2)	$ml \cdot dl^{-1}$	$Hb \cdot 1.34 \cdot SaO_2$
Mixed venous oxygen content ($C\bar{v}O_2$)	$ml \cdot dl^{-1}$	$Hb \cdot 1.34 \cdot S\bar{v}O_2$
Oxygen delivery (DO_2)	$ml \cdot min^{-1} \cdot m^{-2}$	$CI \cdot Hb \cdot 13.4 \cdot SaO_2$
Oxygen consumption rate (VO_2)	$ml \cdot min^{-1} \cdot m^{-2}$	$CI \cdot Hb \cdot 13.4 \cdot (SaO_2 - S\bar{v}O_2)$
Oxygen extraction ratio (O_2ER)	%	VO_2/DO_2
Physiologic shunt fraction (Q_s/Q_t)	%	$\dfrac{(CcO_2 - CaO_2)}{(CcO_2 - C\bar{v}O_2)}$†
Ventilation-perfusion index (VQI)	%	$\dfrac{(1 - SaO_2)}{(1 - S\bar{v}O_2)}$

*MAP: mean arterial pressure; MPAP: mean pulmonary artery pressure; RAP: right atrial pressure; Hb: hemoglobin.

†CcO_2 is calculated using estimated oxygen content for oxygen tension equal to alveolar oxygen tension.

catheter permits central venous, pulmonary vascular, and pulmonary artery wedge pressure measurement. When combined with thermodilution cardiac output, myocardial and vascular performance variables can be readily calculated. With the addition of mixed venous saturation monitoring (via blood sampling or catheter hemoximetry), oxygen transport and utilization variables can be readily monitored.

CALCULATION OF HEMODYNAMIC PARAMETERS

The basic measurements just listed provide significant information on hemodynamic function. A number of derived parameters permit a more precise evaluation of certain aspects, including myocardial performance, vascular resistances, and oxygen transport and utilization. These derived parameters are necessary to achieve the goals of therapy previously outlined. Formulas for calculation of these hemodynamic parameters are given in Table 11–3. Normal values are given in Table 11–4, along with values desirable for prevention and treatment of sepsis and MOFS.

INTERPRETATION OF HEMODYNAMIC PARAMETERS

Although a full discussion of hemodynamic interpretation is beyond the scope of this chapter, a brief review of certain parameters is warranted. Pulmonary artery wedge pressure (PAWP) in general reflects left atrial pressure (LAP). In the absence of mitral valve disease, mean LAP approximates left ventricular end-diastolic pressure, which is the measure of preload we are seeking. However, patients with sepsis and MOFS usually have pulmonary involvement and frequently require mechanical ventilation, which can alter the relationship between PAWP and LAP. Positive end-expiratory pressure (PEEP) at levels of 10 cm H_2O

Table 11–4   Normal and Desired Values of Hemodynamic Parameters

Parameter	Normal Range	Desired Values*	Units
Heart rate	70–90	<120	min^{-1}
Mean arterial pressure	80–100	>70	torr
Mean pulmonary artery pressure	12–16	<20	torr
Pulmonary artery wedge pressure	8–12	12–16	torr
Right atrial pressure	5–8	<8	torr
Cardiac index	3.5–4.5	>4.5	$L \cdot min \cdot m^{-2}$
Stroke volume index	35–45	>45	$mv \cdot m^{-2}$
Left ventricular stroke work	45–65	>45	$g \cdot m \cdot m^{-2}$
Right ventricular stroke work	4–8	>10	$g \cdot m \cdot m^{-2}$
Systemic vascular resistance	1800–2400	1200–2000	$dyne \cdot s \cdot cm^{-5} \cdot m^{2}$
Pulmonary vascular resistance	50–200	<250	$dyne \cdot s \cdot cm^{-5} \cdot m^{2}$
Arterial oxygen tension	90–95	>60	torr
Arterial saturation	95–100	>90	%
Mixed venous oxygen tension	35–50	>35	torr
Mixed venous saturation	70–75	>60	%
Oxygen delivery	550–650	>650	$ml \cdot min^{-1} \cdot m^{-2}$
Oxygen consumption	110–150	>170	$ml \cdot min^{-1} \cdot m^{-2}$
Oxygen extraction ratio	25–30	<30	%
Pulmonary shunt fraction	3–5	<5	%

*Values desirable for treatment of patients with or at risk of developing sepsis and MOFS.

or more result in an overestimation of the true transmural pressure of the atria. This amount of overestimation is dependent on the pulmonary compliance, but averages about one third the PEEP level. The best means of optimizing preload in patients with significant pulmonary involvement is to construct a ventricular response curve during fluid challenge. Stroke work index (or stroke volume index) is calculated as the PAWP is increased by fluid challenges, and preload is considered optimal when left ventricular stroke work index (LVSWI) can no longer be increased. Changes in the level of ventilatory support may require reassessment of preload. When PAWP measurements are made, they should be obtained from the waveform tracing at end-expiration to avoid the influence of changes in pleural pressure during inspiration and expiration.

Ventricular stroke work index is probably an underutilized hemodynamic parameter. Although there is some variability in repeated measures, it perhaps best reflects ventricular performance more than any other measurement. When therapy is introduced to optimize ventricular performance, such as fluid challenges or inotropes, serial measurements of LVSWI or right ventricular stroke work index provide an objective assessment of response to therapy. Stroke volume index provides much the same information as stroke work, but does not take into account the ability of the ventricle to generate pressure as part of its performance.

Continuous measurement of mixed venous oxygen saturation ($S\bar{v}O_2$) is now possible with fiberoptic pulmonary artery catheters. The catheter obviates the need to draw mixed venous blood samples for analysis, facilitating calculations of the oxygen transport variables. The measurement has also been used to follow short-term changes in cardiac output in patients with cardiac disease. However, $S\bar{v}O_2$ is unreliable for following cardiac output in patients with sepsis and MOFS. Oxygen extraction may be dependent on delivery, and oxygen consumption can change rapidly in these patients, so that $S\bar{v}O_2$ is no longer dependent on cardiac output alone.

Another pitfall in the interpretation of $S\bar{v}O_2$ is the assumption that it reflects tissue oxygenation. Because of the complex microvascular changes that occur in MOFS and the dynamics of oxygen release from hemoglobin, $S\bar{v}O_2$ (and mixed venous oxygen tension) may overestimate the state of tissue oxygenation. The best clinical assessment of the adequacy of tissue oxygenation is the oxygen flux test, in which oxygen delivery is increased through fluid loading and inotropic agents or decreased through administration of PEEP. A corresponding increase or decrease in oxygen consumption suggests a covert oxygen debt.

Pulmonary Support

Maintenance of cardiovascular function and oxygen delivery requires support of the pulmonary system. There are two principal goals in support of the pulmonary system for management of sepsis or trauma-induced cardiovascular dysfunction. First and foremost is correction of hypoxemia. Oxygen delivery is directly related to arterial oxygen saturation. Arterial desaturation in the presence of an inability of the cardiovascular system to compensate further results in marked impairment of oxygen delivery. The arterial saturation should be maintained at 90% or higher. Although this corresponds to an arterial oxygen tension (PaO_2) of about 60 torr, measurement of saturation via spectrophotometry is essential. Calculated saturation based on PaO_2 measurement can be influenced markedly by altered 2,3-diphosphoglycerate levels following transfusion and by temperature, and cannot be relied on.

Ventilation-perfusion mismatch occurs in septicemia,[12] resulting in hypoxemia, and usually responds to supplemental oxygen via mask or nasal cannula. It will not, however, correct the intrapulmonary shunting that is present in more severe respiratory insufficiency. If hypoxemia is refractory, the institution of continuous positive airway pressure (CPAP) or mechanical ventilation with PEEP can effectively reduce intrapulmonary shunting via alveolar recruitment and elevation of the functional residual capacity. This is perhaps best accomplished via endotracheal intubation, but selective application of airway pressure therapy via face mask has been successful in our hands as well as others.

The second major role of pulmonary support in sepsis and MOFS is reduction in the work of breathing. The mechanical properties of the lung are significantly altered in acute lung injury, resulting in an increased work of breathing.[13] As a result, the respiratory muscles have been shown to account for as much as 50% of the total oxygen consumption.[14] Institution of a ventilatory support should be made at the earliest signs of increased work of breathing (tachypnea with decreased tidal volume and hyperventilation). Since an intact respiratory drive is present in most of these patients, pressure support ventilation usually provides the necessary reduction in inspiratory work with minimal adverse effects on cardiovascular function.[15] If respiratory drive is insufficient or in question, assisted ventilation or intermittent mandatory ventilation with pressure support is indicated.

Fluid Therapy

A cornerstone in the management of septicemia and trauma is rapid restoration of intravascular volume and expansion of the extracellular space. A decrease in intravascular volume is almost universal in untreated sepsis and trauma. Volume losses in sepsis result from transudation of fluid out of the vascular space and increases in vascular capacitance. In the trauma patient, blood loss is partially compensated for by transcapillary refill from the interstitial space. An obligate increase in extracellular space capacitance occurs in both conditions, from both changes in the extracellular matrix as well as a generalized increase in microvascular permeability.

One has a choice of crystalloid and colloid solutions for initial fluid therapy. Although considerable debate has been held over which fluid is most appropriate, there is still no consensus. Rational fluid administration requires a thorough understanding of the responses to each type of fluid. A brief discussion of the effects of each type of fluid will be given, followed by a recommended approach to fluid resuscitation based on these principles.

CRYSTALLOIDS

The distribution space of isotonic crystalloid solutions is the interstitial and intravascular spaces. These solutions have several advantages over colloids, including proved effectiveness in restoration of volume loss and lesser expense. Since only about 22% of administered volume stays intravascular,[16] larger volumes are required and significant expansion of the interstitial space results. Interstitial space expansion is desirable, since it is an obligatory response in trauma and septicemia, yet overexpansion can lead to excessive edema, potentially compromising gas exchange in the lungs and in the peripheral tissues. Human studies have demonstrated an increased incidence of pulmonary edema when crystalloids alone were used for volume expansion,[17] but this is probably transitory, and it is unclear if there are any long-term adverse effects.

COLLOIDS

Iso-oncotic colloid solutions (plasma and plasma protein fractions, 5% albumin, 6% hetastarch, and dextrans) have the advantage of more rapid restoration of intravascular volume, since they are better retained within the intravascular space, and better maintenance of colloid oncotic pressure. Volume expansion can occur with less total volume than with crystalloids.[17] Colloid administration better supports microcirculatory flow, as is evident from improvements in tissue oxygen utilization. This effect is not found with crystalloids.

Disadvantages include cost and relative lack of expansion of the interstitial space in the presence of an increased capacitance of that space. An impairment of urine output and renal excretion of sodium and water was demonstrated when albumin solutions alone were used in resuscitation from hemorrhagic shock.[18] A frequently raised concern is that flux of oncotically active particles into the interstitium could worsen or prolong tissue edema, but no data as yet exist to support this concept.

FLUID RESUSCITATION PROTOCOL

Fluid resuscitation is perhaps best governed by the application of principles based on the available data. The goal of resuscitation is restoration of tissue perfusion and oxygen consumption. A combination of crystalloid and colloid is usually required to meet this goal. With this goal in mind, one must follow indicators of adequate perfusion. In simple hemorrhagic shock, clinical signs are generally adequate. When sepsis, capillary leak, and signs of multiple organ impairment complicate the picture, then invasive hemodynamic monitoring and lactate measurements permit more critical assessment of response to therapy.

The initial fluid should be crystalloid. It is readily available, and expands the interstitial space as well as the vascular space. It frequently is the only fluid necessary to restore tissue perfusion. Glucose-containing fluids should be used only for maintenance fluids, not for rapid fluid administration during resuscitation.

Colloid administration should commence when crystalloids alone either fail to achieve the goal of tissue oxygenation or are associated with adverse effects such as excessive pulmonary or peripheral edema. In severe septicemia, crystalloids alone may be insufficient for rapid restoration of tissue perfusion, and colloids are added to the regimen. In addition, once interstitial expansion has occurred, crystalloids may be inadequate for maintenance of tissue oxygenation. Peripheral perfusion and oxygen consumption are better maintained with colloid than crystalloid in high-risk patients.[19,20]

The end points of fluid administration in sepsis and MOFS are best determined through hemodynamic monitoring. In general a PAWP of 12 to 15 torr is optimal, but this can vary with coexistent cardiac disease. We recommend monitoring ventricular performance (stroke work index or stroke volume index) because the PAWP is raised during fluid resuscitation. The end point would be that PAWP above which no further increases in stroke volume index or LVSWI result. Any further fluid loading will put the patient at increased risk of pulmonary edema without improving ventricular performance. If other therapies are subsequently instituted that can alter performance, such as PEEP, or if the patient's condition changes, then repeat challenge may be indicated.

Burn shock represents a special situation.[21] Significant increases in capillary permeability develop in the first 24 hours after a major burn, and colloids may result in more edema if used during this initial period. Crystalloids alone should be used until the permeability defect begins to resolve, after which colloids may be more effective at maintaining intravascular volume. Hypertonic saline solutions are also being used with increasing frequency in the initial 24 hours.[22]

Hematocrit and Blood Transfusion

Effective oxygen transport depends on an adequate concentration of hemoglobin. In the normal subject, a decreased oxygen content in anemia can be compensated for through an increased cardiac output, so that oxygen delivery is maintained. In the critically ill patient with cardiovascular dysfunction, full compensation cannot usually be achieved, and inadequate delivery results.

However, blood transfusion increases blood viscosity in addition to increasing oxygen content. Viscosity is a nonlinear function of hematocrit, and hematocrit levels above 35 to 40% result in marked viscosity increases. Microcirculatory blood flow is compromised at higher viscosities. The optimal hematocrit, that is, that hematocrit that provides the best oxygen content-microcirculatory blood flow match to maximize tissue oxygen availability, has yet to be adequately determined. Reasons for the difficulties are several. Capillary hematocrit is less than large vessel hematocrit and cannot be easily measured. Viscosity in capillaries is not determined solely by the determinants of large vessel hematocrit, in part because of the alignment of red cells in capillaries. Capillary blood flow is difficult to measure and is not feasible in humans. It is also very likely that an optimal hematocrit may depend on a multitude of factors that can be quite variable. These factors include the cause and degree of maldistribution of capillary blood flow.

In the absence of direct microcirculatory measurements, investigators have attempted to determine optimal hematocrit on the basis of indirect data, such as survival. Czer and Shoemaker[23] studied a series of critically ill surgical patients and suggested survival to be maximal at a hematocrit of 30 to 32%. The work of Messmer et al.[24] suggests optimal tissue oxygenation takes place at 25 to 30% hematocrit. In the gut, however, a hematocrit on the order of 45% may be optimal.[25] Each organ therefore may have a hematocrit at which oxygen availability is optimal, which may differ from organ to organ. The role of red cell transfusion in sepsis and MOFS has yet to be fully elucidated. In a study of the oxygen utilization response to red cell transfusion in sepsis following adequate volume resuscitation, we found that as a group, the rate of oxygen consumption ($\dot{V}O_2$) did not improve, but individual patients did demonstrate increased $\dot{V}O_2$.[26] No pretransfusion variable consistently predicted a beneficial response. Gilbert et al.[27] found that elevated lactate levels predicted an improvement in $\dot{V}O_2$ in response to red cell transfusion, but their data suggest that their patients were not fully volume resuscitated. It is currently our practice to transfuse to attain a hemoglobin of 10 to 12 $g \cdot dl^{-1}$ while monitoring the cardiopulmonary response. In the absence of an improvement in cardiovascular performance or oxygen consumption, we limit further transfusion.

Inotropic and Vasoactive Drugs

Although fluid resuscitation remains the first line of therapy for restoration and maintenance of tissue perfusion, inotropic and vasoactive drugs can provide cardiovascular support when fluid therapy is insufficient to achieve adequate perfusion. The mainstays of pharmacologic support of the circulation are the

Table 11–5   Adrenergic Receptor Profiles of Catecholamines

Drug	β_1	β_2	α_1	α_2	*DA-1*
Dobutamine	+++	0→+	0	0	0
Dopamine*	+→+++	++	0→+++	+	+++
Norepinephrine	+++	+++	+++	+	0
Epinephrine	+++	+++	+++	+++	0

*Dose-dependent effects.
Note: + = minimal, ++ = moderate, +++ = major effects.

catecholamines, which mediate their effects via the adrenergic receptors. The phosphodiesterase inhibitors have also demonstrated efficacy in septic shock.

ADRENERGIC RECEPTORS

A brief review of adrenergic receptor actions helps in the selection of catecholamines for the management of cardiovascular failure in sepsis and trauma. The three major adrenergic receptor classes are the α receptors, mediating primarily peripheral vascular effects, the β receptors, mediating cardiac, vascular, and endocrine effects, and dopaminergic receptors. Although there are only two subclasses of each receptor group, their actions are quite variable because of the variations in receptor locations in different tissues. α_1 receptors are postsynaptic and mediate calcium-dependent vasoconstriction of the peripheral vasculature. The presynaptic α_2 receptor is thought to feed back negatively on norepinephrine release from neuron endings. β_1, receptors affect the force of myocardial contraction, heart rate, and conduction velocity. β_2 receptors produce peripheral vasodilation.

Dopaminergic-1 (DA-1) receptors mediate dilation of renal, splanchnic, cerebral, and coronary vessels via the adenylate cyclase system. A dopaminergic-mediated inhibition of aldosterone secretion may have a beneficial effect in the hyperaldosteronism of critical illness. DA-2 receptors are inhibitory in nature and are located in the central nervous system and various other tissues.

Sepsis has modulating effects on the adrenergic receptors that can influence the action of catecholamines. Down-regulation of peripheral α-adrenergic receptors has been noted in experimental models of sepsis.[28] Myocardial depression is associated with a blunted response to β_1 stimulation. The acidosis that frequently accompanies sepsis can attenuate the action of catecholamines.

ADRENERGIC PROFILES OF THE CATECHOLAMINES

Each catecholamine has a specific effect on the various adrenergic receptors. The adrenergic receptor agonist profiles of the presently available catecholamines are summarized in Table 11–5.

OTHER CARDIOVASCULAR PHARMACOLOGIC AGENTS

The phosphodiesterase inhibitors, of which amrinone is the prototype, are non-catecholamine inotropic drugs. The mechanism of action is not fully understood, but inhibition of phosphodiesterase F-III with increases in cyclic adenosine mon-

Table 11–6 Hemodynamic Effects and Dosages of Cardiovascular Drugs

Drug	Dose	HR	PAWP	CI	MAP	SVRI
Dobutamine	5–30 $\mu g \cdot kg^{-1} \cdot min^{-1}$	→↑	↓	↑	→	↓
Dopamine	2–3 $\mu g \cdot kg^{-1} \cdot min^{-1}$	→	→	→	→	→
	5–10 $\mu g \cdot kg^{-1} \cdot min^{-1}$	→	→	↑	→↑	→
	>10 $\mu g \cdot kg^{-1} \cdot min^{-1}$	↑	↑	↑	↑	↑
Norepinephrine	>0.05 $\mu g \cdot kg^{-1} \cdot min^{-1}$	↓	↑	→↑	↑↑	↑↑
Epinephrine	0.005–0.05 $\mu g \cdot kg^{-1} \cdot min^{-1}$	↑	→	→↑	→	→↓
	>0.05 $\mu g \cdot kg^{-1} \cdot min^{-1}$	↑	↑	↑	↑	↑
Amrinone	5–30 $\mu g \cdot kg^{-1} \cdot min^{-1}$	→↑	↓	↑	→↓	↓

Note: HR: heart rate; CI: cardiac index; SVRI: systemic vascular resistance index; →: no change; ↑: increased; ↓: decreased; ↑ ↑: large increase.

ophosphate (cAMP) may play a major role. Amrinone is capable of improving oxygen delivery in septic shock.[29] Since it has vasodilator properties, hypotension may limit its use as a single agent, but it has been shown to be effective in combination with adrenergic agents.[30] Since it does not depend on the adrenergic system, it may be useful when response to catecholamines is poor.

Glucagon has inotropic effects that result from elevation of cAMP levels independently of the β receptors. Its role at present is usually restricted to the need for inotropic action in the presence of previously administered β-blockers. The dose is 5 to 6 mg intravenously followed by 2 to 10 mg.hr^{-1} infusion.

CARDIOVASCULAR DRUG ADMINISTRATION

There is no universally accepted regimen for pharmacologic support of the patient with cardiovascular failure in sepsis or multiple organ failure. The choice of inotropic and vasoconstrictor agents in the management of sepsis and early multiple organ failure is influenced largely by the mechanisms of the underlying cardiovascular dysfunction. The hemodynamic effects of the commonly used drugs are summarized in Table 11–6, along with recommended dosage regimens. It should be emphasized that pharmacologic support is indicated only after expansion of the intravascular space with fluids is complete, but insufficient for maintenance of organ perfusion and oxygen consumption.

The following are guidelines for selection of cardiovascular pharmacologic agents:

1. Our initial approach in patients without marked hypotension is the administration of inotropes without significant peripheral vascular effects. We attempt first to support the cardiac output as a means of maintaining blood pressure, since the use of agents with peripheral vascular effects may impair organ perfusion and worsen microcirculatory blood flow distribution. Dobutamine provides this mechanism of action and has been found superior to dopamine alone for maintaining tissue perfusion and oxygen consumption

in critically ill postoperative patients.[31] In patients with established sepsis, however, this effect was less pronounced. The dose is 5 to 30 $\mu g \cdot kg^{-1} \cdot min^{-1}$ continuous infusion. Amrinone is an alternative to dobutamine. We administer it as a bolus dose of 1 $mg \cdot kg^{-1}$ followed by 10 $\mu g \cdot kg^{-1} \cdot min^{-1}$. If the response is inadequate, we repeat the bolus dose once or twice, and raise the infusion to 20 or 30 $\mu g \cdot kg^{-1} \cdot min^{-1}$, respectively. We have noted in some patients that the combination of both drugs provided a response when either drug alone resulted in inadequate responses. Lower doses of epinephrine, which provide primarily β stimulation (0.005 to 0.05 $\mu g \cdot kg^{-1} \cdot min^{-1}$), has been used, but not extensively studied in this circumstance.

2. When significant hypotension (mean arterial pressure [MAP] less than 60 torr) from low systemic vascular resistance (less than 500 $dyne \cdot s \cdot cm^{-}5 \cdot m^2$) is present or cannot be overcome by inotropic agents, α-adrenergic agents may be useful. Norepinephrine has been shown to be beneficial in sepsis. Although this agent has α-adrenergic effects, it is also has β_1 and β_2 effects, so that oxygen delivery is well maintained. Because of its β effects, it may be used alone, but we preferably add it to an inotropic agent such as dobutamine. This permits us to adjust relative α and β effects to maintain an adequate cardiac output and oxygen delivery while assuring an adequate perfusion pressure (MAP more than 65 torr). Dopamine in higher doses (5 to 20 $\mu g \cdot kg^{-1} \cdot min^{-1}$) is an alternative to norepinephrine, but the dopaminergic effects seen at lower doses are lost in the presence of the α-adrenergic effects. Epinephrine in moderate doses (above 0.05 to 0.1 $\mu g \cdot kg^{-1} \cdot min^{-1}$) can provide α and β support, but has not been as extensively studied as the other agents. We have noted more significant ectopy and tachycardia with epinephrine than with the other agents.

3. Dopamine, when not used in vasoconstrictor doses, is added in low doses (2 to 3 $\mu g \cdot kg^{-1} \cdot min^{-1}$) to augment renal and mesenteric perfusion in all patients. This drug has been demonstrated to enhance renal blood flow even during the administration of norepinephrine[32] and has diuretic properties independent of renal blood flow.[33]

4. We avoid pure α-agonists such as phenylephrine hydrochloride, since they tend to reduce cardiac output without improving peripheral blood distribution and oxygen availability.

Reduction of Oxygen Demand

Oxygen delivery is limited when cardiovascular failure complicates critical illness. Fluid and pharmacologic therapy can usually improve oxygen availability, but an equally important therapeutic consideration is the reduction in oxygen demand. The beneficial influence of mechanical ventilation in reducing oxygen requirements has already been discussed. Administration of anxiolytic or analgesic agents, or both, can reduce oxygen consumption. Pain results in a cardiovascular response that can be detrimental to oxygen supply to utilization balance and should be well controlled. Neuromuscular blockade in association with sedation can reduce the dosage of sedative required and reduce the chance of adverse cardiovascular effects from large sedative doses. Mechanical ventilatory support in a closely monitored situation is required for neuromuscular blockade. Hyperthermia increases oxygen consumption by about 7% for each degree centigrade increase in body temperature and should be controlled.

Other Factors Affecting Cardiovascular Function

A number of etiologic factors for cardiovascular dysfunction and failure have been presented herein. By and large, treatment of these is based on treatment of the underlying disorder. There are a number of other factors that, although not part of MOFS, can certainly contribute to worsening of ventricular function. Many of these can be prevented or minimized, but this requires recognition of the contributing factors.

Positive Pressure Ventilation and PEEP

It is now well recognized that PEEP has adverse effects on cardiovascular function. These effects include an increase in RV afterload, increase in RV diameter, and decrease in LV diastolic compliance. Both ventricles are thus affected, but the right ventricle is the most sensitive. A direct myocardial depressant effect has been noted, but the mechanism is not clear.

Since PEEP has been shown to be extremely beneficial in reducing intrapulmonary shunting and improving arterial saturation, it is almost universally applied. One must not only be aware of the adverse effects of PEEP, but should routinely consider the beneficial and adverse effects of PEEP in making management decisions involving the cardiovascular system.

The application of PEEP should be systematic and its cardiovascular effects assessed when adjusting it. We choose a level of PEEP that offers the best compromise between improved arterial oxygenation and diminished cardiac output, that is, offers the best oxygen delivery. Intrapulmonary shunt (Q_s/Q_t), and oxygen delivery (or mixed venous saturation) are measured at several levels of PEEP. The lowest level at which either shunt fraction is minimal or oxygen delivery or $S\bar{v}O_2$ is maximal is chosen. The ventilation-perfusion index is an easily calculated estimate of shunt fraction and can be used in place of Q_s/Q_t. Because of the increased RV afterload induced by PEEP, it may be necessary to volume load the patient to improve RV function in order that higher levels of PEEP may be applied with preservation of cardiac output.

In addition to adjustment of PEEP, the mode of positive pressure ventilation also influences cardiovascular function. The modes provide a spectrum of the degree of positive pressure that is delivered to the patient. Continuous mandatory ventilation (CMV), such as assist or control, provides the greatest mean positive pressure. Intermittent mandatory ventilation (IMV) provides less and is associated with improved renal and hemodynamic function in comparison with CMV. Pressure support (pressure assist) ventilation, since it only assists the patient's inspiratory effort, provides the least but is dependent on the level of support required. In general, the modes that reduce cardiovascular embarrassment, however, are associated with greater work of breathing for the patient, so both of these factors must be considered. Our preference is to use IMV initially, then change to pressure support when the patient's respiratory drive becomes reliable, since the latter mode has less cardiovascular effect at lower levels of support.[15]

Anesthetic and Medication Effects

As a result of impairment of myocardial performance in MOFS, one should minimize further depression when using pharmacologic agents. A brief review of the basic cardiovascular actions of these drugs will help to guide the clinician in administration of these drugs. These drugs are used in both the operating suite, often with continued effects into the postoperative period, or they may be administered in the postoperative period. Essentially all anesthetic agents in use today produce some degree of myocardial depression, thus further blunting the cardiovascular response. Halothane and enflurane cause a reduction in blood pressure and cardiac output. Isoflurane reduces systemic vascular resistance, so that even though blood pressure is reduced, cardiac output is better maintained. Barbiturates, used as induction agents, depress contractility and cause arteriolar and venous vasodilation, resulting in a lowering of blood pressure and tachycardia. Narcotics, with the exception of meperidine, produce no significant myocardial depression but can cause hypotension, at least in part mediated by histamine release. Meperidine has been shown to have some myocardial depressant activity. Since narcotics are an important adjunct in the management of trauma and surgical patients, they are frequently used. Hypotension can be limited by slow administration of the drugs, concomitant administration of fluid, or by pretreatment with histamine receptor blockers. Bradycardia can also result from narcotic administration and can be blocked with atropine if problematic. Benzodiazepines have relatively little effect on the cardiovascular system when used alone, but administration in conjunction with narcotics have been shown to produce an additive effect on myocardial contractility, so close monitoring is required.

Hypothermia

Hypothermia frequently accompanies major trauma and operative procedures and can be compounded by administration of large volumes of fluid and blood at room or refrigerated temperatures. A number of cardiovascular effects result from hypothermia. In the anesthetized patient the compensatory responses to hypothermia are blunted, exaggerating the dysfunction. Cardiac output falls from bradycardia and increases in systemic vascular resistance. Anesthetic agents inhibit to some degree this increase in vascular resistance. A mild metabolic acidosis develops and prolongation of intracardiac conduction can occur. The heart is at increased risk for ventricular fibrillation.

Summary

The systemic response that characterizes sepsis, major tissue injury, and early MOFS frequently results in cardiovascular dysfunction. Myocardial depression, decrease in ventricular preload, variable changes in afterload, and complex microvascular changes result in decreased systemic oxygen delivery and tissue oxygen utilization. A therapeutic protocol aimed at achieving a mild to moderately hyperdynamic cardiovascular state and maximizing oxygen delivery and consumption may improve survival in high-risk patients. These goals are attained through appropriate fluid resuscitation with crystalloids and colloids, inotropic support, blood transfusion, and reduction in oxygen demand. Other factors adversely affecting cardiovascular function such as positive pressure ventilation are minimized. Keys to successful prevention of multiple organ failure include early recognition and rapid institution of goal-directed therapy.

References

1. Frank O. Die Grundform des arteriellen Pulses. Z Biol 1898; 37:483.
2. Patterson SW, Piper H, Starling EH. The regulation of the heart beat. J Physiol (Lond) 1914; 48:465.
3. Parrillo JE, Burch C, Shelhamer JH, Parker MM, Natanson C, Schuette W. A circulating myocardial depressant substance in humans with septic shock. Septic shock patients with a reduced ejection fraction have a circulating factor that depresses in vitro myocardial cell performance. J Clin Invest 1985; 76:1539–1553.
4. Reilly JM, Burch-Whitman C, Parker MM, et al. Characteristics of a myocardial depressant substance in patients with septic shock. Circulation 1987; 76:165.
5. Dhainaut JF, Huyghebaert MF, Monsallier JF, Lefevre G, Dall'Ava-Santucci J, Brunet F, Villemant D, Carli A, Raichvarg D. Coronary hemodynamics and myocardial metabolism of lactate, free fatty acids, glucose, and ketones in patients with septic shock. Circulation 1987; 75:533–541.
6. Ellrodt AG, Riedinger MS, Kimchi A, Berman DS, Maddahi J, Swan HJ, Murata GH. Left ventricular performance in septic shock: reversible segmental and global abnormalities. Am Heart J 1985; 110:402–409.
7. Bersten A, Hersch M, Neal A, et al. Adequate myocardial O$_2$ transport fails to prevent LV failure in a non-hypotensive model of sepsis. Chest 1988; 94:473.
8. Sibbald WJ, Driedger AA, Myers ML, Short AIK, Wells GA. Biventricular function in the acute respiratory distress syndrome: hemodynamic and radionuclide assessment with special emphasis on right ventricular function. Chest 1983; 84:126–134.
9. Sibbald WJ, Prewitt RM. Right ventricular function. Crit Care Med 1983; 11:321–322.
10. Bland RD, Shoemaker WC, Abraham E, Cobo JC. Hemodynamic and oxygen transport patterns in surviving and nonsurviving postoperative patients. Crit Care Med 1985; 13:85–90.
11. Shoemaker WC, Appel P, Bland R. Use of physiologic monitoring to predict outcome and to assist in clinical decisions in critically ill postoperative patients. Am J Surg 1983; 146:43–50.
12. Siegel JH, Giovanni I, Coleman B: Ventilation: Perfusion maldistribution secondary to the hyperdynamic cardiovascular state as the major cause of increased pulmonary shunting in human sepsis. J Trauma 1979; 19:432–460.
13. Milic-Emili J, Ploysongsang Y. Respiratory mechanics in the adult respiratory distress syndrome. Crit Care Clin 1986; 2:573–584.
14. Roussos C, Macklem PT. The respiratory muscles. N Engl J Med 1982; 307:786–797.
15. Wissing DR, Romero MR, Houston M, Owens M, Lambert RS, Kinasewitz GT. Hemodynamic effects of pressure support ventilation (PSV). [Abstr.] Respir Care 1987; 32:892.
16. Weil MH, Rackow EE. A guide to volume repletion. Emerg Med 1984; 16:101.
17. Rackow EC, Falk JL, Fein IZ, Siegel JS, Packman MI, Haupt MT, Kaufman BS, Putnam D. Fluid resuscitation in circulatory shock: a comparison of the cardiorespiratory effects of albumin, hetastarch and saline solutions in patients with hypovolemic and septic shock. Crit Care Med 1983; 11:839–850.
18. Lucas CE, Weaver D, Higgins RF, Ledgerwood AM, Johnson SD, Bouwman DL. Effects of albumin versus non-albumin resuscitation on plasma volume and renal excretory function. J Trauma 1978; 18:564–570.
19. Hauser CJ, Shoemaker WC, Turpin I, Goldberg SJ. Oxygen transport responses to colloids and crystalloids in critically ill surgical patients. Surg Gynecol Obstet 1980; 150:811–816.

20. Appel PL, Shoemaker WC. Evaluation of fluid therapy in adult respiratory failure. Crit Care Med 1981; 9:862–869.
21. Demling RH. Fluid resuscitation after major burns. JAMA 1983; 250:1438–1440.
22. Monafo WW, Chuntrasekul C, Ayvazian VH. Hypertonic sodium solutions in the treatment of burn shock. Am J Surg 1973; 126:778–783.
23. Czer LS, Shoemaker WC. Optimal hematocrit value in critically ill postoperative patients. Surg Gynecol Obstet 1978; 147:363–368.
24. Messmer K, Sunder-Plassmann L, Jesch F, Gornandt L, Sinagowitz E, Kessler M. Oxygen supply to the tissues during limited normovolemic hemodilution. Res Exp Med (Berl) 1973; 159:152–166.
25. Shepherd AP, Riedel GL. Optimal hematocrit for oxygenation of canine intestine. Circ Res 1982; 51:233–240.
26. Conrad SA, Dietrich KA, Hebert CA, Romero MD. Failure of red cell transfusion to improve oxygen consumption in human septic shock. Circ Shock 1989; 27:346.
27. Gilbert EM, Haupt MJ, Mandanas RY, Huaringa AJ, Carlson RW. The effect of fluid loading, blood transfusion, and catecholamine infusion on oxygen delivery and consumption in patients with sepsis. Am Rev Respir Dis 1986; 134:873–878.
28. McMillan M, Chernow B, Roth RL. Hepatic alpha-1 adrenergic receptor alteration in a rat model of chronic sepsis. Circ Shock 1986; 19:185–193.
29. Domb M, Van der Linden P, Azimi G, Motte S, de Boelpaepe C, Vincent JL. Amrinone administration in septic shock. Intensive Care Med 1986; 12(Suppl):262.
30. Vincent JL, de Boelpaepe C, Luyaert P, Contempre B, Schmartz D, Coussaert E. Association of amrinone with norepinephrine in endotoxin shock in dogs. [Abstr.] Crit Care Med 1988; 16:403.
31. Shoemaker WC, Appel PL, Kram HB, Duarte D, Harrier HD, Ocampo HA. Comparison of hemodynamic and oxygen transport effects of dopamine and dobutamine in critically ill surgical patients. Chest 1989; 96:120–126.
32. Schaer GL, Fink MP, Parrillo JE. Norepinephrine alone versus norepinephrine plus low-dose dopamine: enhanced renal blood flow with combination pressor therapy. Crit Care Med 1985; 13:492–496.
33. Hilberman M, Maseda J, Stinson EB, Derby GC, Spencer RJ, Miller DC, Oyer PE, Myers BD. The diuretic properties of dopamine in patients after open-heart operation. Anesthesiology 1984; 61:489–494.
34. Shoemaker WC. Hemodynamic and oxygen transport patterns in septic shock: physiologic mechanisms and therapeutic implications. In Sibbald WC, Sprung CL (eds): Perspectives on sepsis and septic shock. Fullerton, CA: Society of Critical Care Medicine, 1986.

12

Pulmonary Failure and Acute Respiratory Distress Syndrome

DAVID N. HERNDON
DANIEL L. TRABER

Parenchymal lung injury frequently accompanies multiple organ failure.[1,2] This damage has been given the name "adult respiratory distress syndrome" (ARDS) (Table 12–1). There were and are many different titles for this syndrome, such as shock lung or wet lung, which occurs in children as well as adults (Table 12–2). This syndrome is grossly characterized by an intensive pulmonary edema and hypoxemia. Although bacterial infections are the most common cause of the syndrome,[1] it is also associated with other risk factors, such as multiple trauma,[3] disseminated intravascular coagulation,[4] acid aspiration,[5,6] and inhalation injury[7,8] (Table 12–3). These risk factors all have certain common pathophysiologic elements (Table 12–4). In each case, as a result of the initial insult, humoral or cellular mediators, or both, are activated that subsequently induce microvascular damage and pulmonary edema (Fig. 12–1). It has been suggested that bacteremia or endotoxemia may be the common factor to all of these forms of injury.[9] However, the fact that there are subtle differences in the response to each of these injuries would argue for a differing basis for the lung lesions in each of these situations.

192

Table 12–1   Criteria for Diagnosing ARDS*

Clinical Setting
  Catastrophic event
    Pulmonary
    Nonpulmonary, such as shock
  Exclusions
    Chronic pulmonary disease
    Left heart abnormalities
  Respiratory distress (judged clinically)
    Tachypnea >20, usually greater
    Labored breathing

Chest Radiograph: Diffuse Pulmonary Infiltrates
  Interstitial (initially)
  Alveolar (later)

Physiologic
  PaO_2 <50 mmHg with FiO_2
  Overall compliance <50 ml/cm H_2O (usually 20 to 30 ml/cm H_2O)
  Increased shunt fraction Qs/Qt and dead space ventilation V_D/V_T

Pathologic
  Heavy lungs, usually >1000 g
  Congestive atelectasis
  Hyaline membranes
  Fibrosis

*From Petty.[139] Reprinted with permission.

Table 12–2   Synonyms for ARDS*

Adult hyaline membrane disease
Adult respiratory insufficiency syndrome
Congestive atelectasis
DaNang lung
Hemorrhagic atelectasis
Hemorrhagic lung syndrome
Hypoxic hyperventilation
Postperfusion lung
Post-traumatic atelectasis
Post-traumatic pulmonary insufficiency
Progressive pulmonary consolidation
Progressive respiratory distress
Pump lung
Shock lung
Traumatic wet lung
Transplant lung
White lung
Wet lung

*From Taylor and Duncan.[140] Reprinted with
permission.

Table 12–3   Conditions Associated with ARDS*

Shock
  Hemorrhagic
  Septic
  Cardiogenic
  Anaphylactic

Trauma
  Burns
  Fat emboli
  Lung contusion
  Nonthoracic trauma (especially head trauma)
  Near-drowning

Infection
  Viral pneumonia
  Bacterial pneumonia
  Fungal pneumonia
  Gram-negative sepsis
  Tuberculosis

Inhalation of toxic gases
  Oxygen
  Smoke
  Nitrogen dioxide, ammonium, chlorine
  Cadmium
  Phosgene

Aspiration of gastric contents (especially with a pH <2.5)

Drug ingestion
  Heroin
  Methadone
  Barbituates
  Ethchlorvynol
  Thiazides
  Fluorescein
  Propoxyphene
  Salicylates
  Chlorodiazepoxide
  Colchicine
  Dextran 40

Metabolic
  Uremia
  Diabetic ketoacidosis

Miscellaneous
  Pancreatitis
  Postcardiopulmonary bypass
  Postcardioversion
  Multiple transfusions
  Disseminated intravascular coagulation
  Leukoagglutinin reaction
  Eclampsia
  Air or amniotic fluid emboli
  Bowel infarction
  Carcinomatosis

*From Taylor and Duncan.[140] Reprinted with permission.

Table 12–4   Risk Factors Associated with Development of ARDS*

Definite Risk Factors	*Probable Risk Factors*
Systemic sepsis	Severe pancreatitis
Pulmonary contusion	Diffuse pneumonia
Aspiration	Multiple emergency blood transfusions
Inhalation of toxic substances	
Near drowning	
Fractures of long bones	

*From Norwood and Civetta.[141] Reprinted with permission.

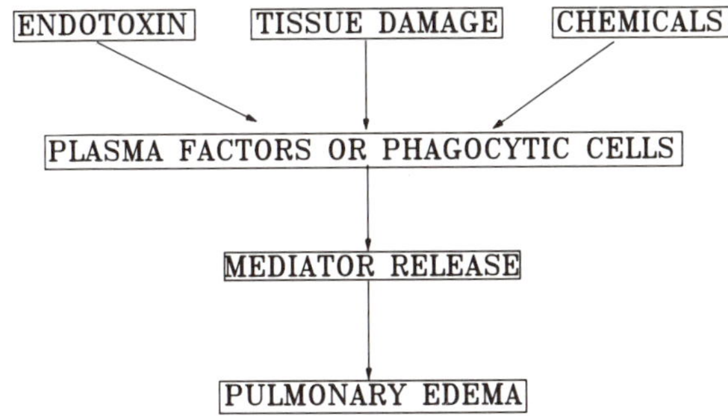

Figure 12–1. We have found these data to be as indicated above (unpublished data).

Pathophysiology

Triggering Events

The pathophysiology of ARDS involves a cascade of events that ultimately leads to lung damage. It has been suggested that the activation of coagulation Factor XII may be the trigger that initiates the cascade of events that culminates in ARDS (Fig. 12–2).[10] Factor XII can be activated by endotoxin,[11] injured surfaces,[12] as well as other agents.[13,14] Activation of Factor XII will lead to the conversion of prekallikrein to kallikrein,[15,16] which in turn is responsible for the formation of bradykinin. Bradykinin can increase microvascular permeability to protein[17] and is thus an additional putative mediator of ARDS. Likewise the activation of complement occurs with formation of Factor XIIa.[18] Since certain chemotactic complement components, such as C3a and C5a, both prime phagocytic cells and attract them to the site of injury,[19,20] complement activation may also lead to pulmonary injury.

Endotoxin may also have a direct effect on phagocytic cells, especially macrophages, causing the release of chemotactic materials, such as leukotriene (LT) B_4. In addition, platelets and leukocytes release products of the eicosanoid pathway, such as thromboxane A_2 (TXA_2) and the peptide leukotriene LTC_4/D_4. Both affect an increase in microvascular to interstitial fluid flux, the former by increasing microvascular pressure and the latter by changing permeability to pro-

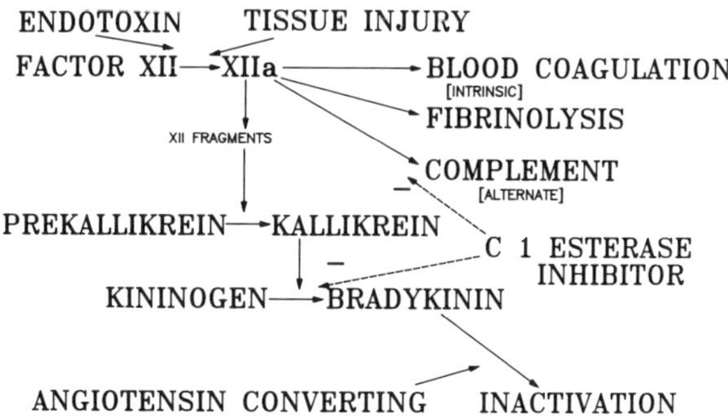

Figure 12–2. We have found these data to be as indicated above (unpublished data).

tein.[21,22] Thus, endotoxin may induce pulmonary damage through the activation of macrophages, leukocytes, and platelets. In addition, bacteria and endotoxin may produce direct effects on pulmonary vascular endothelial cells by causing them to express receptor sites for binding leukocytes[23] and thus leading to leukocyte-mediated endothelial injury. In fact, endotoxin may directly injure endothelial cells by causing the endothelial cells to produce increased amounts of oxygen-free radicals.[24]

Phagocytic Cells

POLYMORPHONUCLEAR CELLS

The traditional, postulated mechanism for ARDS has been that locally generated complement products attract polymorphonuclear (PMN) cells to the lung parenchyma where they release proteolytic enzymes and oxygen-free radicals that result in lung injury.[25–27] The demonstration that depletion of PMN cells with hydroxyurea reduces the lung injury seen with endotoxin challenge in sheep supports this hypothesis.[28,29] A similar scenario has been noted in which leukocyte depletion diminishes lung damage following inhalation injury.[30] PMN cells release oxygen-free radicals and proteolytic enzymes when activated and these are present in the injured lung and tissue fluids draining the pulmonary areas.[31–33] A role for oxygen-free radicals in the pathogenesis of ARDS is supported by studies documenting that the extent of pulmonary edema seen in animal models of ARDS is reduced by oxygen radical scavengers[25,34,35] and that there is an association between the presence of lipid peroxidation materials formed from the release of free radicals and tissue injury.[25,30] Endotoxin-induced lung injury also is associated with the release of both proteolytic enzymes and oxygen radicals by neutrophils.[32,36–39] The biologic activity of the proteolytic enzymes is increased in this situation, since there is a concomitant reduction in antiprotease activity due to its destruction by the liberated oxygen-free radicals.[32,38,39] In fact, the degree of lung injury can be decreased by the administration of an antiprotease.[40]

Although these data are strong evidence that the neutrophil is important in the pathogenesis of ARDS, recent findings contradict the role of PMN in the pathophysiology of ARDS. For example, depletion of leukocytes in goats does not affect the lung response to endotoxin,[41] whereas sheep depleted of their neutrophils actually show an exacerbated lung response to lipopolysaccharide.[42] In addition, ARDS is often seen in patients with an absence or near absence of circulating neutrophils.[43–46] Thus, the exact role of the PMN cell in ARDS requires further evaluation.

MACROPHAGES

The data relating to PMN cells have caused a renewed interest in the role of the macrophage in lung injury. The recent discovery of a pulmonary intravascular macrophage in many animal species,[47–49] including man,[50] have added to this interest. These cells may play a very important part in ARDS, especially in those situations in which there is a reduction or absence of PMNs in the circulation. The pulmonary alveolar macrophages may also be vectors of injury, since they release proteolytic enzymes and oxygen radicals.[51,52] They appear more adept at doing so than neutrophils. The macrophage is also the source of tumor necrosis factor (TNF)[53] as well as the chemotactic material LTB_4,[54] both of which may be important in triggering ARDS.

PLATELETS

The role of platelets in ARDS is not clear. They are a major source of TXA_2 and TXA_2 may contribute to microvascular fluid flux by increasing capillary hydrostatic pressure.[36,55,56] However, the lung damage in experimental models of ARDS is uneffected by depletion of these cells.[57–59] Platelets may be important in the reparative processes that take place during recovery from ARDS.[60]

LYMPHOCYTES

Few studies have linked lymphocytes with ARDS. Bohs et al.[61] reported that the pulmonary hypertensive response to endotoxin in sheep was reduced in animals depleted of their T lymphocytes, thus implicating these cells as a possible source of TXA_2. However, since lymphocytes are a source of interleukin-2, they may play a role in ARDS.[62] In addition, the C3H-HEJ mouse, which is resistant to endotoxin, apparently has defective lymphocyte function.[63]

ENDOTHELIAL CELLS

The vascular endothelial cell has historically been considered to be an entropic contributor to ARDS. These cells have been shown to contain contractile materials,[64,65] which may be important in the changes in vascular permeability that occur with ARDS.[64] Additionally, since endothelial cells can produce oxygen-free radicals in response to endotoxin administration,[66] they may play an important part in ARDS. Lastly, the triggering phenomenon that initially attracts cells to the lung may have its origin in the endothelium.

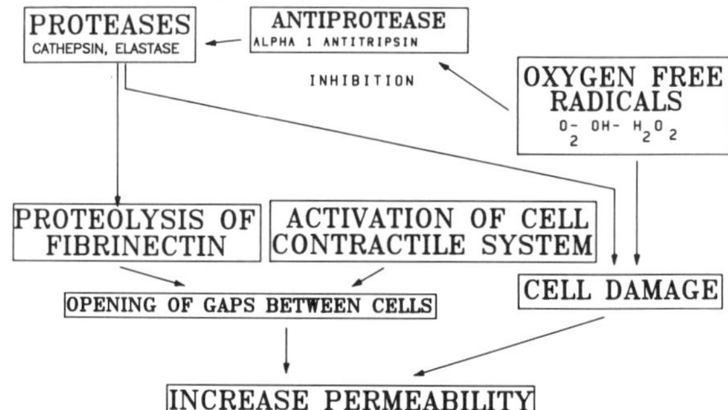

Figure 12–3. We have found these data to be as indicated above (unpublished data).

Humoral Mediators

OXYGEN-FREE RADICALS

Oxygen-free radicals (H_2O_2, $O2^-$, OH^-), can be released from a number of sources during ARDS. These are extremely reactive compounds and probably exist for only a fraction of a second. Therefore they must be released in close proximity to the lung parenchymal areas in order to produce an injury. They produce injury by a number of actions (Fig. 12–3). They induce a contraction of the fibrils within the endothelial cells causing them to become more spherical. This opens gaps between cells to allow for the passage of protein from the vascular to the interstitial compartments.[67] The radicals also inactivate alpha$_1$-antiprotease,[26] and loss of this important inhibitor allows proteases to produce damage to the parenchyma of the lung. The oxygen-free radicals also can cause the formation of chemotactic materials, thereby attracting leukocytes to the area of injury where these recruited cells may further amplify the injury in a positive feedback reaction.[68] The free radicals may likewise damage the basement membranes of the microvasculature as a result of lipid peroxidation.[69] The evidence for the involvement of oxygen radicals in ARDS is extensive. For example, plasma lipid peroxidation products are elevated following endotoxemia[70,71] and smoke inhalation,[30] whereas the pulmonary edema seen with these two forms of experimental ARDS can be blocked by the use of oxygen-free radical scavengers.[25,72]

PROTEOLYTIC ENZYMES

Proteolytic enzymes are released from phagocytic cells following their activation.[27] Elastase is elevated in the plasma of patients with ARDS,[73] whereas protease inhibitors have been shown to be effective in minimizing the extent of pulmonary damage in several forms of experimental ARDS.[40] These proteolytic enzymes, especially elastase, are very destructive to the pulmonary microvascular integrity,[74] since they destroy the endothelial cell membrane.[75] The cells are joined to one another by fibronectin, which is a preferential substrate of elastase.[72] Proteases can also destroy the endothelial cells themselves. These actions of the proteases are augmented by the release of oxygen-free radicals, since these latter materials inactivate alpha$_1$-antiprotease, the major antiprotease for serine elastase, which is released by activated PMN cells.[26]

COMPLEMENT

Evidence exists that complement is activated in association with ARDS.[18] Patients with ARDS are found to have reduced levels of native complement in their blood,[12] whereas the levels of complement breakdown products, especially C3a and C5a, are elevated.[76] However, recent studies question the importance of complement in ARDS. Animal models of ARDS in which complement was depleted using viper venom[77] showed pulmonary changes in response to bacteremia[78] and endotoxemia[76] that were similar to those seen in the intact animals. In addition to these in vivo studies, in vitro studies by Meyrick et al.[79] have shown that, although PMN cells can penetrate endothelial cell membranes in response to complement stimulation, the permeability of the membrane to albumin remained unchanged. These data support the idea that, although complement activation occurs in association with ARDS and may be important in the attraction of cells to the pulmonary areas, complement activation alone is not responsible for the activation of phagocytic cells and the release of oxygen radicals and proteolytic enzymes, which are prominent features of the syndrome.

EICOSANOIDS

The catabolites of arachidonic acid have been closely identified with ARDS. The stable metabolite of TXA_2 has been shown to be present in the plasma and lung lymph in experimental forms of ARDS[36,56] and some aspects of the syndrome can be alleviated by the administration of cyclooxygenase inhibitors.[55,79] However, this material is not elevated consistently throughout ARDS[36,80] and TXA_2 blockade has little effect on the pulmonary permeability associated with ARDS.[55] Thus, the exact importance of TXA_2 in ARDS is questionable. The leukotrienes have likewise been shown to be elevated [81–83] in patients with ARDS and in experimental models of lung injury. The potent chemotactic material LTB_4 also has been reported to be elevated during endotoxemia.[84] We have made a similar observation in experimental ARDS produced by endotoxin or inhalation injury (unpublished data). The significance of these reports becomes even more important, since the role of complement as the key mediator of lung damage has been questioned. LTB_4 may indeed be primal in initiating ARDS.

The precursor of the leukotrienes, 5-hydroxyeicosatetraenoic acid, was reported to be increased following endotoxin administration to sheep.[85,86] We have found an elevation of LTC_4 /LTD_4 in lung lymph following both inhalation injury and endotoxin challenge (unpublished data). The LTs may be responsible for some of the edema formation noted with ARDS, since these materials may induce changes in microvascular permeability.[83,87] Conclusive proof that ARDS can be blocked by agents that block the LTs or their synthesis is not yet available. There are reports in which an inhibitor of lipooxygenase, the enzyme responsible for the synthesis of LTs, was administered prior to endotoxemia and the pulmonary response was essentially unchanged.[88,89] Unfortunately, the investigators did not demonstrate that they used a pharmacologically effective dose of the blocking drug in these studies. Thus, it is still possible that agents, such as LTC$_4$/LTD$_4$ antagonists, may be effective in the treatment of ARDS, since these compounds have been shown to be effective in reducing some of the cardiopulmonary sequelae of sepsis.[90,91]

TUMOR NECROSIS FACTOR

TNF is a monokine that is released from macrophages and other monocytes in response to a number of substances, including endotoxin.[53,92] This material produces a response similar to endotoxin when injected into man.[93,94] TNF induces pulmonary edema,[95] which may be secondary to TNF-mediated activation of PMN cells. PMN cells stimulated by TNF demonstrate increased adherence, produce increased amounts of oxygen-free radicals, and have a reduced chemotactic response.[96] As a consequence, TNF has been proposed as a major triggering agent in sepsis and thus TNF is a potential cause of ARDS.[53] The development of recombinant technologies may make it possible to create antibodies to TNF and thus offer the possibility for a new concept of treatment for the syndrome.

Cellular Adherence

Studies of children deficient in leukocytic and endothelial surface materials have shown that in order for leukocytes and monocytes to damage endothelial cells they must first adhere to them.[97–99] The receptor complexes on the surface of the macrophages and leukocytes, which mediate binding of these cells to the endothelial surface are the Mac-1, LFA-1, and P150,95 binding sites.[100–102] Mac-1 and P150,95 are stored within the cells and expression is increased (up-regulated) by chemotactic factors.[99–101] Up-regulation of these receptors can be induced by TNF.[101] Similarly, there are binding sites on the endothelial cells, which are up-regulated by a number of substances, including endotoxin, TNF, and chemotactic factors.[103] Perhaps the single most important development in the treatment of ARDS will be the development of monoclonal antibodies directed against these surface-binding proteins, since by blocking or disrupting margination of leukocytes within the pulmonary circulation, tissue injury can be reduced.

Hepatic Interaction

The liver plays a very important role in ARDS. In man, under normal circumstances, 90% of the functional reticuloendothelial mass is present in the liver.[104,105] The majority of this hepatic function resides in the Kupffer cells.[107] Thus, bacteria and their toxins, which may enter the circulation especially from the gut, are removed from the circulation by the liver. The liver's position in the circulation as a bypass filter and its large blood flow make it unique in this regard. Consequently, hepatic dysfunction will enhance systemic blood levels of these organisms or their toxins. With chronic failure of the liver, this clearance function may be assumed by other organs, including the lung, which have been shown to have significant reticuloendothelial function.[47,48]

An additional function of the liver in injury and infections is to produce acute-phase reactants, which may limit lung damage. For example, the liver is the principal source of fibronectin.[106] Since reduced levels of fibronectin are associated with impaired hepatic phagocytic function, decreased circulating fibronectin levels may result in elevations of pulmonary microvascular permeability. Neihaus et al.[107] have shown that sheep depleted of fibronectin have a much more severe reaction to bacteremia than intact animals. Hepatic cells are also an important source of alpha$_1$-antiprotease,[108] which is important in the neutralization of several proteases released by activated PMN cells.[109] Some serum lipoproteins of hepatic origin may also inactivate circulating materials responsible for the toxicity of endotoxin.[110]

Thus, hepatic damage appears to be important in the development of ARDS, since the liver is both a site of synthesis and detoxification of many of the putative mediators of lung injury. Examples of endogenous mediators synthesized or detoxified by the liver are: TNF,[111,112] platelet-activating factor,[113] interleukin-1,[114] and the catabolites of arachidonic acid,[115] especially the peptides LTC$_4$ and LTD$_4$.[116,117] The injured liver may release these putative mediators into its lymphatic or venous drainage and these mediators can subsequently promote lung injury, either directly or through interactions with other mediators.[118] Also, since Kupffer cells also remove toxic materials released into the circulation,[104,119] liver dysfunction may potentiate ARDS by increasing the duration of action of these mediators.

Intestine

Acute intestinal ischemia may lead to an increase in the permeability of the gut wall to intestinal endotoxin.[120] This can lead to further lung damage as a result of the entrance of these materials into the circulation.[121] Mesenteric vasoconstriction may be important in the development of endotoxemia,[122] since intestinal vasoconstriction is associated with the translocation of endotoxin into the circulation. We have demonstrated that mesenteric vasoconstriction and translocation will occur following inhalation injury.[123,124] Thus, the intestinal track can contribute to lung damage and lung damage may contribute to intestinal dysfunction. These positive feedback loops may be important in the pathogenesis of multiple organ system failure.

Other Organs

Damage to other organ systems may cause ARDS through failure of intestinal barrier function leading to endotoxemia and bacterial translocation. For example, burn injury to the skin produces both mesenteric vasoconstriction and bacterial translocation,[123,124] whereas the release of bacteria and products of inflammation from damaged or infected tissues can lead to damage or an exacerbation of damage to the lung.[125,126] This phenomenon has been reported to occur after a myocardial infarction.[127] Damage to the heart will not only predispose the lung to injury, as a result of the elevated left atrial pressure secondary to myocardial depression, but the injured myocardium releases proteases and mediators of inflammation into the coronary sinus and thus the pulmonary circulation where they cause further damage to the lung microvasculature.[128]

The lung can likewise injure other organs. We have shown both a myocardial depression and an increase in systemic microvascular permeability following inhalation injury.[129–131] Iatrogenic injury may also result from the use of positive end-expiratory pressure (PEEP) as a treatment for ARDS. Patten et al.[132] have reported the release of mediators from the lung with the use of PEEP. Increased intrathoracic pressure, associated with PEEP or intermittent mandatory positive pressure ventilation, may also compromise blood flow to systemic organs as a result of a decrease in cardiac output and an increase in central venous pressure. The liver is especially sensitive to damage under these situations, since the portal circulation is a low pressure system.[133] The lung also has a number of other important functions that may be impaired when it is injured. Thus, ARDS may lead to the failure of other organ systems. For example, the angiotensin-converting enzyme is present on the endothelial surface of the pulmonary vasculature.[134] This enzyme is important in the conversion of angiotensin I to II[135] and the degradation of bradykinin.[136] These functions may not be carried out in ARDS, since this enzyme may be destroyed. Thus, in ARDS electrolyte imbalance and systemic microvascular permeability changes may occur.

Diagnosis

ARDS is a clinical syndrome that follows trauma, infection, acid aspiration, near drowning, or septic shower by as much as 24 hours. It is characterized by the onset of tachypnea and tachycardia in the absence of hypoxemia or acidosis and is associated with disorientation or agitation (Table 12–1). In the early stages, chest radiographs will be normal. Subsequently, perivascular edema develops that proceeds to diffuse intra-alveolar edema. That is, early chest radiographs demonstrate very subtle increases in interstitial markings, which proceed to a diffuse whiting of the lung fields over a 4- to 5-day period. Kunkel et al.[137] have described a clinically useful system for grading the chest radiographic findings that correlates extremely well with the amount of pulmonary extravascular fluid (Figs. 12–4 through 12–8). Early intervention with the institution of definitive therapy should be initiated as soon as grade 1 chest radiographic findings are identified.

The primary differential diagnosis is between ARDS and hydrostatic pulmonary edema caused by cardiac failure or fluid overload. Causes of cardiac failure include infarction, ischemia, pericardial effusion, or myocardial depression. Physical examination focusing on cardiac failure looks for neck vein distention with the patient elevated at 30°, bibasilar rales, a new third or fourth heart sound, and liver enlargement. An electrocardiogram should be obtained to determine whether or not myocardial ischemia or infarction has occurred. The importance of an early accurate differentiation between ARDS and pump failure almost always requires institution of invasive Swan-Ganz catheter monitoring (Table 12–5). In cases of hydrostatic pulmonary edema, left-sided cardiac filling pressures, as determined by catheter wedge measurements, will be elevated.

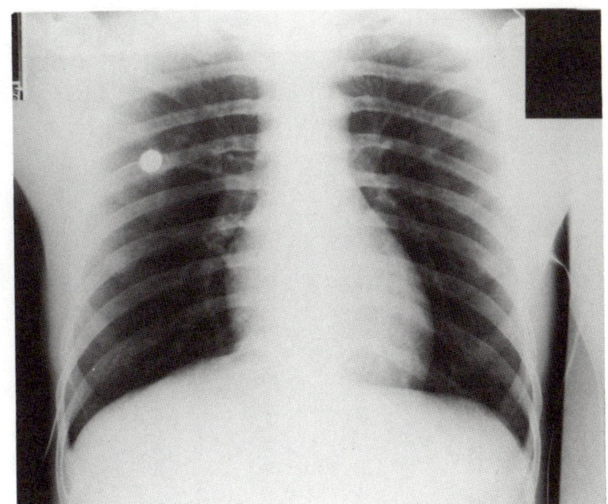

Figure 12–4. Normal chest radiograph. Extravascular lung water (EVLM) 3 to 7 ml/kg. Grade 0.

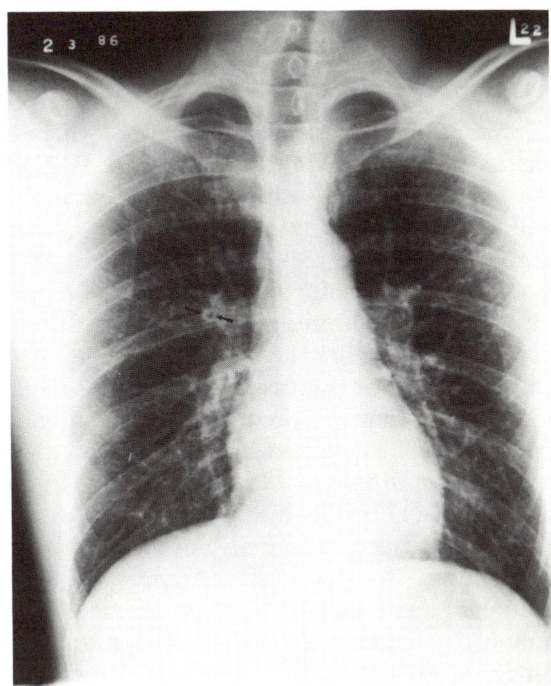

Figure 12–5. Peribronchial cuffing (indicated by arrows). EVLM, 6 to 9 ml/kg. Grade 1.

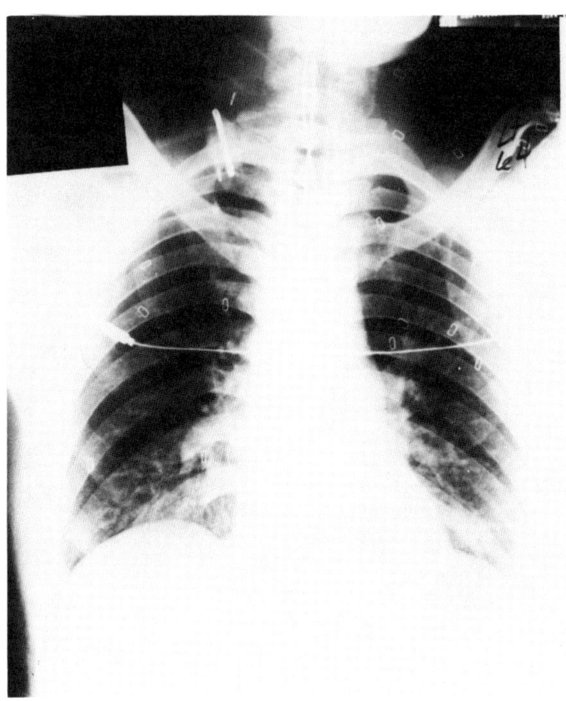

Figure 12–6.   Mild interstitial edema.
EVLM 8 to 12 ml/kg. Grade 2.

Cardiac output in cases of pump failure will be lower than normal and peripheral vascular resistance will be elevated. In ARDS, associated with sepsis or endotoxemia, the cardiac output will be high and the peripheral vascular resistance will be low. Pure fluid overload may occur from overadministration of fluid during complicated operative procedures or due to the development of acute renal failure. In both these situations, wedge pressures will be elevated, but cardiac output and peripheral vascular resistance will be closer to normal. Urinary to plasma ratios of osmolality, creatinine, urine to blood urea nitrogen ratio, and creatinine clearance will identify the development of renal failure. Pulmonary edema can also occur from cerebral edema with normal hemodynamics; this should be suspected in cases of head injury, tumor, or stroke.

As the syndrome of ARDS progresses, frequent and intermittent obstruction of the airways results in areas of atelectasis and emphysema. Alveoli collapse and shunting occurs as a result of pulmonary blood flow to unventilated areas of the lung. The result is hypoxemia and dyspnea with an arterial oxygen saturation of less than 80 mmHg on a fractional inspired oxygen (FiO_2) of 0.6 or an arterial oxygen tension (PaO_2) to FiO_2 ratio of less than 100. As the lungs become progressively stiffer, the amount of pressure required to inflate them increases from 25 to approximately 50 ml/cm H_2O. Between 5 and 13 days from the onset

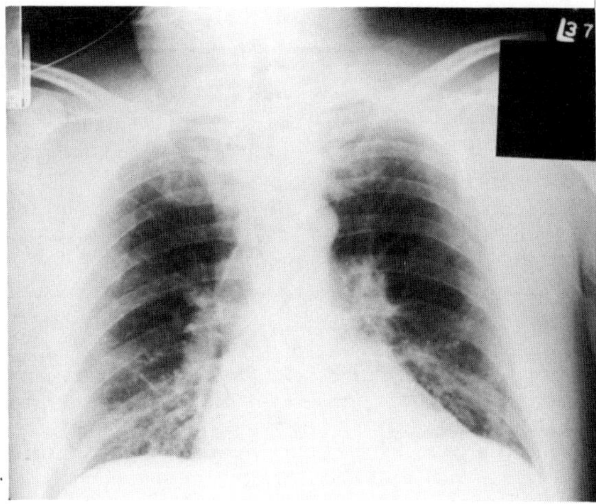

Figure 12–7. Severe interstitial edema. EVLM 12 to 18 ml/kg. Grade 3.

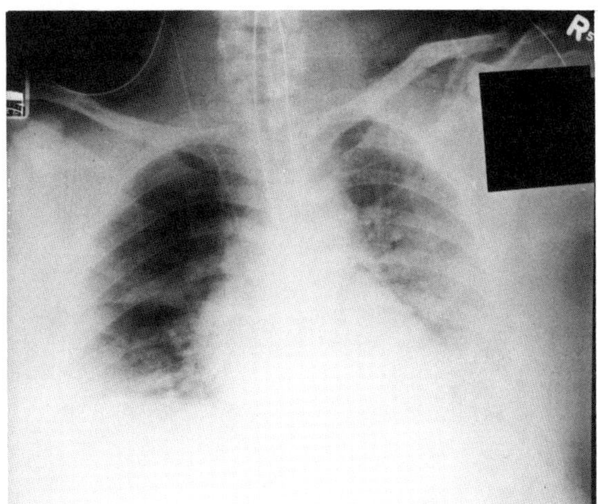

Figure 12–8. Alveolar infiltrates. EVLM 16 to 22 ml/kg. Grade 4.

of the initial episode, bronchopneumonia usually develops and complicates therapy. Initially, these pneumonias are caused by staphylococcal organisms, but later gram-positive organisms are replaced by gram-negative bacteria. Chest radiographic changes at this point frequently reveal definitive pneumonic infiltrates (Fig. 12–9).

Clinical Treatment

Diagnosis and treatment are directed toward definitive management of the underlying pathologic entity. For example, drainage of an abscess is the most rewarding of all treatments for a patient with ARDS.

Table 12–5   Changes in Cardiac Index (CI), Pulmonary Arterial (PAP) and Pulmonary Arterial Wedge Pressure (PWP)*

	Normal	*Septic*	*Heart Failure*	*Volume Overload*
CI 1/min/m^2	3(2–5)†	8(4–10)	1.5(1–3)	4(3–6)
PWP mmHg	9(3–12)	10(3–14)	25 (13–30)	11(10–14)
PAP mmHg	18(16–20)	20(18–22)	27 (16–30)	18(17–20)
MAP mmHg	93(80–100)	60(50–90)	60 (50–80)	96(80–100)
SVR dyne-sec/cm^5/m^2	2480	600	3200	1920

*The patient with sepsis usually demonstrates a very high cardiac output with only a slight elevation of pulmonary wedge pressure. This latter is dependent on the degree of resuscitation. The opposite is true in the patients with congestive heart failure. In this case, the cardiac output is low and the wedge pressure is high. Although the arterial pressure (MAP) is reduced in both situations, the patient with sepsis is hypotensive as a result of a decreased vascular resistance (SVR). In a patient with fluid overload there is a moderate increase in cardiac output and a reduced vascular resistance. ARDS is most commonly seen in the patient with sepsis and is a rare occurrence in the patient in congestive heart failure. The pulmonary edema in these patients is secondary to an increased pulmonary microvascular hydrostatic pressure.

†Average (range).

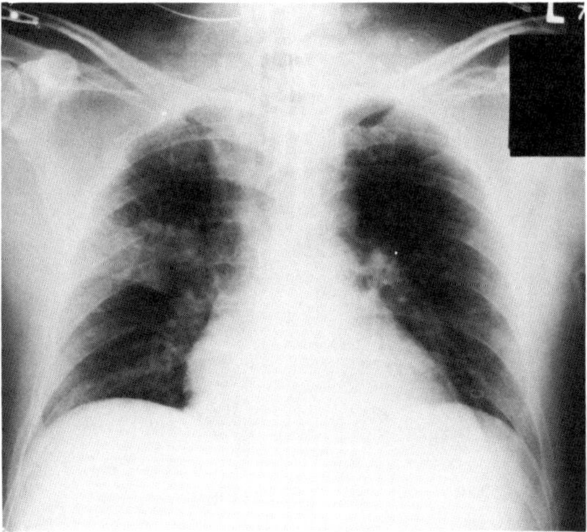

Figure 12–9. Right upper lobe pneumonia.

Currently, other care is supportive, since pharmacologic manipulations of the previously described mediators that increase pulmonary microvascular permeability have not been demonstrated to be clinically efficacious. Steroids have clearly been demonstrated to be of no use.[8]

Ventilatory support becomes necessary when the PaO_2 to FiO_2 ratio is less than 200, when an FiO_2 of 0.4 cannot maintain an arterial oxygen level of greater than 80, when a 50% decrease in lung compliance occurs, or when the respiratory rate exceeds 30 to 40 breaths/min. Another indication for ventilatory support is when the resting minute ventilation becomes less than 10 L/min and the maximum voluntary ventilation falls below a safe level of 20 L/min ventilation because of the obligatory tachypnea as the patient tires. ARDS is characterized by decreased thoracic compliance as the lung becomes stiffened by excess extravascular pulmonary water, but this increase in extravascular water cannot be easily measured until after intubation has been successfully completed.

Treatment consists of intubation at the first hint of respiratory distress. Initially, an inspired oxygen concentration of greater than 0.6 may be required to reverse arterial hypoxia. The debate over performing a tracheostomy versus prolonged nasotracheal intubation in this setting has not been scientifically resolved. However, the great majority of centers initially use nasotracheal intubation with low pressure endotracheal tubes to prevent complications such as tracheoesophageal fistula or late tracheal stenosis, which occur more frequently with high pressure cuffed tubes. Some centers perform tracheostomies after 2 to 3 weeks of nasotracheal intubation if further prolonged ventilatory support is envisioned.

Usual ventilator settings are a tidal volume of 10 to 15 ml/kg or more precisely (height [cm] $\times$ 10) $-$ 800 for men and (height[cm] $\times$ 10) $-$ 900 for women. The initial respiratory rate is set at 10 and varied to ensure adequate ventilation based on the arterial carbon dioxide tension. The FiO_2 is initially established at 100% and PEEP at 5 to 7.5 cm H_2O. The inspiratory to expiratory ratio is kept at less than 1:1 to prevent retention of air in the lung. Arterial blood gasses are measured every 15 minutes to adjust the ventilator until a return to normal values is attained. The basic concept is to intervene maximally and then gradually pull back once a stable level of support has been achieved. Blood gasses are obtained every 6 hours plus 15 minutes after any ventilator change or during any episode of distress.

PEEP or continuous positive airway pressure (CPAP) are the mainstay of treatment of the syndrome. They are used to decrease alveolar collapse. Both techniques have been shown to restore the reduced levels of alveolar volume or functional residual capacity to normal. By opening up collapsed alveoli and restoring the functional residual capacity of the lung to normal, pulmonary compliance is improved and the work of breathing is reduced. PEEP is increased to restore ventilation to perfusion ratios to more normal levels and to allow the FiO_2 to be maintained at levels of 0.5 or less. In this way, PEEP reduces the incidence of oxygen toxicity associated with high FiO_2 values while maintaining a PaO_2 of 60 mmHg. The indications for starting PEEP or CPAP include hypoxemia with a PaO_2 of less than 60 torr with an FiO_2 greater than 0.5 or when the calculated shunt fraction is greater than 20%. PEEP is also used prophylactically for hydrostatic pulmonary edema, congestive heart failure, flail chest, aspiration of gastric contents, smoke inhalation injury, and other etiologies that are associated with ARDS.

The best level of PEEP beyond the usual starting point of 5 to 7.5 cm H_2O has been hotly debated, but is usually agreed to be that level of PEEP that allows maintenance of an adequate arterial oxygen saturation when ventilating with an FiO_2 of less than 0.5. Cardiac output monitoring should be undertaken and PEEP increased in 2 to 3 cm H_2O increments (Table 12–5). If cardiac output falls before a nontoxic FiO_2 can be achieved by increasing PEEP, the filling pressure of the ventricle should be increased by the administration of balanced salt solution or a combination of fluid administration and intropic agents, such as dopamine or dobutamine. These techniques may allow a further increase in PEEP without compromising cardiac output. It is important to remember that the ultimate goal is to improve oxygen delivery to the peripheral tissues and that oxygen delivery is determined by the product of the arterial oxygen content and the cardiac output. Most clinicians will also optimize hematocrit around 30%.

Fluid resuscitation must be titrated at all times to maintain cardiac output, since a decrease in pulmonary blood flow will cause worsening of microvascular permeability changes due to a build-up of toxic mediators. The common practice of running patients with ARDS dry must be assiduously avoided.[138] Strikingly large amounts of fluid are required for otherwise similar injuries when the lung is injured.[8] Fluid overload that would superimpose a hydrostatic pulmonary edema on the permeability lesion must be avoided, making Swan-Ganz monitoring advisable in most circumstances.

Antibiotics are only given for documented infections based on positive chest radiographic findings and the results of deep bronchial brush cultures. Many investigators studying patients with ARDS with concurrent pneumonias report that tracheal cultures alone are inadequate to diagnose the causative pathogens of pneumonias apparent on chest radiographs. These investigators advocate deep brush bronchoscopy cultures or even skinny needle lung biopsy cultures in rare cases. Problems with pneumothorax may occur when this technique is used.

Judicious antimicrobial treatment of pulmonary or unlocalizable infectious sources are the most important treatment modalities in the syndrome, after surgical drainage of localized abscesses or fixation of unstable fractures. Since eradication of ongoing bacteremia or endotoxemia may represent the only possibility for survival in some patients, daily attempts at identifying potential sources of infection must be made. Quantitative wound or urine cultures can be of particular help. Broad-spectrum, systemic antimicrobials are administered if signs of sepsis are present even in the absence of an identifiable source. A patient is treated for sepsis if four of the following criteria are observed: (1) temperature less than 36.5°C or greater than 38.5°C; (2) respiratory rate greater than 30 breaths/min; (3) serum glucose greater than 150 mg/dl^{-1}; (4) platelet count less than 1×10^5; (5) white blood cells greater than 15×10^3 or less than 5×10^3; (6) volume of nasogastric residual greater than 200 ml/hr$^-$1 (or ileus on radiographs; (7) pneumonia or urine or wound culture with greater than 10^5 bacteria/ml or other identifiable source of infection. When specific organisms are not found, vancomycin, an aminoglycoside, and clindamycin or vancomycin, an aminoglycoside, and metronidazole are instituted presumptively.

Nasotracheal suctioning at frequent intervals and selective bronchoscopic drainage of inspissated materials are standard practice when clinically indicated by chest radiographic findings. Daily chest radiographs are required. Inspired air must be humidified to prevent inspissation of secretions. Mucolytic agents such as N-acetylcysteine have been used frequently.

Every 2 hours specially trained ventilatory support service personnel and nurses should perform nasotracheal suction and lavage with small quantities of normal saline in ventilator-dependent patients. They should roll the patient from side to side and have him assume an erect position at least once every 2 hours. Chest physiotherapy consisting of physical percussion and utilization of vibrators is also suggested. Due to the nature of the pathologic changes of ARDS, which is characterized by intermittent areas of atelectasis, pneumothorax is a frequent complication. Whenever a pneumothorax is suspected, a large bore needle should be inserted immediately into the side in question to allow decompression. When chest radiographic confirmation is available, chest tubes are placed under stable conditions.

Nasogastric tubes are placed routinely to maintain decompression of the gastrointestinal tract, to deliver hourly enteral feedings, to measure gastric residuals, and to prevent gastric dilation, which can result in aspiration pneumonitis and secondary pneumonia. Gastric residuals are measured every hour to assure that gastric distension is not occurring. Antacid prophylaxis through the nasogastric tube should be guided by hourly pH measurements. It should be noted that some evidence indicates that neutralization of gastric pH allows bacteria to proliferate in the stomach that would normally be destroyed. Clinical trials comparing sucralfate, a nonacid-reducing agent, against traditional pH lowering techniques are under way.

Sedation is necessary to prevent dislodgement of endotracheal tubes or their blockage, which are a primary cause of death. However, overdosing with narcotics leads to a decrease of gastrointestinal motility, which can contribute to the lower gastrointestinal ileus and thus exacerbate pulmonary failure. Narcotics are rarely indicated in children, since their use as sedatives in this situation produces an ileus that almost always prevents adequate enteral feeding. Paralyzing patients is rarely required to improve compliance. However, caution should be taken when paralyzing patients, since if the tube becomes obstructed or dislodged and the patient cannot breath spontaneously, a cardiopulmonary arrest is likely. Succinylcholine is specifically contraindicated in burn patients and those with neurologic trauma because this depolarizing agent can produce massive hyperkalemia. Sedation with antianxiety medications, such as diazepam, hypnotics, or other relaxation therapies are of paramount importance. Bronchodilators are of assistance when bronchoconstriction occurs. Maintenance of uninterrupted periods of sleep markedly improves ventilatory management.

Under fortunate circumstances, the patient's condition will gradually improve. He will have intact reflexes, circulatory stability, no excessive pulmonary secretions, and the criteria for which intubation was started will have been reversed. In this circumstance, a gradual weaning from the respirator becomes possible. If nutritional support and intermittent exercise of the respiratory system as well as other body muscles has been achieved, extubation may usually be achieved when the following criteria are met: an FiO_2 of 0.4 provides adequate arterial oxygenation, spontaneous tidal volume is greater than 5 ml/kg, vital capacity is greater than 10 ml/kg, maximum inspiratory force is at least -30 cm H_2O pressure, upper airway protective reflexes are present, and the condition requiring intubation has been corrected. Maintenance of positive nitrogen balance minimizes muscle wasting and is an important factor in the patient's ability to tolerate the work of breathing following extubation.

Currently, mortality from ARDS remains high. It is hoped that survival can be increased by the development of new pharmacologic agents that correct the basic pathophysiologic processes leading to ARDS.

References

1. Seidenfeld JJ, Pohl DF, Bell RC, Harris GD, Johanson WG Jr. Incidence, site, and outcome of infections in patients with the adult respiratory distress syndrome. Am Rev Respir Dis 1986;134:12–16.
2. Carrico CJ, Meakins JL, Marshall JC, Fry D, Maier RV. Multiple-organ-failure syndrome. Arch Surg 1986;121:196–208.
3. Lauwers LF, Rosseel P, Roelants A, Beeckman C, Baute L. A retrospective study of 130 consecutive multiple trauma patients in an intensive care unit. Intensive Care Med 1986;12:296–301.
4. el Kassimi FA, Al-Mashhadani S, Abdullah AK, Akhtar J. Adult respiratory distress syndrome and disseminated intravascular coagulation complicating heat stroke. Chest 1986;90:571–574.
5. Stothert JC, Winn R, Nadir B, Hildebrandt J, Carrico CJ. Acid aspiration: mechanism of injury in awake goats. Surg Forum 1982;32:313–315.
6. Winn R, Nadir B, Stothert JC, Hildebrandt J. Lung fluid balance and gas exchange following acid aspiration in awake goats. J Appl Physiol 1984;56:979–985.
7. Traber DL, Herndon DN. Pathophysiology of smoke inhalation. In Haponik EF, Munster AM (eds): Respiratory sequelae of burns. New York: McGraw Hill, chapter 4. 1990.
8. Herndon DN, Barrow, RE, Traber DL, Rutan TC, Rutan RL, Abston S. Extravascular lung water changes following smoke inhalation and massive burn injury. Surgery 1987;102:341–349.
9. Coridis DT, Ishiyama M, Woodruff PWH, Fine J. Role of the intestinal flora in clearance and detoxification of circulating endotoxin. J Reticuloendothel Soc 1972;14:513–521.
10. Traber DL. Endotoxin: the causative factor of mediator release during sepsis. Prog Clin Biol Res 1987;236A:377–392.
11. Kalter ES, van Dijk WC, Timmermann A, Verhoef J, Bouma BN. Activation of purified human plasma prekallikrein triggered by cell wall fractions of Escherichia coli and Staphylococcus aureus. J Infect Dis 1983;148:682–691.
12. Heidman M. Complement activation in vitro induced by endotoxin and injured tissue. J Surg Res 1979;26:670–673.
13. Van der Graaf F, Keus FJA, Vlooswijk RAA, Bouma BN. The contact activation mechanism in human plasma: activation induced by dextran sulfate. Blood 1982;59:1225–1222.
14. Kluft C. Determination of prekallikrein in human plasma: optimal conditions for activating prekallikrein. J Lab Clin Med 1978;91:645–653.
15. Schachter M, Barton S. Kallikreins (kininogenases) and kinins. In Cahill G Jr, deGroot LJ (eds): Endocrinology: metabolic basis of clinical practice. New York: Grune & Stratton, 1979.
16. Carvalho AC, DeMarinis S, Scott CF, Silver LD, Schmaier AH, Colman RW. Activation of the contact system of plasma proteolysis in the adult respiratory distress syndrome. J Lab Clin Med 1988;112:270–277.
17. Godin DV, Wright JM, Tuchek JM, Scudamore CH. Plasma lysosomal enzymes in experimental and clinical endotoxemia. Clin Invest Med 1983;6:319–325.
18. Aasen AO, Mellbye OJ, Ohlsson K. Complement activation during subsequent stages of canine endotoxin shock. Scand J Immunol 1986;8:509–513.
19. Weigelt JA, Chenoweth DE, Borman KR, Norcross JF. Complement and the severity of pulmonary failure. J Trauma 1988;28:1013–1019.
20. Heideman M, Bengtson A. Complement activity in shock. Prog Clin Biol Res 1987;236A:3–9.
21. Letts LG. Leukotrienes: role in cardiovascular physiology. (Review.) Cardiovasc Clin 1987;18:101–113.
22. Samuelsson B. Leukotrienes: mediators of immediate hypersensitivity reactions and inflammation. Science 1983;220:568–575.
23. Schleimer RP, Rutledge BK. Cultured human vascular endothelial cells acquire adhesiveness for neutrophils after stimulation with interleukin 1, endotoxin, and tumor-promoting phorbol diesters. J Immunol 1986;136:649–654.

24. Shiki Y, Meyrick BO, Brigham KL, Burr IM. Endotoxin increases superoxide dismutase in cultured bovine pulmonary endothelial cells. Am J Physiol 1987;252:C436–440.
25. Seekamp A, Lalonde C, Zhu D, Demling R. Catalase prevents prostanoid release and lung lipid peroxidation after endotoxemia in sheep. J Appl Physiol 1988;65:1210–1216.
26. Carp G, Janoff A. In vitro suppression of serum elastase-inhibitory capacity by reactive oxygen species generated by phagocytizing polymorphonuclear leukocytes. J Clin Invest 1979;63:793–801.
27. Janoff A, White R, Carp H, Harel S, Dearing R, Lee D. Lung injury induced by leukocytic proteases. Am J Pathol 1979; 97:111–136.
28. Hinson JM Jr, Hutchinson AA, Ogletree ML, Brigham KL, Snapper JR. Effect of granulocyte depletion on altered lung mechanics after endotoxemia in sheep. J Apply Physiol 1983;55:92–99.
29. Heflin AC, Brigham KL. Prevention by granulocyte depletion on altered lung mechanics after endotoxemia in sheep. J Clin Invest 1981;68:1253.
30. Basadre JO, Sugi K, Traber DL, Traber LD, Neihaus GD, Herndon DN. The effect of leukocyte depletion on smoke inhalation injury in sheep. Surgery 1988;104:208–215.
31. Meyrick B, Brigham KL. Acute effects of *Escherichia coli* endotoxin on the pulmonary vascular responses to endotoxin in unanesthetized sheep. Structure : functional relationship. Lab Invest 1983;48:458–470.
32. Traber DL, Herndon DN, Stein MD. Traber LD. Flynn JT, Niehaus GD. The pulmonary lesion of smoke inhalation in an ovine model. Circ Shock 1986;18:311–323.
33. Herndon DN, Traber LD, Linares H, Flynn JT, Niehaus G, Kramer G, Traber DL. Etiology of the pulmonary pathophysiology associated with inhalation injury. Resuscitation 1986;14:43–59.
34. Bernard GR, Lucht WD, Neidermeyer ME, Snapper JR, Ogletree ML, Brigham KL. Effect on n-acetylcysteine on the pulmonary function. J Clin Invest 1984;73:1772–1784.
35. Kimura R, Mlcak R, Richardson J, Desai M, Herndon D, Traber L, Traber D. Treatment of smoke-induced pulmonary injury with nebulized dimethylsulfoxide. Circ Shock 1988;25:333–341.
36. Demling RH, Smith M, Gunther R, Flynn JT, Gee MH. Pulmonary injury and prostaglandin production during endotoxemia in conscious sheep. Am J Physiol 1981;240:H348–H353.
37. Traber DL, Schlag G, Redl H, Traber LD. Pulmonary edema and compliance changes following smoke inhalation. J Burn Care Rehabil 1985;6:490–494.
38. Herndon DN, Traber DL, Niehaus GD, Linares HA, Traber LD. The pathophysiology of smoke inhalation injury in a sheep model. J Trauma 1984;24:1044–1051.
39. Kimura R, Traber LD, Herndon DN, Linares HA, Lubbesmeyer HJ, Traber DL. Increasing duration of smoke exposure induces severe lung injury in sheep. J Appl Physiol 1988;64:1107–1113.
40. Traber DL, Adams T Jr, Sziebert L, Traber LD. Effect of a proteolytic enzyme inhibitor on the cardiopulmonary response to endotoxin. Resuscitation 1986;14:91–104.
41. Winn R, Mauder R, Harlan J. Neutrophils depletion does not prevent lung edema following endotoxin infusion in goats. J Appl Physiol 1986;62:116–121.
42. Basadre JO, Singh H, Herndon DN, Stothert J, Traber LD, Horn K, LeBlanc K, Flynn JT, Traber DL. Effect of antibody mediated neutropenia on the cardiopulmonary response to endotoxemia. J Surg Res 1988;45:266–275.
43. Maunder RJ, Hackman RC, Riff E, Albert RK, Springmeyer SC. Occurrence of the adult respiratory distress syndrome in neutropenic patients. Am Rev Respir Dis 1986;133:313–316.
44. Laufe MD, Simon RH, Flint A, Keller JB. Adult respiratory distress syndrome in neutropenic patients. Am J Med 1986;80:1022–1026.
45. Ognibene FP, Martin SE, Parker MM, Schlesinger T, Roach P, Burch C, et al. Adult respiratory distress syndrome in patients with severe neutropenia. N Engl J Med 1986;315:547–551.
46. Braude S, Krausz T, Apperley J, Goldman JM, Royston D. Adult respiratory distress syndrome after allogenic bone-marrow transplantation: evidence for a neutrophil-independent mechanism. Lancet 1985;1:1239–1242.
47. Warner AE, Brain JD. Intravascular pulmonary macrophages: a novel cell removes particles from blood. Am J Physiol 1986;250:R728–R732.
48. Warner AE, Barry BE, Brain JD. Pulmonary intravascular macrophages in sheep: morphology and function of a model constituent of the mononuclear phagocyte system. Lab Invest 1986;55:276–288.
49. Dehring DJ, Wismar BL. Animal models of sepsis. In Staub NC (ed): Biology of the pulmonary intravascular macrophages. Mt. Kisco, New York: Futura, 1989.
50. Dehring DJ, Wismar BL. Intravascular macrophages in pulmonary capillaries of man. Am Rev Respir Dis 1989;139:1027–1029.

51. McLeish KR, Stelzer GT, Wallace JH. Regulation of oxygen radical release from murine peritoneal macrophages by pharmacologic doses of PGE2. Free Radic Biol Med 1987;3:15–20.
52. Winkler GC. Pulmonary intravascular macrophages in domestic animal species: review of structural and functional properties. Am J Anat 1988;181:217–234.
53. Dinarello CA, Mier JW. Current concepts—lymphokines. N Engl J Med 1987;317:940–945.
54. Fels AO, Powlowski NA, Cramer EB, King TK, Cohn ZA, Scott WA: Human alveolar macrophages produce leukotriene B$_4$. Proc Natl Acad Sci USA 1982;79:7866–7870.
55. Adams T Jr, Traber DL. The effects of prostaglandins synthetase inhibition on the cardiopulmonary response to endotoxin in sheep. Circ Shock 1982;9:681–689.
56. Huttemeier PC, Watkins WD, Peterson MB, Zapol WM. Acute pulmonary hypertension and lung thromboxane release after endotoxin. Circ Res 1984;50:688–694.
57. Myrvold HE, Brandberg A, Lindquist O, Busch C, Lewis DH. Hemodynamic changes in thrombocytopenic dogs after endotoxin. Eur Surg Res 1976;8:124–125.
58. From AHL, Fong JSC, Chiu T, Good RA. Role of platelets in the pathogenesis of canine endotoxin shock. Infect Immun 1976;13:1591–1594.
59. Brindenbaugh GA, Flynn JT, Lefer AM. Effect of induced thrombocytopenia in experimental circulatory shock. Physiologist 1976;19:138.
60. Lo SK, Burhop KE, Kaplan JE, Malik B. Role of platelets in maintenance of pulmonary vascular permeability to protein. Am J Physiol 1988;254:H763–H771.
61. Bohs CT, Fish JC, Miller TH, Traber DL. Pulmonary vascular response to endotoxin in normal and lymphocyte depleted sheep. Circ Shock 1979;6:13–21.
62. Reuben JM, Hersh EM, Murray JL, Munn CG, Mehta SR, Mansell PW. IL-2 production and response in vitro by the leukocytes of patients with acquired immune deficiency syndrome. Lymphokine Res 1985;4:103–116.
63. Gurtler LG, Rank WR. Genetic differences between endotoxin-sensitive and resistant C3 H mice. Z Immunitaetsforsch 1976;151:420–429.
64. Svensjo E, Grega GJ. Evidence for endothelial cell-mediated regulation of macromolecular permeability by postcapillary venules. Fed Proc 1986;45:89–95.
65. Miller FN, Sims DE: Contractile elements in the regulation of macromolecular permeability. Fed Proc 1986;45:84–88.
66. Brigham KL, Meyrick B, Berry LC Jr, Repine JE. Antioxidants protect cultured bovine lung endothelial cells from injury by endotoxin. J Appl Physiol 1987;63:840–850.
67. Grega GJ, Adamski SW, Dobbins DE. Physiological and pharmacological evidence for the regulation of permeability. Fed Proc 1986;45:96–100.
68. Petrone WF, English DK, Wong K, McCord JM. Free radicals and inflammation: superoxide-dependent activation of a neutrophil chemotactic factor in plasma. Proc Natl Acad Sci USA 1980;77:1159–1163.
69. Sakaguchi S, Kanda N, Hsu C, Sakaguchi O. Lipid peroxide formation and membrane damage in endotoxin-poisoned mice. Microbiol Immunol 1981;25:229–244.
70. Demling R, Lalonde C, Jin LJ, Ryan P, Fox R. Endotoxemia causes increased lung tissue lipid peroxidation in unanesthetized sheep. J Appl Physiol 1986;60:2094–2100.
71. Demling RH, Lalonde C, Ryan P, Zhu D, Liu Y. Endotoxemia produces an increase in arterial but not venous lipid peroxides in the adult sheep. J Appl Physiol 1988;64:592–598.
72. Brown M, Desai M, Traber LD, Herndon DN, Traber DL. Dimethylsulfoxide with heparin in the treatment of smoke inhalation injury. J Burn Care Rehabil 1988;9:22–25.
73. Cochrane CG, Stragg R, Revak SD. Pathogenesis of the adult respiratory distress syndrome. J Clin Invest 1983;71:754–761.
74. Janoff A. Elastases and emphysema: current assessment of the proteases-antiprotease hypothesis. Am Rev Respir Dis 1985;132:417–433.
75. Janoff A, Weissmann G, Zweifach B, Thomas L. Pathogenesis of experimental shock IV. Studies on lysosomes in normal and tolerant animals subjected to lethal trauma and endotoxemia. J Exp Med 1962;116:451–466.
76. Heideman M, Kauser F, Gelin LE. Complement activation early in endotoxin shock. J Surg Res 1979;26:74–78.
77. Huttemeier PC, Berry D, Bloch KJ, Watkins WD, Zapol WM. Pulmonary vasoconstriction and profound leukopenia in two sheep experimental models: effects of complement depletion. Chest 1983;83:24S–25S.
78. Dehring DJ, Steinberg SM, Wismar BL, Lowery BD, Carey LC, Cloutier CT. Complement depletion in a porcine model of septic acute respiratory disease. J Trauma 1987;27:615–625.
79. Meyrick B, Hoffman LH, Brigham KL. Chemotaxis of granulocytes across bovine pulmonary study intimal explants without endothelial cell injury. Tissue Cell 1984;16:1–16.

80. Godsoe A, Kimura R, Herndon D, Flynn JT, Schlag G, Traber L, Traber D. Cardiopulmonary changes with intermittent endotoxin administration in sheep. Circ Shock 1988;25:61–74.
81. Ratnoff WD, Matthay MA, Wong MY, Ito Y, Vu KH, Weiner-Kronish J, Goetzl EJ. Sulfido-peptide-leukotriene peptidases in pulmonary edema fluid from patients with the adult respiratory distress syndrome. J Clin Immunol 1988;8:250–258.
82. Shapiro JM, Mihm FG, Trudell JR, Stevens JR, Feeley TW. Leukotriene D_4 increases extravascular lung water in the dog. Circ Shock 1987;21:121–128.
83. Knoller J, Schonfeld W, Joka T, Sturm J, Konig W. Generation of leukotrienes in polytraumatic patients with adult respiratory distress syndrome (ARDS). Prog Clin Biol Res 1987;236:311–316.
84. Fujimoto K, Kobayashi T. The role of leukotriene B_4 in endotoxin-induced lung injury in unanesthetized sheep. Respir Physiol 1988;71:259–268.
85. Ogletree M, Oates J, Brigham KL, Hubbard W. Evidence of pulmonary release of 5-hydroxyeicosatetraenonic acid (5-HETE) during endotoxemia in sheep. Prostaglandins 1982;23:459–468.
86. Ogletree M, Begley C, King G, Brigham KL. Influence of steroidal and nonsteroidal antiinflammatory agents on accumulation of arachidonic acid metabolites in plasma and lung lymph after endotoxemia in awake sheep. Measurements of prostacyclin and thromboxane metabolites and 12-HETE. Am Rev Respir Dis 1986;133:55–61.
87. Noonan TC, Asrar BM. Pulmonary vascular response to leukotriene D_4 in unanesthetized sheep: role of thromboxane. J Appl Physiol 1986;60:765–769.
88. Zadoff AD, Kobayashi T, Brigham KL, Newman JH. Diethylcarbamazine on pulmonary vascular response to endotoxin in awake sheep. J Appl Physiol 1986;60:1380–1385.
89. Morel DR, Huttemeier PC, Skoskiewicz MJ, Nguyenduy T, Melvin C, Robinson DR, Zapol WM. Dose-dependent effects of a pyridoquinazoline thromboxane synthetase inhibitor on arachidonic acid metabolites and hemodynamics during E. coli endotoxemia in anesthetized sheep. Prostaglandins 1987;33:879–902.
90. Smith EF, Kinter LB, Jugus M, Wasserman RD, Eckardt RD, Newton JF. Beneficial effects of the peptidoleukotriene receptor antagonist, SK&F 104353, on the responses to experimental endotoxemia in the conscious rat. Circ Shock 1988;25:21–31.
91. Etemadi AR, Tempel GE, Farah BA, Wise WC, Halushka PV, Cook JA. Beneficial effects of a leukotriene antagonist on endotoxin-induced acute hemodynamic alterations. Circ Shock 1987;22:55–63.
92. Tabor DR, Burchett SK, Jacobs RF. Enhanced production of monokines by canine alveolar macrophages in response to endotoxin-induced shock. Proc Soc Exp Biol Med 1988;187:408–415.
93. Michie HR, Spriggs DR, Manogue KR, Sherman ML, Revhaug A, O'Dwyer ST, Arthur K, Dinarello CA, Cerami A, Wolff SM, Kufe DW, Wilmore DW. Tumor necrosis factor and endotoxin induce similar metabolic responses in human beings. Surgery 1988;104:280–286.
94. Michie HR, Mangue KR, Spriggs DR, Revhaug A, O'Dwyer S, Dinarello CA, Cerami A, Wolff SM, Wilmore DW. Detection of circulating tumor necrosis factor after endotoxin administration. N Engl J Med 1988;318:1481–1486.
95. Gashill HV. Continuous infusion of tumor necrosis factor: mechanisms of toxicity in the rat. J Surg Res 1988;44:664–671.
96. Warren JS, Kunkel SL, Cunningham TW, Johnson KJ, Ward PA. Macrophage-derived cytokines amplify immune complex-triggered responses by rat alveolar macrophages. Am J Pathol 1988;130:489–495.
97. van-Noesel C, Miedema F, Brouwer M, de-Rie MA, Aadren LA, van-Lier RA. Regulatory properties of LFA-1 alpha and beta chains in human T-lymphocyte activation. Nature 1988;333:850–852.
98. Anderson DC, Springer TA. Leukocyte adhesion deficiency: an inherited defect in the Mac-1, LFA-1 and p150,95 glycoproteins. Annu Rev Med 1987;38:175–194.
99. Schmalstieg FC. Leukocyte adherence defect. Pediatr Infect Dis J 1988;17:867–872.
100. Anderson DC, Miller LJ, Schmalstieg FC, Rothlein R, Springer TA. Contribution of the Mac-1 glycoprotein family to adherence-dependent granulocyte functions: Structure function assessments employing subunit specific monoclonal antibodies. J Immunol 1986;137:15.
101. Petrequin PR, Todd RF, Devall LJ, Boxer LA, Curnutte JT. Association between gelatinase release and increased plasma membrane expression of Mol glycoprotein. Blood 1987;69:605–610.
102. Todd RF, Arnaout RE, Rosine CA, Peters WA, Babior BM. Subcellular location of the large subunit of Mol (formerly gp110), a surface glycoprotein associated with neutrophil adhesion. J Clin Invest 1984;74:1280–1290.

103. Pohlman TH, Stannass KA, Beatty PG, Ochs HD, Harlan JM. An endothelial cell surface factor(s) induced in vitro by lipopolysaccharide, interleukin-1 and tumor necrosis factor increases neutrophil adherence by a CDw18 (LFA)-dependent mechanism. J Immunol 1986;136:45–48
104. Wardle EN. Kupffer cells and their function. Liver 1987;7:63–75.
105. Saba TM. Physiology and physiopathology of the reticuloendothelial system. Arch Intern Med 1970;126:1031–1052.
106. Owens MR, Cimino CD. Synthesis of fibronectin by the isolated perfused rat liver. Blood 1982;59:1305–1309.
107. Niehaus GD, Schumacker PT, Saba TM. Influence of opsonic fibronectin on lung fluid balance during bacterial sepsis. J Appl Physiol 1980;49:693–699.
108. Sganga G, Siegal JH, Brown G, Colemen B, Wiles CE, Belzberg H. Reprioritization of hepatic plasma protein release in trauma and sepsis. Arch Surg 1985;120:187–199.
109. Blackwood RA, Moret J, Mandl I, Turino GM. Emphysema induced by intravenously administered endotoxin in an alpha-1-antitrypsin deficient rat model. Am Rev Respir Dis 1984;130:231–236.
110. Warren HS, Chedid LA. Strategies for the treatment of endotoxemia: Significance of the acute phase responses. Rev Infect Dis 1987;9:5630–5638.
111. Beutler B, Cerami A. Cachectin: more than a tumor necrosis factor. N Engl J Med 1987;316:379–385.
112. Tracy KJ, Beutler B, Lowry SF, Merryweather J, Wolpe S, Milsark W. Shock and tissue injury induced by recombinant human cachectin. Science 1986;234:470–474.
113. Bessin P, Bonnet J, Thibaudeau D, Agier B, Beaudet Y, Gilet F. Pathophysiology of shock states cause by PAF-acether in dogs and rats, In Benveniste J, Arnous B (eds): Platelet-activating factor (INSERM symposium No. 23). Amsterdam: Elsevier Science Publishers BV, 1983:343–355.
114. Dinerello CA. Interleukin-1. Rev Infect Dis 1984;6:51–95.
115. Cook JA, Halushka PV, Wise WC. Modulation of macrophage arachidonic acid metabolism: potential role in the susceptibility of rats in endotoxic shock. Circ Shock 1982;9:605–617.
116. Beutler BA, Milsark IW, Cerami A. Cachectin/tumor necrosis factor: production, distribution, and metabolic fate in vivo. J Immunol 1985;135:3972–3977.
117. Hagman W, Denzlinger C, Keppler D. Role of peptide leukotrienes and their hepatobiliary elimination in endotoxin action. Circ Shock 1984;14:223–235.
118. Movat HZ, Cybulsky, MI, Colditz IG, Chan W, Dinarello CA. Acute inflammation in gram-negative infection: endotoxin, interleukin 1, tumor necrosis factor, and neutrophils. Fed Proc 1987;46:97–104.
119. Schumaker PR, Saba TM. Pulmonary gas exchange abnormalities following intravascular coagulation: reticuloendothelial involvement. Ann Surg 1980;192:95–102.
120. Bounous G. Acute necrosis of the intestinal mucosa. Gastroenterology 1982;82:1457–1467.
121. Cuevas P, Fine J. Demonstration of a lethal endotoxemia in experimental occlusion of the superior mesenteric artery. Surg Gynecol Obstet 1971;133:81–83.
122. Deitch EA, Berg R, Specian R. Endotoxin promotes the translocation of bacteria from the gut. Arch Surg 1987;122:185–190.
123. Herndon DN, Morris SE, Coffey JA, Milhoan RA, Barrow RE, Traber DL, Townsend DM. Enteric translocation of microorganisms in cutaneous thermal injury. Progress in Clinical and Biological Research G. Schlag, H. Reidle, eds. New York: Alan R. Liss, Inc., 1989
124. Morris SE, Navaratnam N, Traber DL, Herndon DN. Bacterial translocation and mesenteric blood flow in a large animal model after cutaneous thermal and smoke inhalation injury. Surg Forum 1988;39:189.
125. Demling RH, Lalonde C, Jin LJ, Katz A, Ryan P. Comparison of the postburn hyperdynamic state and changes in lung function (effect of wound bacterial content). Surgery 1986;100:828–835.
126. Lalonde C, Demling RH. Lung dysfunction after thermal injury in relation to prostanoid and oxygen radical release. J Appl Physiol 1986;61:103–112.
127. Toyofuku T, Kobayashi T, Kubo K, Koyama S, Kusama S. Effects of coronary ischemia on lung fluid balance in conscious sheep. J Appl Physiol 1988;65:617–624.
128. Harris TR, Collins JC, Rosselli RJ. Effects of coronary flow reduction on lung vascular tissue transport in sheep. J Appl Physiol 1983;55:1906–1915.
129. Sugi K, Newald J, Traber LD, Maguire JP, Herndon DN, Schlag G, Traber DL. Correlation between lung injury and myocardial depression after endotoxin (LPS) in sheep. Circ Shock 1988:24:251.
130. Sugi K, Newald J, Traber LD, Maguire JP, Herndon DN, Schlag G, Traber DL. Endotoxin causes myocardial depression in sheep. Fed Proc 1988;2:A1691.
131. Montero K, Lubbesmeyer HJ, Traber DL, Kimura R, Traber LD, Herndon DN. Inhalation injury increases systemic microvascular permeability. Surg Forum 1987;38:303–305.

132. Patten MT, Liebman PR, Hecktman HB. Humorally mediated deceases in cardiac output associated with positive end expiratory pressure. Microvasc Res 1977;13:137–139.
133. Johnson EE, Hedley-Whyte J. Continuous positive pressure ventilation and choledochoduodenal flow resistance. J Appl Physiol 1975;39:937–942.
134. Antonaccio MJ: Angiotensin converting enzyme (ACE) inhibitors. Annu Rev Pharmacol Toxicol 1982;22:57–87.
135. Skeggs LT Jr. Historical review of the renin-angiotensin system. In Doyle AE, Bearn AG (eds): Hypertension and the angiotensin system: therapeutic approaches. New York: Raven Press, 1984:31–45.
136. Ryan JW. Processing of the endogenous polypeptides by the lungs. Annu Rev Physiol 1982;44:241–255.
137. Kunkel KR, Barrow RE, Rubin SA, Noss PJ, Herndon DN. Significance of changes in chest x-rays and extravascular lung water in burned patients without inhalation injury. In preparation.
138. Herndon DN, Traber DL, Traber LD. Effect of resuscitation on inhalation injury. Surgery 1986;100:248–251.
139. Petty TL. Adult respiratory distress syndrome: definitions and historical perspective. Clin Chest Med 1982;3:3.
140. Taylor RW, Duncan CA. The adult respiratory distress syndrome. Res Med 1983;1:17.
141. Norwood SH, Civetta JM. Ventilatory support in patients with ARDS. Surg Clin North Am 1985;65:895.

13

Acute Renal Failure

RICHARD L. GAMELLI
GEOFFREY M. SILVER

The kidney is responsible for maintaining homeostasis in the setting of severe injury, sepsis, and multiple organ failure while responding to increasing metabolic demands. The kidney is a complex organ. It produces erythropoietin, participates in vitamin D metabolism, and is the site of gluconeogenesis during periods of starvation. It continuously performs these tasks in a dynamic environment of neural, hormonal, hemodynamic, and metabolic signals. During the adverse conditions imposed by injury, sepsis, and organ failure, the kidney responds predictably and effectively in order to maintain homeostasis. In the event that metabolic or hemodynamic limits are exceeded, or renal parenchymal damage occurs, the renal homeostatic response is impaired or lost and acute renal failure (ARF) ensues.

ARF in the setting of critical illness both with and without other organ failure is relatively frequent with an associated mortality rate of 50% or greater.[1] The mortality and morbidity is directly related to the severity of the underlying disease, the presence of infection, and the number of other organ systems involved.[2,3] In those patients who develop ARF the prevention of associated complications and the early institution of therapy are critical to improving patient outcome. In order to understand the therapy of ARF, it is necessary to be familiar with the normal renal anatomy and physiology.

Anatomy

The structural arrangement of the vascular and tubular elements of the functioning human kidney has a profound effect on the integrity of renal homeostatic functions. The renal arteries arise directly from the abdominal aorta at the second

216

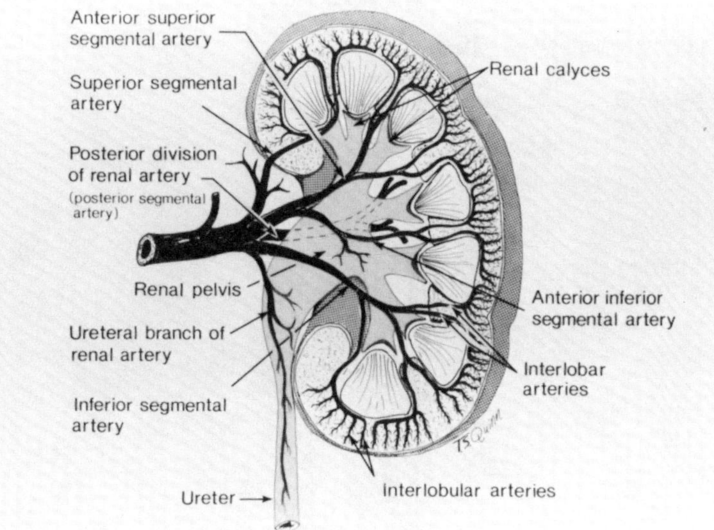

Figure 13–1. At the level of the hilum each renal artery divides into an anterior and posterior division supplying separate vascular segments of the kidney. There are five segments: the apical, the upper anterior, the middle anterior, the lower, and the posterior. The anterior division of the renal artery gives rise to the upper, middle, and lower segmental arteries. The posterior division supplies the posterior segment. The apical segment is supplied by either the anterior or posterior division.

lumbar vertebrae. The origin is approximately 1 cm below the origin of the superior mesenteric artery. The right renal artery is longer and passes behind the inferior vena cava and right renal vein, posterior to the head of the pancreas and the second part of the duodenum. The left renal artery passes behind the renal vein posterior to the body of the pancreas and splenic vein. Prior to entering the renal parenchyma, the renal arteries give off an inferior suprarenal artery. Branches of this artery supply the inferior portion of the suprarenal gland as well as the perinephric tissue, the renal capsule, the renal pelvis, and the proximal ureter. At the level of the renal hilum, each artery divides into an anterior and posterior division supplying separate vascular segments of the kidney. There are five segments: the apical, the upper anterior, the middle anterior, the lower, and the posterior. The anterior division of the renal artery gives rise to the upper, middle, and lower segmental arteries. The posterior division supplies the posterior segment. The apical segment is supplied by either the anterior or posterior division. Arising from these primary branches are the lobar, interlobar, arcuate, and interlobular arteries. The lobar arteries are distributed one to each pyramid. These divide just prior to entering the parenchyma into two or three interlobar arteries that run toward the cortex along the renal pyramids. At the junction between the cortex and the medulla, the interlobar arteries divide at right angles into several arcuate arteries that course between the cortex and medulla (Fig. 13–1). These in turn branch and form the nonanastomosing interlobular arteries that give rise to the afferent arterioles. The glomerulus, which is a system of branching capillaries, lies between the afferent and efferent arteriole.

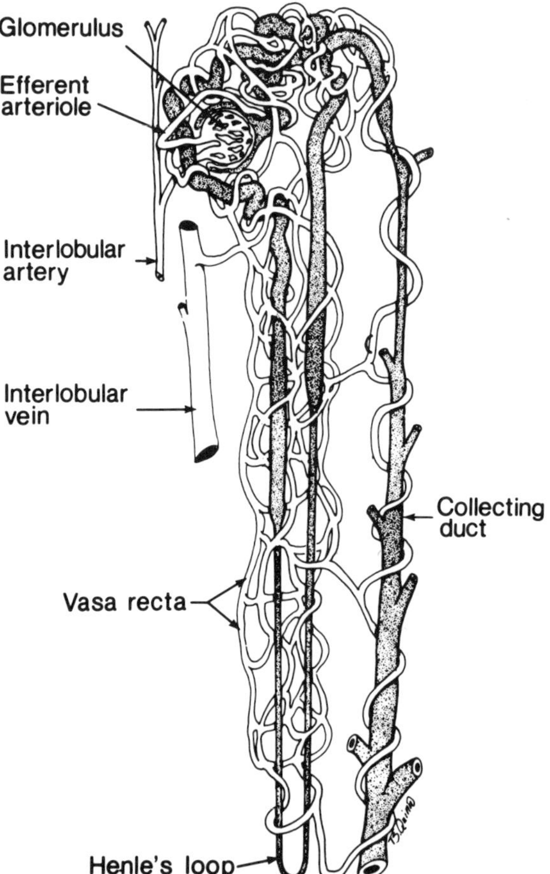

Figure 13–2.   The vasa recta are shown arranged in close proximity to the nephron and descending deep into the medulla. This anatomic arrangement facilitates the preservation of medullary hypertonicity via the countercurrent exchange mechanism. This relationship may break down during conditions of increased plasma flow, such as during sepsis, causing loss of medullary hypertonicity and resulting in decreased ability to concentrate the urine.

The nephron is considered to be the functional unit of the kidney. This unit consists of the glomerular capillaries connected to a continuum of specialized tubular segments spatially oriented to each other, to vascular elements, and to other nephrons. The afferent arterioles, the glomerular capillaries, and the efferent arterioles are in intimate contact with the nephron. The peritubular capillaries of the renal cortex are derived from the efferent arterioles. Efferent arterioles that are located within the inner third of the cortex are the origin of the descending and ascending vasa recta. The vasa recta are arranged in dense parallel hairpin-shaped loops that are in close proximity to the nephron and descend deep into the medulla (Fig. 13–2). This anatomic arrangement facilitates the preservation of medullary hypertonicity through the countercurrent exchange mechanism.[4,5]

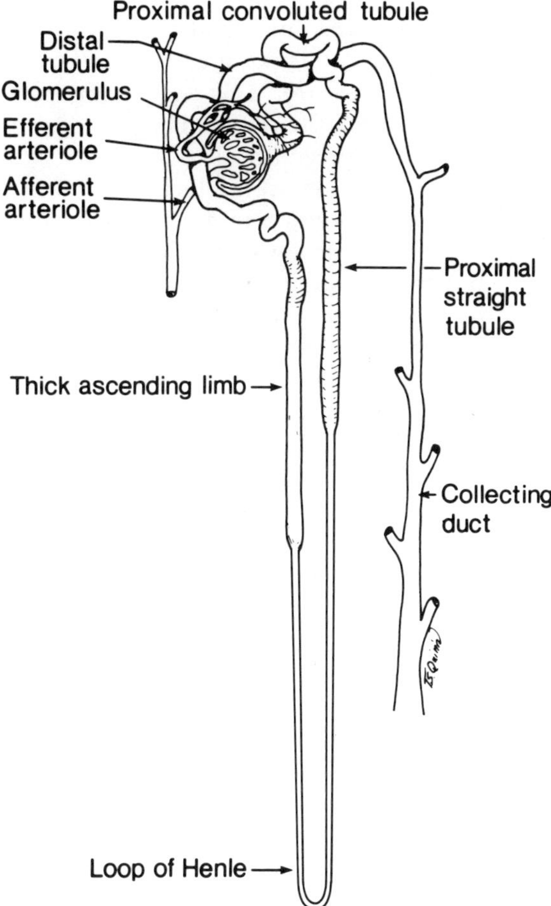

Figure 13–3. The anatomic arrangement of the nephron, the functional unit of the kidney, is diagramed. Note the position of the afferent and efferent arterioles in relation to the proximal convoluted tubule.

The segmental divisions of the nephron, often the source of controversy, are based on both structure and function. The divisions are the glomerulus, the proximal tubule, the loop of Henle, and the distal nephron. Each of these segments can be further subdivided, based on structure and function.

Renal Structure and Function

Glomerulus

The glomerulus is surrounded by Bowman's space, which is the beginning of the proximal tubule (Fig. 13–3). The glomerulus is a set of specialized capillaries situated between the tonically active afferent and efferent arterioles. These arterioles are regulated by several factors, including neural and hormonal influences, which assist in maintaining hydrostatic pressure to drive glomerular filtration. The glomerular hydrostatic pressure is maintained to between 30 and 50% of systemic mean arterial pressure.[6] This relationship generally is operative until mean arterial pressure approaches 80 mmHg. At this pressure, glomerular filtration and urine output drop precipitously.[7]

The basics of glomerular filtration were elucidated by Starling in the 19th century. Starling proposed that filtration was the net result of opposing hydrostatic and oncotic forces. Forces that favor filtration are the glomerular capillary hydrostatic pressure and the oncotic pressure of Bowman's space. Forces opposing filtration are the hydrostatic pressure within Bowman's space and the oncotic pressure of the glomerular capillary. For any single nephron, this relationship can be expressed quantitatively by the following equation:

$$SNGFR = K_f[(Pgc-Pb)-(pgc-pb)] \tag{1}$$

Where: SNGFR is the single nephron glomerular filtration rate; K_f is the filtration coefficient; Pgc is the glomerular capillary hydrostatic pressure; Pb is the hydrostatic pressure of Bowman's space; pgc is the oncotic pressure of the glomerular capillary; and pb is the oncotic pressure of Bowman's space.

The K_f is dependent on the permeability of the membrane and the total glomerular surface area available for filtration.[8] The glomerular capillary membrane acts as a filter allowing molecules to pass into Bowman's space on the basis of size and charge.[9] The glomerular membrane is normally permeable to neutral solutes up to a molecular weight of 50,000 d. It is negatively charged and therefore less permeable to polyanions, such as albumin.[10,11]

Proximal Tubule

The proximal tubule can be subdivided into the proximal convoluted tubule and the proximal straight tubule (Fig. 13–3). Approximately 180 L of filtrate enter the sum of proximal tubules in a normal person each day. Two thirds of the filtrate volume and half the sodium is reclaimed by the proximal tubule isotonically. Sodium is actively transported from the tubular lumen by a sodium and potassium activated adenosine triphosphatase (ATPase).[12,13] This is followed by passive reabsorption of water and other solutes driven to maintain osmotic and electrostatic equilibrium as the plasma flows toward the loop of Henle.

Fifty to 70% of the total filtered calcium is reabsorbed in the proximal tubule under the control of parathyroid hormone (PTH).[14] The remaining filtered calcium is reabsorbed in the ascending limb of Henle and the collecting duct, with less than 3% excreted. The principal function of PTH is the regulation of calcium in the extracellular fluid compartment. In the kidney the overall effect of PTH is the summation of the differential effects of the hormone across the entire nephron.[15] Through a cyclic adenosine monophosphate (cAMP) mechanism, PTH increases Ca^{++} reabsorption and decreases sodium-dependent phosphate, bicarbonate, and fluid reabsorption in the proximal tubule, the thick ascending

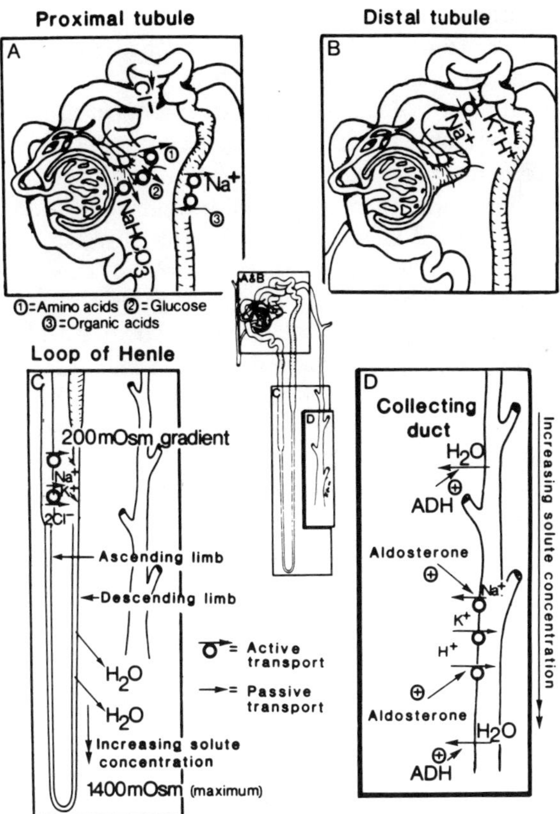

Figure 13–4.   The solute transportation function of each segmemental division is depicted. Arrows indicate the direction of transport. Arrows coupled to circles indicate active transport. D: ⊕ indicates increased activity of the coupled event.

limb of Henle, and the collecting duct.[16] This decreased absorption of solute can be compensated for by increased reabsorption more distally.

Loop of Henle

There are three types of Henle's loops: cortical, short, and long. The cortical loops originate from superficial glomeruli and do not enter the medulla. The other two types of loops arise from juxtamedullary glomeruli and can be further characterized by the extent to which they penetrate the medulla. The loop of Henle can be divided into descending and ascending limbs. The ascending limb has both a thin and a thick portion. The descending limb receives the isotonic filtrate from the proximal tubule. In the descending limb the functional characteristics of the tubular cells change. Sodium is no longer transported actively and the cells are more permeable to water and less permeable to solute (Fig. 13–4). The net result is the passive movement of water out of the lumen into the medullary interstitium rendered hypertonic by the proximal tubules of surrounding nephrons and the thick ascending limb. The luminal filtrate is therefore concentrated. As the descending limb changes to the ascending limb, the permeability of solutes increases and permeability to water decreases abruptly.[17] This causes solutes to diffuse out of the lumen, thereby deceasing the tonicity of the filtrate. As the thick segment is reached, the active transport of sodium resumes while the tubule remains impermeable to water. This has two consequences: further dilution of the luminal filtrate and maintenance of medullary hypertonicity.[18] Calcium is reabsorbed in the thick segment as well.

The structural and functional aspects of Henle's loop allow for the production of high intramedullary tonicity by countercurrent multiplication. The necessary components of this system are: (1) the production of osmotic pressure differences between the ascending and descending limbs of the loop; (2) differential permeability allowing solute diffusion from the ascending limb to the descending limb; and (3) sufficient length along which small concentration changes can be multiplied and maintained. The loop of Henle has all of these characteristics inherent in its structure. The thick ascending limb transports sodium actively and is able to maintain a gradient of 200 mOsm (Fig. 13–4).[19] The descending limb is freely permeable to water and slightly permeable to solute. Together these two features allow the production of a concentration gradient that causes successive increases in descending solute concentration by both equilibration and net solute flow from the thick ascending limb to the thin descending limb. As successively higher concentrations reach the site of transport in the thick ascending limb, the same 200 mOsm concentration gradient is maintained, thereby establishing higher medullary tonicity. The mechanism is extremely effective, permitting maximal concentrations near the hairpin portion of Henle's loop to reach 1400 mOsm. This high tonicity is supported by a second countercurrent multiplication system provided by the anatomic arrangement of the vasa recta. The ascending and descending vasa recta run parallel and in close proximity to each other and the loop of Henle. The capillary membranes of the vasa recta are freely permeable to solute, allowing passive flow of solute from the highly concentrated plasma of the ascending vasa recta to the lower concentration of the descending vasa recta. This arrangement supports and maintains the concentration gradient from the cortex to the deep medulla created by the loop of Henle.

Juxtaglomerular Apparatus

The end portion of the thick ascending limb returns to the cortex where it comes in close proximity to its own glomerulus. The thick ascending limb passes through the angle formed by the afferent and efferent arterioles and makes intimate contact with each as well as with the capillaries of the glomerular tuft. This site is the location of the juxtaglomerular apparatus. The juxtaglomerular apparatus consists of the macula densa, the extraglomerular mesangial cells, which fill the angle between the afferent and efferent arterioles, the afferent arteriole, and the efferent arteriole (Fig. 13–5).[20] The macula densa is a group of densely packed cells, found at the site of contact between the ascending limb and the afferent and efferent arterioles, that are different from the usual epithelial cells of the thick ascending limb. The macula densa is believed to function as a

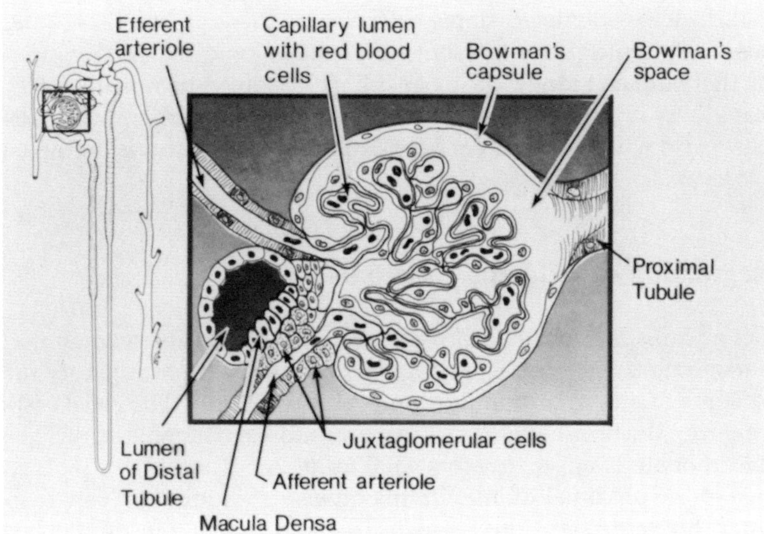

Figure 13–5. The cross-sectional anatomy of the glomerulus is shown. The juxtaglomerular apparatus consists of the macula densa, the extraglomerular mesangial cells, which fill the angle between the afferent and efferent arterioles, the afferent arteriole, and the efferent arteriole. The macula densa is shown as a group of densely packed cells, found at the site of contact between the ascending limb and the afferent and efferent arterioles.

tubular sensor capable of responding to changes in the luminal flow rates of the thick ascending limb by influencing the glomerular filtration rate (GFR).[21] This mechanism is known as tubuloglomerular feedback.

Distal Convoluted Tubule

The filtrate reaching the distal convoluted tubule is hypotonic by virtue of the active transport along the length of the thick ascending limb of Henle's loop. This filtrate represents 20% of the original protein-free filtrate. At the level of the distal convoluted tubule, additional sodium is reabsorbed actively, the rate being regulated by the influence of aldosterone. Potassium is also secreted in the distal convoluted tubule and is linked with both the rate of sodium reabsorption and hydrogen ion secretion (Fig. 13–4).

Collecting Duct

Nearly 30 L of hypotonic filtrate reach the collecting ducts per day. Under the influence of antidiuretic hormone (ADH) the cells of the distal convoluted tubule and the collecting duct become more permeable, allowing passive water reabsorption and concentration of urine. This passive reabsorption of water is driven by the high tonicity of the medullary interstitium created by countercurrent multiplication. The deeper the collecting tubule penetrates the medulla, the higher the medullary tonicity allowing maintenance of a concentration gradient between the increasing tonicity of the luminal contents of the collecting duct

(Fig. 13–4). In water-depleted states urine osmolarity can reach 1400 mOsm by this process. This number represents the physiologic maximal concentrating ability of the human kidney. With an obligate solute turnover of 600 to 800 mOsm/day, there is therefore an obligate urine volume of 500 ml/day. Less urine production per day will result in accumulation of solutes and is defined as renal failure.

Renal Regulation of Acid and Base Balance

Both renal and respiratory mechanisms are responsible for maintaining blood pH. The respiratory response is through alterations in the ventilatory rate causing rapid adjustments in carbon dioxide pressure (PCO_2). The renal response is through altering the bicarbonate pool and excretion of titratable acid. The filtered load of bicarbonate is approximately 4500 mEq/day. The bulk of bicarbonate is reabsorbed in the proximal tubule. In this process sodium is actively reabsorbed in exchange for hydrogen ions, which are buffered in the tubule lumen by available bicarbonate. The water and carbon dioxide formed are reabsorbed into the cell where the formation of bicarbonate is catalyzed by carbonic anhydrase. Factors causing increased bicarbonate reabsorption are extracellular fluid (ECF) volume depletion, increased PCO_2, and hypokalemia. The distal nephron is also responsible for the regulation of acid-base balance by reabsorption of bicarbonate, formation of titratable acidity, and production of ammonium ion.

As nonvolatile acids are formed from metabolic processes, bicarbonate is consumed by buffering the acid in the ECF. The sodium salt of the acid anions are filtered at the glomerulus. In the distal nephron, hydrogen ions are secreted into the tubular lumen and a bicarbonate ion is formed for each acid anion filtered. Sodium is reabsorbed from the tubular lumen and bicarbonate is secreted by the tubular cell into the bloodstream. Secreted protons form ammonium ions in combination with ammonium and in turn combine with acid anions to be excreted. Approximately 50 to 70 mEq of acid is produced in this fashion each day.

Renal Responses to Decreased Perfusion

The renal responses to injury and sepsis are primarily due to changes in renal perfusion. The integration of systemic and renal responses to decreased perfusion is an adaptive spectrum of survival events initiated through changes in renal vascular resistance, changes in blood flow distribution, glomerular filtration, solute reabsorption, and water excretion. This response is a graded continuum in which progressively severe perfusion deficits are counteracted by increased renal and systemic responses. In the euvolemic state an equilibrium is established by a balance of vasoconstrictors, vasodilators, prostaglandins, and neural tone.[22,23] In mild states of hypovolemia, or less than 15% hemorrhage, the kidney responds to restore effective plasma volume while at the same time preserving renal function. The initial response is a decrease in afferent arteriolar tone allowing maintenance of flow to the glomerulus. This is a remarkably effective process of autoregulation that maintains GFR over a significant range of perfusion pressures. Eventually progressive perfusion deficits cause progressive increases in renal vascular resistance in order to maintain systemic perfusion. As 20 to 30% of cardiac output is directed to renal perfusion, substantial gains to systemic perfusion are available. During this process intrinsic renal blood flow is shunted from the outer cortex to the juxtamedullary region and medulla in an effort to maintain GFR.[24,25] As renal vascular resistance increases, deficits in renal function occur manifested by oliguria as a result of diminished glomerular filtration.[26] This begins to occur at moderate volume deficits equivalent to 15 to 30% hemorrhage.[27] As mean arterial pressure falls below 80 mmHg., renal blood flow and GFR fall precipitously. In severe (more than 40%) hemorrhage renal blood flow will virtually cease and cell damage will result if the situation is not quickly reversed.

The responses just discussed are mediated by the interaction of the sympathetic nervous system, locally and systemically released hormones and locally released prostaglandins.[28] Reductions in perfusion pressure at the glomerulus cause reductions in filtration. This results in decreased sodium delivery to the thick ascending limb of Henle. The change in sodium delivery is monitored at the macula densa, which in turn stimulates renin release from the granular epithelial cells of the juxtaglomerular apparatus. Renal renin production causes the conversion of angiotensin I to angiotensin II, which in turn triggers release of aldosterone, augmenting sodium reabsorption. Angiotensin II also works to increase arteriolar tone both systemically and at the efferent arteriole.[29] Angiotensin II will preferentially increase efferent arteriolar tone, thereby increasing renal vascular resistance while maintaining GFR.[30-32]

A decrease in perfusion pressure is also the stimulus for increased systemic release of ADH by the posterior pituitary. Vasopressin will cause both systemic and renal vasoconstriction. The renal effects of vasopressin appear to be modified by the local release of vasodilator prostaglandins, which inhibit vasoconstriction of the arterioles in the juxtamedullary region.[33] The overall result of this complex interaction is the finely controlled progressive response of the renal vasculature to decreasing perfusion. This is a dynamic response allowing the progressive increase of renal vascular resistance and the preservation of glomerular filtration (Fig. 13–6).

As already described, both ADH and aldosterone are released during ECF volume depletion. Aldosterone release is triggered by increasing levels of angiotensin II and decreasing levels of atrial natriuretic factor.[34,35] Aldosterone and ADH function together to restore ECF volume by increasing sodium and free water reabsorption respectively.

Pharmacologic Manipulation of Renal Function: Diuretics

Diuretics are drugs that increase the rate of urine formation. In addition, diuretics have a wide variety of both renal and systemic effects. Diuretics may be classified

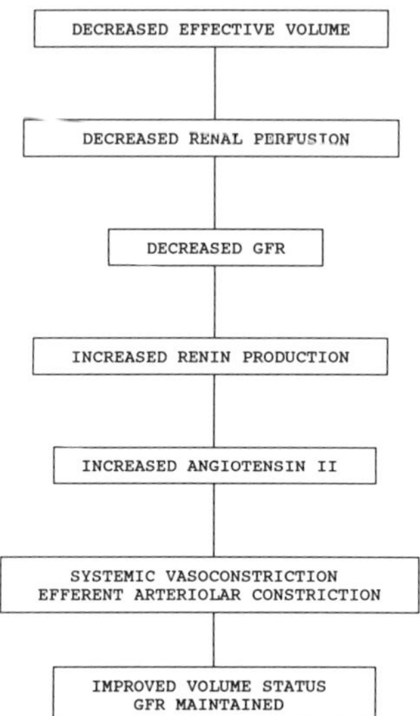

Figure 13–6.   The sequence of events in the homeostatic response to decreased effective volume. In minor hemorrhage or volume depletion this sequence will reestablish the GFR. In more severe volume disturbances increased angiotensin II will cause constriction of the afferent arteriole resulting in progressive deterioration of the GFR.

based on the site of their proposed action, which provides a rationale for their use.

The osmotic diuretics, such as mannitol, exert primary effects throughout the nephron. They are freely filtered at the glomerulus and are poorly reabsorbed by the renal tubule. In addition, they are pharmacologically inert and can therefore be administered in quantities sufficient to increase the osmolality of the plasma and the osmotic load of the filtrate reaching the nephron.[36] The increased osmotic load causes an increase in urine volume, thereby increasing the rate of excretion of sodium, potassium, and chloride. The filtrate volume is subject to modification by the action of ADH on the collecting tubule.

Carbonic anhydrase inhibitors such as acetazolamide, have multiple sites of action including the kidney, intraocular structures, gastrointestinal tract, and central nervous system. In the kidney inhibition of carbonic anhydrase causes reduced reabsorption of bicarbonate ion in the proximal tubule. Micropuncture studies of isolated nephrons also show decreased reabsorption of sodium and chloride. The overall mechanism is poorly understood but clearly the net effect is increased solute load in the tubule lumen. The effects of this decreased reabsorption are partially compensated for by an increase in solute reabsorption by the distal nephron, thereby limiting the efficiency of the diuretic effect.

The thick ascending limb of Henle is the site of action of the so-called loop diuretics. This class of potent agents contains furosemide, ethacrynic acid, and bumetanide. At usual therapeutic doses these diuretics do not have appreciable systemic effects. Higher doses have been known to cause hearing loss. Their potency is the product of at least two different effects: they block active transport of chloride and inhibit tubuloglomerular feedback.[37] In so doing, they increase the solute load reaching the distal tubules without decreasing the GFR. This dual effect greatly increases their diuretic efficiency. Administration of furosemide or ethacrynic acid does not alter renal oxygen consumption despite reducing the sodium reabsorption by approximately one third.[38]

The distal tubule is the site of action of the thiazide diuretics, chlorthalidone, and metolazone. These diuretics decrease sodium reabsorption in the cortical portion of the ascending limb and distal convoluted tubule. The overall effects of the thiazides are similar to the loop diuretics except with respect to calcium. The loop diuretics are calciuric while the thiazides are hypocalciuric and will cause elevated serum calcium levels with prolonged use.

The distal tubule is the site of action of the potassium-sparing diuretics. The triamterine group causes the formation of a positive potential difference in the distal tubule, which inhibits secretion of potassium ion. In addition, this diuretic decreases sodium permeability inhibiting reabsorption. The spironolactone group acts by competitive inhibition of aldosterone activity at the receptor level.[39] This inhibits sodium reabsorption and in turn potassium secretion.

Lithium and demeclocycline are agents that have diuretic effects at the collecting duct. These diuretics induce a water diuresis by antagonizing the effects of ADH. Their clinical value is limited by their toxicity.

Acute Renal Failure

ARF can be defined as a syndrome characterized by an abrupt reduction in renal function that results in the accumulation of nitrogenous wastes.[40–42] The origins of the syndrome are diverse and often multifactorial. Renal failure is generally classified as oliguric or nonoliguric. The oliguric form is associated with 24-hour urine volumes of less than the obligate minimum output of approximately 500 cc. The nonoliguric form may have urine outputs as high as 2 L/day.[43] The combined incidence is reported to be as high as 4.9% of all hospital admissions.[44] Certain groups of patients exhibit incidences of renal failure significantly higher. The associated mortality rate from ARF after severe trauma, prolonged surgery, burns, and sepsis is greater than 50%. The most common cause of death is infection.

Etiology

The origin of ARF can be viewed as secondary to prerenal, renal, and postrenal causes. Prerenal causes are attributed primarily to decreases in effective plasma volume, impaired cardiac output, or renal vascular obstruction. Renal causes are due to parenchymal lesions of the glomerulus or tubules caused by numerous factors, including nephrotoxins and prolonged prerenal or postrenal states. Thus, it is important to identify prerenal causes early because improved intravascular volume may prevent or significantly attenuate an episode of ARF. Postrenal causes are related to an obstructed excretory system

Pathophysiology

The renal manifestations associated with parenchymal disease are the result of four broad categories of pathophysiologic events: renal ischemia, chemical injury, blood vessel diseases, and glomerular diseases. The lesions caused by ischemic and chemical injury are commonly referred to as acute tubular necrosis (ATN), although the pathologic processes may not be limited to this site or may not be identifiable. Postischemic injury is the most common form of ARF found in surgical patients. This can be caused by several factors and generally includes those factors responsible for prerenal azotemia.

The difference between prerenal azotemia and renal failure due to ischemia is one of severity and the distinction between the two is not always clear. Prerenal azotemia is generally reversible by correcting the underlying pathologic mechanism. When the causative state is allowed to persist, the resulting pathologic damage is more severe and may progress to cell injury and necrosis. The renal medulla is susceptible to ischemic damage because of the high metabolic rate and subsequent high oxygen consumption of the resident cells.[45] Also, medullary blood flow remains reduced after resuscitation, further aggravating the acute injury.[46] When blood flow is no longer adequate to maintain metabolic demands, as in shock, ischemic damage follows.

The pathologic lesions of nephrotoxic ATN are similar to those found in ischemic ATN. There is proximal tubule cell necrosis and obstruction of the lumen by casts. Unlike ischemic injury, the distribution of the lesions is different and the mechanism of induction varies from agent to agent. In ischemic ATN the lesions are primarily medullary and juxtamedullary, whereas in nephrotoxic ATN the lesions are evenly distributed throughout the nephron population.[47]

Differential Diagnosis of Acute Renal Failure

A systematic approach facilitates the diagnosis and management of altered renal function. Impaired renal function can result from diminished renal blood flow, parenchymal damage, or obstruction of urine outflow. A useful first step in assessing the cause of altered renal function is in determining the primary defect, that is, prerenal, renal, or postrenal causes. Prerenal, renal, and postrenal causes of ARF all produce azotemia differently and these differences can be quantitated and allow the clinician to discriminate between the various anatomic locations. Unfortunately, it may not be possible to identify a single cause and in a substantial number of patients the cause will be multifactorial.

HISTORY AND PHYSICAL EXAMINATION

A thorough history, physical examination, and chart review are essential in evaluating the patient developing ARF. The clinician must determine the presence of preexisting renal disease, risk factors, exposure to nephrotoxins, infection, cardiac failure, and hemodynamic instability. Physical examination may yield information relevant to the patient's volume status, cardiac dysfunction, or the presence of sepsis. Pelvic and rectal examinations may show a large obstructing mass or an enlarged prostate as potential causes of postrenal obstruction.

URINALYSIS

The chemical and microscopic analysis of the urine will yield diagnostic information in the majority of patients with new onset renal dysfunction. In prerenal azotemia the urine is concentrated (urine osmolarity of more than 350 mOsm). The microscopic examination is unremarkable, containing few findings except for hyaline casts, and the urine sediment is normal.

Patients with intrinsic renal failure will demonstrate greater than 2 to 3 red cells/high-powered field. Brown pigmented casts and renal tubular epithelial cells are observed in the majority of these cases. Both hemolysis and rhabdomyolysis cause positive testing for occult blood but will contain no red cells. Patients with hemoglobinuria will have pink-colored plasma. The presence of urate crystals is diagnostic of uric acid nephropathy.

In obstructive uropathy the urine will not be concentrated and the urine will usually be unremarkable. The sediment will be normal as well. A sterile catheterization of the bladder should be performed early because this will resolve a bladder obstruction. Dilation of the collecting system is also detectable by ultrasonography, which is easily performed and poses no further risk to the patient.

URINE FLOW RATE

Oliguria is defined as a total urine output of less than 400 ml/day. Anuria is defined as an output of less than 50 ml/day or by the absence of urine on catheterization. The presence of sustained anuria suggests obstructive uropathy, mechanical obstruction of the renal arteries, or renal cortical necrosis.

Progressive azotemia can occur without oliguria. This syndrome, aptly called nonoliguric renal failure, is relatively common. Anderson et al.[43] in 1977 showed that greater than 59% of the ARF patients in their study population had progressive azotemia and nonoliguria. It occurs quite frequently after traumatic injuries and burns.[48,49] In patients with severe burns the incidence may approach 40%.[50] Patients with nonoliguric ARF have significantly better prognosis in terms of morbidity and mortality, less morbidity from infection, and gastrointestinal bleeding.[43]

URINE CHEMISTRY

Spot urine sodium samples aid in the diagnosis of renal failure. In prerenal states the kidney will avidly retain sodium in an attempt to correct the volume deficit. Therefore urine concentration will be less than 10 mEq/L. A more accurate expression is the fractional excretion of sodium (FE_{Na}). The FE_{Na} is:

$$Fe_{Na} = \frac{\text{Urine Na}}{\text{Plasma Na}} \div \frac{\text{Urine Cr}}{\text{Plasma Cr}} \times 100\% \qquad (2)$$

where Cr is creatinine. In prerenal states the FE_{NA} will be less than 1 (Table 13–1). In renal parenchymal injury the concentrating ability of the kidney will be lost and FE_{Na} will be greater than 1. This analysis is about 90% sensitive and specific in differentiating between prerenal azotemia and ATN.[51]

Table 13–1   Laboratory Assessment of Acute Renal Failure

	Prerenal	*Renal*	*Postrenal*
Urinalysis	—	2–4+	–
Protein	—	2–4+	1+
RBC	—	2–4+	±
Casts	Few hyaline	Pigmented, epithelial, WBC	–
Chemistry			
Urine (U) Osm	>500 mOsm/L	Equals plasma	Variable
U_{Osm}/P_{Osm}	<1.5	<1.5	Variable
U_{Na}	20 mOsm/L	50 mOsm/L	Variable
FE_{Na}	<1%	>3%	Variable

WBC: white blood cells; RBC: red blood cells; Osm: osmoles.

BLOOD CHEMISTRY

Decreased GFR causes accumulation of nitrogenous wastes with an increase in the blood urea nitrogen (BUN) and serum creatinine concentration. The rate of increase will depend on the catabolic rate of the patient. An elevated BUN is commonly seen in patients with trauma, infection, rhabdomyolysis, or gastrointestinal hemorrhage. In patients who have had severe muscle necrosis, as in crush injuries or burns, an inordinate increase in creatinine will be observed as well. This is because creatine is released from injured muscle and converted to creatinine spontaneously in the bloodstream.

Hyperkalemia is one of the most severe complications of ARF and occurs most frequently in patients with both oliguria and tissue injury.[52] Diabetics and patients with myonecrosis are at the highest risk level for hyperkalemia.

CLINICAL COURSE

The clinical course can be subdivided into three phases; initiation, maintenance, and recovery. The initial phase corresponds to the period during which renal function begins to deteriorate but prior to the onset of irreversible renal damage. It is within this period that preventive or therapeutic measures may have a significant impact. This phase is often heralded by decreasing urine output and, if recognized, immediate therapeutic measures may result in reversal and avoidance of more serious injury. Unfortunately, this period is often unrecognized because nonoliguric forms of ARF often precede oliguric renal failure and additionally this phase is often of short duration.

The maintenance phase begins at the point when the renal insult is no longer readily reversible and parenchymal damage has occurred. The duration of this phase is variable and depends on the severity of the insult. In oliguric renal failure this may vary from a few days to several months, whereas nonoliguric renal failure typically lasts for 5 to 7 days.

The onset of the recovery phase is marked by stabilization of BUN and creatinine levels and improvement in GFR. In oliguric patients the onset of this phase will be associated with improved urine output. In nonoliguric patients this phase will be associated with stabilization of BUN and creatinine levels.

Management of Acute Renal Failure

Management of Azotemia and Oliguria

The goal of the therapeutic plan should be to restore renal blood flow, increase tubular urine flow, and stop ongoing injury (Fig. 13–7). Reversible causes of renal damage should be treated or excluded immediately. All prerenal factors must be corrected and attempts made to establish a urine output. Regardless of the effectiveness of the therapeutic plan, certain patients will require dialysis for variable periods of time, depending on the severity of the insult.

Prevention of ARF is an important aspect of treatment. Early intervention in the ischemic process may prevent or decrease renal injury. Establishment of hemodynamic stability is of primary importance at the outset. Hemodynamic monitoring is necessary and may be facilitated by the use of a Swan-Ganz catheter for measurement of cardiac index and wedge pressures as a guide to adequate restoration of effective volume status. Different patients will have different requirements, such as a cardiac index of 3.0 will be adequate for postoperative patient without sepsis but will be well below requirements for the patient with a burn or sepsis.

After resuscitation is complete and prerenal causes have been excluded or treated, potential nephrotoxins discontinued, and obstructive uropathy ruled out, diuretics should be used in an attempt to restore urine output. Caution is advised at this point; if the patient is not adequately resuscitated, then the administration of diuretics will aggravate the volume deficit and worsen the ARF. If resuscitation is complete then the aggressive use of diuretics early during the clinical course may cause reversal of ARF and restoration of urine output. In this process oliguric renal failure may be converted to nonoliguric renal failure, a situation that is easier to manage and carries a lower mortality.[53] The use of mannitol in doses of 12.5 to 25 g with or without furosemide has met with some success. Several uncontrolled trials have shown reversal of oliguria in about two thirds of patients overall.[54,55] The response to loop diuretics is similar.[56] Combinations of high-dose mannitol (25 g) and furosemide (100 to 300 mg) may be beneficial. However, studies of diuretic use in patients with established renal failure and in patients requiring dialysis do not show convincing evidence of being able to decrease the need for dialysis or in decreasing the overall mortality.[57]

Dopamine is known to cause selective renal vasodilation and increased renal blood flow through stimulation of dopaminergic receptors.[58] Low-dose dopamine (2 to 5 μ/kg/min) increases cortical perfusion, GFR, and urine output. For these reasons, dopamine is thought to be beneficial in both treatment and prevention of ARF. Several investigators have studied the impact of dopamine both with and without diuretics. Many of these studies noted improved urine output and improved sodium excretion. Graziani et al.[59] studied the efficacy of dopa-

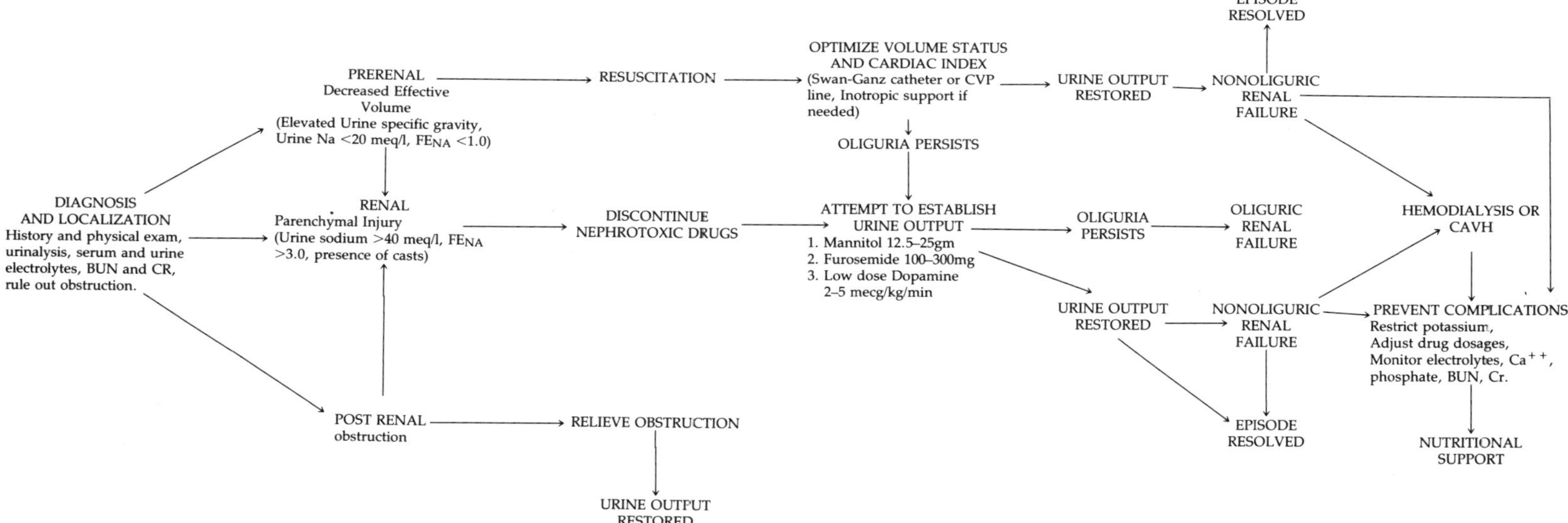

Figure 13–7. The management of oliguria from diagnosis to treatment. Cr: creatinine; CVP: central venous pressure

mine in combination with continuous furosemide infusion in 24 patients who had failed to respond to mannitol infusion. Of these patients, 19 responded with significantly increased urine output.[59] At this point, the evidence for using low-dose dopamine as an agent for treatment of ARF is acceptable. The evidence for the use of dopamine for prophylaxis is sparse and remains controversial.

If resuscitation, diuretics, and low-dose dopamine are ineffective in reestablishing urine output, dialysis may be required. There are three forms of dialysis in common use: hemodialysis, continuous arteriovenous hemofiltration (CAVH), and peritoneal dialysis. The use of peritoneal dialysis has some important limitations in that it requires the use of the peritoneal cavity and is associated with protein loss. In patients requiring total parenteral nutrition (TPN), CAVH is an excellent means of adjusting volume status. Hemodialysis remains the treatment of choice in the hypercatabolic patient with ARF. The use of hemodialysis for ARF in battle casualties in the Korean war diminished mortality from 95 to approximately 65%.[60] Although hemodialysis will require a vascular access procedure and periodic anticoagulation, the benefits are clearly worthwhile. Dialysis should be instituted early to avoid uremic complications. Severely catabolic patients requiring parenteral nutrition should be dialyzed as often as necessary to maintain chemical balance.

In the patient with established renal failure requiring dialysis it is extremely important to prevent severe perturbations in volume status. Calculation of accurate fluid input and output will help prevent complications. Losses from nasogastric tubes, drainage catheters, fistulas, open wounds, open peritoneal cavities, and burns must be accounted for and appropriate adjustments carried out.

Nutritional Supplementation in Acute Renal Failure

Nutritional therapy in the patient with ARF and multiple organ failure represents a difficult clinical challenge. In such patients adequate nutritional support is especially important because of a high catabolic rate and increased susceptibility to infection. In patients with ARF, plasma total protein, albumin, and free amino acid levels are depressed. If patients with trauma, thermal injury, or multiple organ failure have ARF, the metabolic derangements are compounded. The results are a fragile host defense and poor wound healing.

Adequate calories must be supplied to match the metabolic rate. Inadequate caloric supplements will exacerbate the protein catabolism. In the absence of specific measurements 30 to 35 Kcals/kg/day are recommended for surgical patients in ARF. The caloric requirement should be based on the predicted energy needs. Estimation of the resting metabolic energy expenditure, as recommended by Long,[61] is helpful for predicting caloric requirements in injured patients. Also, the use of bedside indirect calorimetry techniques will more precisely predict individual patient needs. Combinations of glucose and lipid may be used. Excess carbohydrate administration will result in excess carbon dioxide production and should be avoided.

Amino acids must be supplied to ensure positive nitrogen balance. The catabolic patient may require 1 to 1.5 g of protein/kg/day. This should be a solution containing both essential and nonessential amino acids. Although the capability to synthesize the nonessential amino acids may be present, this may be impaired in the patient with multiple organ failure. Dialysis should be used to prevent uremic complications, volume overload, and electrolyte abnormalities. Wherever possible enteral feeding should be used.

Metabolic derangements are common in the patient with ARF receiving TPN. Electrolyte abnormalities, hyperglycemia, hypophosphatemia, and hypomagnesemia most often occur at the beginning of TPN therapy. Hyperglycemia can be managed by adding insulin to the TPN solution or by an insulin drip. Enough insulin should be infused to keep the serum glucose level below 200 mg/dl. Patients with sepsis will require substantial amounts of insulin and are most appropriately managed with an insulin drip. The infusion of glucose and insulin will cause shifts of potassium, phosphate, and magnesium intracellularly. This is often to a significant degree and necessitates supplementation between dialysis treatments to avoid complications. Frequent serum levels are therefore mandatory.

Hypophosphatemia in the patient with ARF is often seen after the beginning of TPN infusion. Hypophosphatemia is also common in the patient with extensive burns and is exacerbated by superimposed ARF. Severe hypophosphatemia, or levels below 1.5 mg/dl, may be associated with tissue hypoxia, rhabdomyolysis, myocardial depression, peripheral neuropathy, and respiratory muscle failure. Therapy should be directed toward maintaining serum phosphorus levels between 3 and 4 mg/dl. Phosphorus can be given both orally and intravenously. In severe hypophosphatemia intravenous phosphate can be given at a rate of 1 g over 8 to 12 hours. Frequent levels should be obtained. Care should be taken to avoid hyperphosphatemia.

Management of Complications

Renal excretion of nitrogenous wastes, water, electrolytes, and acids is impaired during ARF. The magnitude of impairment depends on whether the patient is oliguric or nonoliguric. The catabolic state of the patient is important because patients with high catabolic states produce more nitrogenous wastes. For this reason, patients with severe trauma, burns, or sepsis will be difficult to manage if they are oliguric and will require dialysis.

AZOTEMIA

The rate of progression of azotemia is directly proportional to the degree of renal failure and the catabolic rate. In noncatabolic patients the rate of increase of BUN is between 10 and 20 mg/dl/day. In patients who are severely catabolic the rate of increase of the BUN may be extremely rapid. Patients with major thermal burns will catabolize greater than 100 g of protein/day, corresponding to an increase of greater than 40 mg/dl in BUN and 2 mg/dl/day in creatinine. For this reason, early dialysis or CAVH is recommended.

HYPERVOLEMIA

One of the most common complications of ARF is fluid overload.[62,63] Fluid resuscitation during hypovolemic shock is aimed at restoring cardiac output and maintaining renal blood flow. During this process substantial third space accumulation of fluid occurs, particularly in patients with substantial tissue injury. At the point in the patient's clinical course when sequestered fluid is mobilized, symptoms of volume overload occur due to the loss of volume regulatory function by the impaired kidneys. During these fluid shifts, the risk of pulmonary edema is high and warrants the use of invasive monitoring, hemofiltration, or dialysis to avoid volume overload.

HYPONATREMIA

Hyponatremia in ARF is primarily due to free water intake in excess of excretion, not sodium depletion. In addition hyponatremia may arise from water production as a byproduct of metabolism or the release of water from injured cells. Water intake should be restricted when ARF is recognized.

HYPERKALEMIA

Hyperkalemia occurs in 50% of all patients with ARF and is a common cause of death in patients with ARF. Hyperkalemia is caused by impaired excretion, cellular release, and exogenous administration of potassium. Intracellular potassium is in high concentration with muscle cells containing 155 mEq/L of potassium. During cell damage and necrosis, as occurs in crush injury, large amounts of potassium are liberated into the blood. Acidemia will aggravate this complication by causing further shifts of potassium out of the cell in exchange for hydrogen. Acute hyperkalemia usually remains asymptomatic until the serum concentration reaches 6.0 mEq/L. Serum concentrations in this range are associated with electrocardiographic (ECG) abnormalities. The ECG will show characteristic changes beginning with tented or peaked T waves and progressing to prolonged P-R interval, AV block, and ventricular fibrillation. Hyperkalemia must be avoided through restriction, frequent serum determination, ECG monitoring, and the use of hemofiltration or dialysis as often as necessary. Even in this setting hyperkalemia may occur acutely and necessitates immediate treatment. Acute treatment of hyperkalemia is designed to remove excess potassium from the body, restore the transcellular gradient, and reverse membrane abnormalities.[64] In the setting of life-threatening conduction disturbances 10 ml of intravenous 10% calcium gluconate should be administered. This is effective in restoring membrane potential and reversing conduction abnormalities, but only transiently. Administration of 50% dextrose and insulin will cause a shift of potassium toward the intracellular compartment. Neither of these methods will change total body potassium, necessitating the use of dialysis, hemofiltration, or cation exchange resins. Avoidance of hyperkalemia is the most successful treatment and early use of dialysis is advisable.

ACIDOSIS

In catabolic patients with ARF fixed acid production is increased. Sulfuric and phosphoric acids are derived from catabolism at a rate of 50 to 100 mEq/day.[65] The plasma bicarbonate levels will be inversely proportional to the catabolic rate. This relationship will be modified by administration of alkali or through gastric acid loss. Acidosis may be treated with sodium bicarbonate, but this may contribute to hypervolemia. Dialysis will effectively clear excess endogenous acid.

INFECTION

Infectious complications of ARF occur in greater than 50% of patients in association with trauma or surgery.[66] The incidence of infection was 89% in Vietnam casualties who had ARF and accounted for 72% of the deaths.[67] Septicemia, pneumonia, and peritonitis account for the majority of the mortality attributed to infection complicating renal failure.[68] Other causes of infection include wound infection and urinary tract infection. Urinary tract infections are very common and may contribute indirectly to the high mortality rate by causing septicemia.

Prevention of infection is a difficult problem. In the setting of severe trauma and burns immunosuppression is always present. This is further complicated by the addition of renal failure and varying degrees of malnutrition. In addition, the onset of infection is often difficult to diagnose because of the antipyretic effects of uremia and a blunted white cell response.[69] Prevention therefore becomes paramount. Once the patient is stabilized all indwelling catheters should be removed. Those that must remain require constant inspection. Antibiotic treatment should be selective by clinical criteria or by positive sputum, blood, or urine cultures. If an aminoglycoside antibiotic is required, then careful management of dosage via pre- and postdialysis determinations should be performed in order to avoid drug-related complications. In the future it may be possible to use recombinant human hematopoietic factors as an adjunct to antibiotic therapy and thereby reduce the incidence of superimposed nephrotoxicity by reducing the required dose of aminoglycosides.[70]

HEMORRHAGIC COMPLICATIONS

ARF is associated with anemia, hemorrhage, hemolysis, and iatrogenic losses. The primary cause of the anemia is decreased erythropoietin; however, with severe azotemia hemolysis may also occur. The development of severe anemia will exacerbate cardiac, respiratory, and wound healing problems.

Patients who are uremic have an increased incidence of hemorrhage. Uremic patients who have had invasive procedures are at particularly high risk. The primary hemostatic defect is due to platelet dysfunction rather than platelet number. The exact nature of the defect is unclear but it is associated with altered platelet-vessel wall interaction and abnormalities of the von Willebrand factor.[71] Dialysis improves platelet functional abnormalities and reduces the risk of hemorrhage by decreasing the degree of uremia. Platelet transfusions are relatively ineffective because new platelets rapidly acquire the defect. Red cell transfusions are helpful when the hematocrit is less than 25%. Two other effective therapeutic maneuvers in the uremic patient with a prolonged bleeding time are the administration of cryoprecipitate and desmopressin. The use of cryoprecipitate carries the risk of transmitting viral hepatitis and the acquired immune deficiency syndrome. Desmopressin, which induces release of the von Willebrand factor, has been shown to reduce bleeding time in uremic patients when given as a 3 μ/kg infusion over 30 minutes.[72]

Acute gastrointestinal hemorrhage is the second leading cause of death in ARF.[73] The cause of bleeding is due to stress ulceration and gastritis, both of which are increased in ARF. During ARF the clearance of gastrointestinal hormones is also reduced.[74,75] In particular, elevated gastrin levels have been noted.[76] These factors, in addition to platelet dysfunction and the use of anticoagulation during hemodialysis, are in part responsible for the high incidence of hemorrhage in patients with ARF.

HYPERPHOSPHATEMIA

Hyperphosphatemia is a common occurrence in the setting of ARF. This will a greater problem in patients with multiple organ failure in association with trauma, sepsis, dead gut, or necrotic foci because significant amounts of phosphorus is released from dead tissue. Thus, the problem is two-sided; there is increased release of phosphorus as well as diminished excretion. The most effective way to treat hyperphosphatemia is to diminish dietary intake and decrease gastrointestinal absorption by using phosphate binders. Debridement of necrotic tissue will decrease the phosphate load as well.

HYPER- AND HYPOMAGNESEMIA

In the patient with ARF both hyper- and hypomagnesemia may occur. To avoid hypermagnesemia, administration should be controlled by titrating intake to maintain normal serum levels. In the patient with multiple organ system failure, hypomagnesemia occurs after infusions of high caloric solutions, prolonged nasogastric suction, prolonged dietary depletion, and urine losses secondary to nephrotoxic renal damage. Treatment is accomplished empirically by intravenous infusion of magnesium sulfate while monitoring serum magnesium levels.

Prognosis

The overall mortality rate for ARF ranges from 40 to 60%. The nonoliguric form is associated with less mortality (26%) than the oliguric form (50%).[43] Factors associated with increased mortality are the underlying disease, associated multiple organ dysfunction, and the development of complications. Age, sex, length of time on dialysis are less consistently related to mortality. The basic underlying disease is the most important factor in survival. Patients without severe underlying illness and ARF secondary to nephrotoxins may have very low mortality, whereas ARF secondary to trauma and major surgery are associated with a mortality of 62%.[77] The involvement of other organ systems and the addition of complications significantly decreases prognosis.

Acknowledgments. The authors thank their families for their support in this endeavor. In addition we thank our medical artist Anthony Quinn for the illustrations included in this text.

References

1. Cioffi GW, Ashikaga T, Gamelli RL. Probability of surviving postoperative acute renal failure: development of a prognostic index. Ann Surg 1984;200:2.

2. Pine RW, Wertz MJ, Lennard ES, et al. Determinants of organ malfunction or death in patients with intra-abdominal sepsis. Arch Surg 1983:118.
3. DeCamp MM, Demling RH. Posttraumatic multisystem organ failure. JAMA 1988;260:530–534.
4. Gottshalk CW, Lassiter WE, Mylle M. Studies of the composition of vasa recta plasma in the hamster kidney. Exerpta Medica (International Congress Series) 1962;47:375.
5. Thurau K, Levine A. The renal circulation. In Rouiller C, Muller AF (eds): The kidney, morphology, biochemistry, physiology. New York: Academic Press, 1971:1–70.
6. Fried AF, Stein JH. Glomerular dynamics. Arch Intern Med 1983;143:787–791.
7. Navar LG, Marsh DJ, Blantz RC, et al. Intrinsic control of renal hemodynamics. (Symposium Report). Fed Proc 1982;41:3022.
8. Blantz RC. Dynamics of glomerular ultrafiltration in the rat. Fed Proc 1977;36:2602–2608.
9. Rennke HG, Venkatachalam MA. Glomerular permeability: in vivo tracer studies with polyionic and polycationic ferritins. Kidney Int 1977;11:44–53.
10. Brenner BM, Baylis C, Deen WM. Transport of molecules across renal glomerular capillaries. Physiol Rev 1976;56:502.
11. Koushanpour E, Kriz W. Renal physiology: principles, structure, and function, 2nd ed. New York: Springer-Verlag, 1986:86–87.
12. Lorenzen M, Lee CO, Windhager EE. Cytosolic Ca^{++} and Na^+ activities in proximal tubules of Necturus kidney. Am J Physiol 1987;247:F93.
13. Reeves BW, Andreoli TE. Tubular sodium transport. In Shrier RW, Gottschalk CW (eds): Diseases of the kidney, 4th ed. Boston: Little, Brown, 1988.
14. Lassiter WE, Gottschalk CW, Mylle M. Micropuncture study of renal tubular reabsorption of calcium in normal rodents. Am J Physiol 1963;204:771.
15. Morel F. Regulation of kidney function by hormones: a new approach. Rec Prog Horm Res 1983;39:271.
16. Chabardes D, Gagnan-Burnette M, Imbert-Teboul M, et al. Adenylate cyclase responsiveness to hormones in various portions of the human nephron. J Clin Invest 1980;65:439.
17. Jamison RL. Micro puncture studies of segments of thin loop of Henle in the rat. Am J Physiol 1968;215:236.
18. Hebert SC, Andreoli TE. Control of NaCl transport in the thick ascending limb. Am J Physiol 1984;246:F745.
19. Lassiter WE, Gottschalk CW. Regulation of water balance, urine concentration and dilution. In Schrier RW, Gottschalk CW (eds): Diseases of the kidney, 4th ed. Boston: Little, Brown, 1988.
20. Bulger RE, Hebert SC. Structural-functional relationships in the kidney. In Schrier RW, Gottschalk CW (eds): Diseases of the kidney, 4th ed. Boston: Little, Brown, 1988.
21. Guyton AC, Langston JB, Navar G. Theory for renal autoregulation by feedback at the juxtaglomerular apparatus. Circ Res 1964;15(Suppl 1):187.
22. Badr KF, Ichikawa I: Prerenal failure: a deleterious shift from renal compensation to decompensation. N Engl J Med 1988;319:623–629.
23. Laragh JH. Atrial natriuretic hormone, the renin-angiotensin axis, and blood pressure electrolyte homeostasis. N Engl J Med 1988;313:1330–1340.
24. Gransjo G, Wogast M. The pressure flow relationship in renal cortical and medullary circulation. Acta Physiol Scand 1972;85:228.
25. Kelleher SP, Robinette JB, Conger JD. Sympathetic nervous system in the loss of autoregulation in acute renal failure. Am J Physiol 1984;246:F379.
26. Hishaw R, Page G, et al. Mechanism of intrarenal hemodynamic changes following acute arterial occlusion. Am J Physiol 1963;205:1033.
27. Lucas CE. Renal considerations in the injured patient. Surg Clin North Am 1982;62:133–148.
28. Henrich WL, Berl T, McDonald KM, Anderson RJ, Schrier RW. Angiotensin II, renal nerves, and prostaglandins in renal hemodynamics during hemorrhage. Am J Physiol 235:F46–F51.
29. Ichikawa I, Brenner BM. Importance of efferent arteriolar vascular tone in regulation of proximal tubule fluid reabsorption and glomerulotubular balance in the rat. J Clin Invest 1980;65:1192–1201.
30. Yared A, Kon V, Ichikawa I. Mechanism of preservation of glomerular perfusion and filtration during acute extracellular fluid volume depletion. J Clin Invest 1985;75:1477–1487.
31. Kon V, Yared A, Ichikawa I. Role of renal sympathetic nerves in mediating hypoperfusion of renal cortical microcirculation in experimental congestive heart failure and acute extracellular fluid volume depletion. J Clin Invest 1985;76:1913–1920.
32. Dibona G. Prostaglandins and nonsteroidal anti-inflammatory drugs: effects on renal hemodynamics. Am J Med 1986;80(Suppl. 1A):12–21.
33. Chapnick BM, Panstian PW, Klanier E. Influence of prostaglandin synthesis on renal vascular

responses to vasopressor and vasodilator agents in the cat. J Pharmacol Exp Ther 1976;196:44–52.

34. Maack T, Marion DN, Camargo MJF, et al. Effects of auriculin on blood pressure, renal function, and the renin-aldosterone system in dogs. Am J Med 1984;77:1069–1075.
35. Atarashi K, Mulrow PJ, Franco-Saenz R. Effect of atrial peptides on aldosterone production. J Clin Invest 1985;76:1807–1811.
36. Warren SE, Blantz RC. Manitol. Arch Intern Med 1981;141:493–497.
37. Wright FS, Schnermann J. Interference with feedback control of glomerular filtration rate by furosemide, triflocin, and cyanide. J Clin Invest 1974;53:1965–1708.
38. Fleming JS, Rennie DW. Effects of osmotic diuresis on sodium reabsorption and oxygen consumption in the kidney. Am J Physiol 1966;210:751.
39. Corvol P, Claire M, Oblin ME, et al. Mechanism of the antimineralocorticoid effects of spironolactones. Kidney Int 1981;20:1–6.
40. Wilkes BM, Mailloux LU. Acute renal failure: pathogenesis and prevention. Am J Med 1986;80:1129.
41. Anderson RJ, Schrier RW: In Schrier RW, Gottschalk CW (eds) Diseases of the kidney, 4th ed. Boston: Little, Brown 1988.
42. Anderson RJ, Schrier RW: Clinical spectrum of oliguric and non-oliguric acute renal failure. In Brenner BM, Stein JH (eds): Acute renal failure (contemporary issues in nephrology, vol. 6). New York: Churchill Livingstone, 1980.
43. Anderson RJ, Linas SL, Berns AS, et al. Nonoliguric acute renal failure. N Engl J Med 1977;296:1134.
44. Hou SH, Bushinsky DA, Wish JB, et al. Hospital-acquired renal insufficiency: a prospective study. Am J Med 1983;74:243.
45. Brezis M, Rosen S, Silva S, et al. Renal ischemia a new perspective. Kidney Int 1984;26:375.
46. Finn WF, Chevalier RL. Recovery from acute renal failure. Kidney Int 1979;16:113.
47. Kreisberg JI, Venkatachalam MA. Morphologic factors in acute renal failure. In Brenner BM, Lazarus JM (eds): Acute renal failure, 2nd ed. New York: Churchill Livingstone, 1988.
48. Baxter CR, Zelditz WD, Shires GT. High output acute renal failure complicating traumatic injury. J Trauma 1964;4:567.
49. Vertel RM, Knochel JP. Nonologuric acute renal failure. JAMA 1967;200:598–602.
50. Planas M, Wachtel T, Frank H, et al. Characterization of acute renal failure in the burned patient. Arch Intern Med 1982;142:2087.
51. Miller TR, Anderson RJ, Berns AS. Urinary diagnostic indices in acute renal failure. A prospective study. Ann Intern Med 1978;88:47.
52. Knochel, JP. Biochemical, electrolyte, and acid-base disturbances in acute renal failure. In Brenner BM, Lazarus JM (eds): Acute renal failure, 2nd ed. New York: Churchill Livingstone, 1988:683.
53. Barry KG, Malloy JP. Oliguric renal failure: evaluation and therapy by the intravenous infusion of mannitol. JAMA 1962;179:510.
54. Eliahou HE. Mannitol therapy in oliguria of acute onset. Br Med J 1964;1:807.
55. Luke RG, Briggs JD, Allison MEM, et al. Factors determining the response to mannitol in acute renal failure. Am J Med Sci 1970;259:168.
56. Levinsky NG, Bernard BB. Mannitol and loop diuretics in acute renal failure. In Brenner BM, Lazarus JM: Acute renal failure, 2nd ed. New York, Churchill Livingstone, 1988.
57. Kleinknecht D, Ganeval D, Gonzalez-Duque LA, Fermanian J. Furosemide in acute oliguric renal failure: a controlled trial. Nephron 1976;17;51–58.
58. Schwartz LB, Gewertz BL. The renal response to low dose dopamine. J Surg Res 1988;45:574–588.
59. Graziani G, Cantaluppi A, et al. Dopamine and furosemide in oliguric renal failure. Nephron 1984;37:39.
60. Kjellstrand CM, Berkseth RO, et al. Treatment of acute renal. In Schrier RW, Gottshalk CW (eds): Diseases of the kidney. Boston: Little Brown, 1988.
61. Long C. Metabolic response to injury and illness: estimation of energy and protein needs from indirect calorimetry and nitrogen balance. JPEN 1979;3:450.
62. Ledgerwood AM, Lucas CE. Postresuscitation hypertension: etiology, morbidity, and treatment. Arch Surg 1974;108:531–538.
63. Lucas CE, Ledgerwood AM, Shier MR, et al: The renal factor in the post-traumatic "fluid overload" syndrome. J Trauma 1977;17:667.
64. Kunis CL, Lowenstein J. The emergency treatment of hyperkalemia. Med Clin North Am 1981;65.
65. Relman AS. Renal acidosis and renal excretion of fixed acids in health and disease. Adv Intern Med 1964;12:295.

66. McMurray SD, Luft FC, Maxwell DR, et al. Prevailing patterns and predictor variables in patients with acute tubular necrosis. Arch Intern Med 1978;138:950.
67. Lordon RE, Burton JR. Post-traumatic renal failure in military personnel in Southeast Asia. Am J Med 1972;53:137.
68. Routh GS, Briggs JD, Mone JG, Ledingham L. Survival from acute renal failure with and without multiple organ dysfunction. Postgrad Med J 1980;56:244.
69. Kaplow LS, Goffinet JA. Profound neutropenia during the early phase of hemodialysis. JAMA 1968;203:133.
70. Silver GM, O'Reilly M, Mooney DP, Gamelli RL. The beneficial effect of granulocyte colony stimulating factor (G-CSF) in combination with gentamicin on survival following pseudomonas burn wound infection. Surgery 1989;106:452–456.
71. Remuzzi G. Hematopoietic system in uremia part 2; bleeding and coagulation abnormalities. In Massry SG, Glassock RJ (eds): Textbook of nephrology, 2nd ed. Baltimore: Williams & Wilkins, 1989:1205–1206.
72. Mannucci PM, Remuzzi G, Pusineri F, Lombardi R, Valsecchi C, Mecca G, Zimmerman TS. Deamino-8-D-arginine vasopressin shortens the bleeding time in uremia. N Engl J Med 1983;308:8–12.
73. Steinman TI, Lazarus JM. Organ-system involvement in acute renal failure. In Brenner BM, Lazarus JM (eds): Acute renal failure, 2nd ed. New York: Churchill Livingstone, 1988:723.
74. Shapira N, Skillman JJ, Steinman TI, Silen W. Gastric mucosal permeability and gastric acid secretion before and after hemodialysis in patients with chronic renal failure. Surgery 1978;83:528.
75. Hansky J. Effect of renal failure on gastrointestinal hormones. World J Surg 1979;3:463.
76. Wesdorp RI, Falcao H, Banks PB, et al. Gastrin and gastric acid secretion in renal failure. Am J Surg 1981;141:334.
77. Finn WF. Recovery from acute renal failure. In Brenner BM, Lazarus JM (eds): Acute renal failure, 2nd ed. New York: Churchill Livingstone, 1988:878.

14

Hepatic Dysfunction in Multiple Organ Failure

CRAIG WALVATNE
FRANK B. CERRA

Sequential organ failure after injury is now a well-recognized clinical syndrome. Originally described in trauma research units, the failure of lung, kidney, and then liver has been noted to follow septic shock, hypovolemic shock, persistent inflammation such as pancreatitis, the continued presence of dead and injured tissue, and uncontrolled foci of infection. Multiple organ failure syndrome (MOFS) accounts for 75% of surgical intensive care unit (ICU) deaths. Liver failure appears to be the final organ failure in a process that begins at the time of injury, and constitutes the focus of this discussion.

Clinical Presentation and Diagnosis

Patients eventually developing hepatic dysfunction usually have a history of shock after an injury. Treatment with fluids and frequently inotropic support is necessary to achieve hemodynamic stability. Within 3 to 4 days, the patient develops acute lung injury and the signs of persistent hypermetabolism (systemic vascular resistance more than 600 dyne-cm, cardiac index more than 4.5 $L/min/m^2$, and oxygen consumption more than 180 ml/M^2). After several more days, the serum creatinine and then the serum bilirubin levels progressively increase. Death is common after 2 to 3 weeks.

Presentation of hepatic dysfunction usually occurs several days after the onset of hypermetabolism and hyperdynamic physiologic changes. Risk factors thought to predispose patients to the development of hepatic dysfunction include perfusion deficit, persistent focus of dead or injured tissue, uncontrolled focus of infection, or preexisting fibrotic liver disease. Two physical findings are usually associated with developing hepatic failure: encephalopathy and jaundice. Encephalopathy is difficult to attribute purely to hepatic dysfunction, since most critically ill patients have other risk factors besides liver failure that can contribute to encephalopathy, such as medications and sleep deprivation. Thus, jaundice and amino acid clearance appear to be more descriminant characteristics of liver failure than encephalopathy. Elevation of the serum bilirubin levels to greater than 3.0 mg/dl in a setting of no other demonstrable causes of jaundice (such as obstruction, transfusion reaction, or resolving hematoma) and a concomitantly elevated plasma phenylalanine level of greater than 100 µM/L appears to identify those patients who have developed liver insufficiency or failure. In this situation, the transaminase (SGOT, SGPT) and alkaline phosphatase levels are either normal or minimally elevated.[1,2]

The hyperbilirubinemia is predominantly of the conjugated form, suggesting a deficit in excretion rather than impaired hepatocellular uptake.[1,2] Hyperbilirubinemia has been reported to occur anywhere from 1 to 12 days after the onset of hypermetabolism.[1-4] The degree of elevation of the bilirubin and its time course have been suggested as prognostic indicators of patient survival. In their series of trauma patients, Sarfeh and Balint[1] found that the bilirubin levels on day 4 were higher in nonsurvivors (3.6 ± 0.6) than survivors (1.6 ± 0.3). Others have also reported that the pattern of bilirubin elevation appears to be an excellent discriminator of the pattern of MOFS as well as an excellent predictor of outcome (2.2 ± 0.6 mg/dl for survivors versus 8.5 ± 2.2 mg/dl for death).[4]

Hepatic excretory failure is characteristic of the hepatic dysfunction seen in the early phases of MOFS. In contrast, synthetic function appears reasonably well preserved until late in the disease, when protein synthesis fails. Consequently, an early diagnosis of hepatic dysfunction might be made by making use of a marker that can be injected into the blood, and followed as it is taken up by the hepatocytes and excreted by the biliary system. Indocyanine green clearance has been demonstrated by Gottlieb et al.[5] to have the advantage of indicating delayed hepatocyte excretion prior to the appearance of hyperbilirubinemia. Another marker that may be useful in diagnosing early hepatic dysfunction is sulfobromophthalein (BSP). This compound is an organic dye of which 80% is usually excreted in the bile. Additionally, radiolabeled substances are available, such as diisophenin or rose bengal which are excreted in a similar manner. Since extrahepatic biliary obstruction can present with similar findings as those just described, care must be taken not to confuse extrahepatic obstruction for hepatic parenchymal dysfunction. These two clinical entities can usually be differentiated adequately with ultrasound.

Other diagnostic laboratory tests that may be useful include the plasma amino acid clearance and the arterial acetoacetate to β-hydroxybutyrate ratio. The plasma amino acid profile will be discussed more completely later in this chapter. Briefly, the hepatic clearance of aromatic amino acids (phenylalanine, tyrosine, and tryptophan) decreases with decreasing hepatic function. Therefore measurements of aromatic amino acid clearance can be used as a marker of the degree of hepatic dysfunction. The acetoacetate to β-hydroxybutyrate ratio is thought to reflect the hepatic mitochondrial redox potential. With a decreasing redox potential, β-hydroxybutyrate is produced in excess of acetoacetate. Consequently, a progressive decrease in the acetoacetate to β-hydroxybutyrate ratio represents a relative excess of reducing agent and a setting of reduced mitochondrial electron transport capacity. Ozawa et al[6] found that postoperative patients with a ratio of less than 0.4 developed MOFS and that ratios of less than 0.25 were associated with increased mortality.

Pathology

Several authors have published histologic findings from liver biopsies or autopsies taken from patients with MOFS.[1,2,7,8] Their findings are consistent in two areas: (1) there is evidence of centrilobular hepatocellular congestion or necrosis; and (2) there is biliary stasis, with bile noted both intracellularly and inspissated in the canaliculi, without evidence of extrahepatic obstruction. As expected, the presence and degree of biliary stasis seems to correlate with the level of elevation of the serum bilirubin.

In 1950, Mallory et al.[9] noted an additional interesting finding from autopsies of soldiers who had received lethal, shock-producing injuries. Patients who survived less than 12 hours with prolonged shock had no remarkable changes in hepatic histology features. In contrast, 87% of the livers from patients surviving between 12 and 96 hours had histologic evidence of fat vacuolation of the liver parenchymal cells in a centrilobular distribution. Pathologic changes were also seen in other organs (heart, kidney), and were particularly severe in patients who had documented peritonitis.

Pathophysiology

Systemic Effects

Nuytinck et al.[10] attempted to duplicate the histologic findings of MOFS by activating the systemic immune system of hypoxic rabbits with zymosan (a cell wall polyglycan derived from brewers' yeast). They found that this combination of insults caused a picture of hepatocellular damage similar to that seen in MOFS. These and other findings have supported and encouraged much of the immunologic research being performed to explain the mechanisms involved in the process of hepatic failure during MOFS.

Hypermetabolism is a recognized component of MOFS. This process may be defined as an increased requirement for energy and substrate in the presence of altered energy and substrate utilization patterns. There is a change in the catabolic and anabolic functions of the cell, which appear to be mediated by various neurohumoral substances. This change in cellular metabolism can be demonstrated clinically by comparing flow-adjusted arterial and venous concentration differences of substrates with those of normal patients. An easily measured substrate is oxygen. In sepsis or hypermetabolism, oxygen consumption is markedly increased.[11] Since the utilization requirement for oxygen is increased, the delivery of oxygen must also be increased. This is done by maximizing the blood oxygen carrying capacity (by increased FiO_2 and transfusion, if necessary), and increasing the cardiac output (by manipulation of inotropic state and afterload). The body will extract only that amount of substate that it can use, and when the measured oxygen consumption has peaked (will no longer increase with increased cardiac output), there is no need to drive the cardiac output further.

Perfusion Deficit

A deficit in substate delivery to the liver despite elevated cellular demands due to systemic hypermetabolism is thought to be a major initiating factor in the pathophysiologic condition of the hepatic dysfunction of MOFS. Gottlieb et al.[12] measured oxygen consumption and blood flow across the liver in patients without sepsis who had an episode of hypotension (systolic blood pressure less than 90) after severe trauma. They found that there was a significant elevation in the splanchnic oxygen consumption compared with normal. Additionally, they found that the hepatic blood flow was decreased approximately 50% by 12 hours postinjury despite normal or elevated systemic hemodynamics. This deficit in perfusion persisted for about 4 to 5 days after the injury. Evaluation of hepatocellular function by indocyanine green clearance in these patients showed an immediate decrease in the hepatic clearance of the dye, which peaked around day 4 and resolved by day 7. An elevation of the patients' serum bilirubin levels above baseline was usually seen on day 3 and persisted for about 2 weeks.[5] Sarfeh and Balint[13] found similar results in rats after standardized blunt trauma.

Schirmer et al. showed that blunt trauma,[14] sepsis,[15] and immunologic activation by zymosan[16] could all lead to decreased hepatic blood flow despite normal or hyperdynamic systemic hemodynamics. These data suggest that a common pathway exists to decrease blood flow to the liver during the hyperdynamic response. The most likely cause of this decreased hepatic blood flow is decreased blood flow through the portal vein due to systemic shunting of blood from the splanchnic bed during the shock-resuscitation periods. Splanchnic shunting is a normal homeostatic mechanism used by the body and is mediated by the hormones of the neuroendocrine axis. One of the unknowns is to what degree or duration hepatic blood flow must be diminished (inadequate oxygen supply) to impair hepatic function.

Fath et al.[17] showed that 60 minutes of complete hepatic ischemia in dogs was associated with a decrease in the hepatic clearance of amino acids. Becker et al.[18] showed later that this decrease in blood flow could be directly correlated with a decrease in hepatocellular high energy phosphate stores and eventual mortality. Machiedo et al.[19] found that hepatic blood flow was decreased 2 hours after cecal perforation, but it was not until 6 hours after operation that the rats showed signs of hepatocellular dysfunction. Hepatocellular glutathione levels have also been shown to be decreased after 6 hours of sepsis, suggesting that a significant oxidative stress has occurred.[20]

Persistent Focus of Dead or Injured Tissue

A study by Schirmer et al.[14] focused on the question of whether or not adequate debridement will prevent the perfusion deficit seen after trauma. In their study, they compared three groups of animals: those with closed femur fracture, open fracture with tissue debridement, and sham operation. Their results documented that in both the closed and open fracture groups, hepatic blood flow was decreased at 24 hours, but only in the closed fracture group did this decrease in hepatic blood flow persist for 48 hours. These results are consistent with the observations of Seibel et al.[21] and others that immediate treatment of orthopedic patients with open reduction and internal fixation rarely leads to hepatic dysfunction, whereas liver failure is relatively common in patients treated by traction alone. They also noted that bilirubin elevation correlated positively with the duration of femur traction. The studies of Amaral et al.[22] and Morris et al.[23] also indicate that the local wound may release products that regulate hepatic metabolism.

These studies support the concept that systemic metabolism can be regulated by mediators of local tissue injury and that hypermetabolism can be induced by local tissue injury. In this way, tissue injury appears to be able to alter blood flow and hepatocellular function.

Uncontrolled Focus of Infection

Sepsis is common in critically ill patients. Although the overall ratio of gram-negative to gram-positive organisms has been estimated at 2.6:1.0, there is no specific relationship between the type of invading microorganism and the development of MOFS.[24]

The mechanism by which the septic state appears to compromise systemic physiologic responses appears to be related to the uncontrolled activation of the neuroendocrine system and increased cell-cell interactions. Alterations in systemic homeostatic mechanisms appear to be due to the toxic effects of certain bacterial cell wall constituents. The most commonly studied of these is endotoxin (lipopolysaccharide). The endotoxin molecule is a major constituent of the cell wall of gram-negative bacteria and, although its specific characteristics vary from one bacterial species to another, in general all endotoxins induce similar physiologic alterations. Endotoxin activates mononuclear cells and by altering cellular function this induces a hypermetabolic and hyperdynamic state.[25–27] This is not to say that lipopolysaccharide and gram-negative bacteria are the only villains in this story. Quale et al.[28] infused lipopolysaccharide, *Staphylococcus aureus*, or lipoteichoic acid (a staphylococcal cell wall constituent) into rabbits and found delayed BSP excretion in each group.

The source of infection in patients with MOFS is also an issue of some interest. Marshall et al.[29] found that sepsis in patients with MOFS could come from a wide variety of sources. An interesting finding of this study was that the organisms recovered from the blood of these patients was most commonly correlated with the cultures of the upper gastrointestinal tract. It has been widely observed that the upper gastrointestinal tract, although relatively sterile in normal persons, becomes colonized with a number of different organisms in critically ill patients cared for in ICUs. This has been attributed to aggressive prophylaxis against stress ulceration with antacids and H_2 blockers. The mechanism by which these organisms invade the mucosal barrier is still an area of debate. Intestinal compromise because of splanchnic blood flow restriction and loss of mucosal integrity due to inadequate nutrition have been suggested as mechanisms promoting bacterial translocation.[25,30] Recently, O'Dwyer et al.[31] showed that a single intravenous dose of lipopolysaccharide could increase human intestinal permeability to previously excluded substances. This finding suggests that bacteria themselves could trigger a response that could lead to fulminant sepsis.

Preexisting Fibrotic Liver Disease

There are several key features of fibrotic liver disease that predispose these patients to the development of hepatic dysfunction and MOFS. Patients with fibrotic liver disease already have some hepatocellular dysfunction due to their preexisting disease, and the cirrhotic architecture of their livers may predispose them to further damage during a perfusion deficit or a septic insult.[11] Furthermore, since these patients are often malnourished and immune compromised, they are more likely to develop systemic infections. Additionally, one study of cirrhotic patients found that 92.3% of the "healthy" cirrhotics evaluated had a chronic low-grade endotoxemia that was not seen in the noncirrhotic population.[32] This chronic endotoxic state may explain why cirrhotic patients have baseline systemic oxygen consumption levels well above those of normal unstressed noncirrhotic patients. Thus, any further perturbation of the physiologic balance in cirrhotic patients, whether by trauma or sepsis, could lead to MOFS and worsening of hepatic function.

Altered Systemic Metabolism: Carbohydrates

Total body energy expenditure increases 1.5 to 2 times normal (and frequently greater than 2 times normal), whereas substrate preferences change to place greater emphasis on protein as an energy source in critically ill or stressed patients.

The hyperglycemia, which develops in the presence of high insulin levels, is refractory to exogenous insulin. Consequently, whereas there is increased carbohydrate utilization relative to the starvation state, there is decreased glucose utilization relative to the degree of hyperglycemia present. Additionally, catecholamine stimulation of pancreatic alpha and beta islet cells results in a progressive increase in the glucagon to insulin ratio, which is far out of proportion to that predicted from the blood glucose level.

The liver's response to hypermetabolic stimuli is an initial increase in gluconeogenesis and increased glycogenolysis. The substrates of hepatic gluconeogenesis are lactate, alanine, glutamine, glycine, serine, and glycerol. Although much of this response is directed by the neuroendocrine axis, it can be altered in sepsis. Gluconeogenesis was studied in rats subjected to a long-term infusion of endotoxin.[33] Six hours after the initiation of the endotoxin infusion, hepatic gluconeogenesis was increased, but after 24 hours it was depressed. At 48 hours, the level of gluconeogenesis in the endotoxin-treated animals was not significantly different from that of the control animals, despite the fact that the endotoxemic animals manifested hyperglycemia, hyperlactacidemia, and had elevated glucagon and catecholamine levels. It was found on further evaluation that the hepatic conversion of lactate to glucose was no longer sensitive to stimulation from glucagon or norepinephrine. Other studies have shown that, although acute treatment with endotoxin increased glucagon binding to rat liver membrane receptors,[34] chronic therapy decreased the number and affinity of low affinity binding sites.[35] Therefore, although hepatic conversion of lactate to glucose continues, it may not be capable of up-regulating to meet the demands of increased lactate production. In those patients whose hepatic dysfunction worsens to overt failure, serum glucose decreases and lactate increases. This reflects the inability of the liver to maintain even baseline levels of glucose production, an ominous sign followed soon by death.

Altered Systemic Metabolism: Lipids and Ketones

Hypermetabolism is accompanied by hypertriglyceridemia, despite increased peripheral utilization relative to the starvation state. Although much of this increase is caused by the release of lipid stores from adipocytes, increased hepatic lipolysis and lipogenesis also contribute to the hypertriglyceridemic state. Feingold and Grunfeld[36] found that tumor necrosis factor, which is released by macrophages in response to endotoxin stimulation, helps to increase hepatocyte lipogenesis in rats.

Metabolism of lipids to ketones for energy utilization is increased in hypermetabolism, as reflected by an elevation in the total release of ketones. As liver dysfunction develops, the release of β-hydroxybutyrate progressively increases. Since β-hydroxybutyrate is produced predominantly in the liver, this increase demonstrates a decreasing capability of hepatocyte mitochondria to utilize ketones as an energy source. Simultaneously, the serum level of acetoacetate, which is extracted by the peripheral tissues, may decrease to the point of disappearance.[37] This appears to result from decreased hepatic release of acetoacetate as well as increased peripheral utilization. The ratio of acetoacetate to β-hydroxybutyrate has been suggested by some to reflect the hepatic mitochondrial redox potential. Ozawa et al.[6] found that a ratio of more than 0.4 in the arterial blood of postoperative patients was associated with tolerance of the surgical procedure, whereas a level less than 0.4 was associated with the onset of MOFS, and a level of less than 0.25 was associated with eventual mortality.

Altered Systemic Metabolism: Lactate

Lactate production is increased in hypermetabolism.[38,39] This may be due in part to several factors: increased substrate flow down glycolytic pathways with reduced entrance into the Krebs cycle, inadequate gluconeogenic pathways to handle the volume of substrate, decreased oxidative phosphorylation due to down-regulation of the tricarboxylic acid cycle, as from inadequate oxygen delivery. The primary tissue source of lactate is not completely known; postulates include muscle and inflammatory cells. Increased lactate formation in stable hypermetabolism appears to be due to a reduction in the rate of oxidation of pyruvate. Lactate levels also increase when the amount of fat and amino acids (particularly alanine and glutamine) utilized as a source of two carbon fragments in the Krebs cycle increases, or when pyruvate dehydrogenase activity is reduced. This response is best interpreted as consistent with aerobic metabolism (aerobic glycolysis). Since the conversion of pyruvate to lactate is not blocked in sepsis, the ratio of lactate to pyruvate remains normal and is associated stoichiometrically with the release of alanine.[2,37] Thus, an elevated lactate level in the presence of an increased lactate to pyruvate ratio suggests a perfusion defect and in this circumstance the patient should be resuscitated with an adequate volume of intravenous fluids to increase oxygen delivery. Conversely, an increased lactate in the presence of a normal lactate to pyruvate ratio suggests aerobic glycolysis or reduced hepatic clearance, or both.

Altered Systemic Metabolism: Protein

Peripheral protein autocannibalism is an important characteristic of the hypermetabolic response of sepsis. With the decreased ability of tissues to utilize carbohydrates as a complete energy source, the amino acids released from protein catabolism become the primary energy source of the peripheral tissues. The main source of the protein released has been shown to be from skeletal muscle.[40,41] Protein release from skeletal muscle appears to be mediated by hormones, such as cortisol, by cytokines, such as interleukin-1 (IL-1), by autocoids, such as the prostaglandins,[42] and by peptides, such as proteolytic-inducing factor.

Much work has been done analyzing peripheral plasma amino acid concentrations. The main assumption, on which this research is based, is that changes in amino acid concentration from the normal unstressed state reflect a change in the utilization of specific amino acids, which is related to the pathologic processes effecting the patient. For example, data from Cerra et al.[40] implies that there is a preferential utilization in patients with sepsis of branched chain amino acids (BCAA) in the following order of preference: leucine, isoleucine, and valine.

To assess the differential effects of liver dysfunction on the plasma amino acid profile in septic and nonseptic states, Cerra et al.[11] measured the plasma amino acid profile postoperatively in patients with preexistent cirrhosis after elective surgery, and compared this profile to the profiles seen in noncirrhotic patients, noncirrhotic patients with sepsis, and cirrhotic patients with sepsis. This study showed that patients with cirrhosis had increased levels of aromatic amino acids, which are known to be predominantly metabolized by the liver (phenylalanine, tyrosine, and tryptophan), as well as decreased levels of branched chain amino acids. In contrast, these cirrhotic patients did not develop any abnormality of glucose or fat metabolism and recovered satisfactorily from their operations.

Cirrhotic and noncirrhotic patients who developed sepsis had similar responses, with elevated aromatic amino acid levels and decreased branched chain amino acid levels, as well as altered peripheral energy metabolism. Nonsurvivors with sepsis developed increased branched chain amino acid levels as death approached, indicating premorbid peripheral metabolic collapse. Pittiruti et al.[43] compared patients with and without sepsis after trauma and found similar results to those of Cerra et al. They noted a correlation between the development of an increased leucine to tyrosine ratio and eventual death. The degree of elevation of aromatic amino acids, particularly phenylalanine, has also been found to correlate directly with multiple factors, including the degree of hepatic dysfunction, the level of bilirubin, rate of amino acid clearance, and eventual death.[4,11,17,18]

Accumulation of aromatic amino acids in patients with hepatic failure of any cause has been theorized by Fisher and Baldessarini[44] to be the cause of hepatic encephalopathy. They reason that the elevated blood levels of the aromatic amino acids will lead to encephalopathy, since as the blood levels of these aromatic amino acids increase, the rate of transport of these amino acids through the blood-brain barrier also increases. In the central nervous system, these amino acids are metabolized to neuroactive substances, which alter the normal neurotransmitter balance and consequently alter neurologic function.

Altered Cellular Function

Many different cell types make up the substance of the liver, with parenchymal cells (hepatocytes), tissue macrophage (Kupffer cells), endothelial or sinusoidal cells, stromal cells, and canalicular cells being the most prevalent. These cells are positioned in close proximity to each other, facilitating interaction between cell types. This interaction has been shown to alter hepatocellular function with the potential for injury and cell death. This appears to result from the effects of the mediators of cell-cell communications.

Mediators

There are many mediators that are believed to cause some of the changes in physiologic parameters seen in MOFS. An understanding of the actions and interactions of each of these mediators is by no means complete. Current research indicates that the interactions between these mediators are complex, and their effects are wide ranging. This work indicates that key roles are played by IL-1, interleukin-2 (IL-2), tumor necrosis factor (TNF) and the eicosanoids. Several other substances are potentially important; however, evidence implicating them is not quite as strong.

INTERLEUKIN-1

IL-1 is a protein secreted by many cells, including endothelial cells and cells of the monocyte-macrophage line. There are two forms found in humans (alpha and beta), which to date have not been found to have any significant functional differences. Mononuclear cells can be stimulated to produce IL-1 by activated T cells, immune complexes, the C5a component of complement, and cell wall components of microorganisms. In myelohematopoetic tissues, the presence of IL-1 has been shown to be important for optimal cellular activation and proliferation to occur. Other extrahepatic functions of IL-1 include induction of fever, prostaglandin production, fibroblast release of collagenase, and induction of protein autocannibalism in skeletal muscle.[42,45]

INTERLEUKIN-2

IL-2 is also a protein. It is secreted by T lymphocytes on stimulation by IL-1 or by antigen in association with accessory cells (monocytes and B cells). The functions of IL-2 include stimulation of proliferative responses in lymphocytes, mediation of some of the processes leading to antibody production, and induction of lymphokine-activated killer activity by some classes of lymphoid cells.[46,47]

TUMOR NECROSIS FACTOR

The term "tumor necrosis" is based on the observation that this factor can induce hemorrhagic necrosis of tumors in certain experimental models. This factor previously was called cachectin because it was capable of producing anorexia and metabolic disorders leading to cachexia. TNF is produced by activated macrophages, and endotoxin has been identified as one of the most potent stimulators of its production. Receptors for TNF are present on all somatic cells with the exception of erythrocytes. TNF causes a wide range of metabolic alterations, which include enhancement of neutrophil phagocytic and cytotoxic activities, induction of endothelial production of IL-1 and procoagulant factors, augmentation of lymphocyte production of and response to IL-2, and induction of a general shocklike state.[48]

EICOSANOIDS

Eicosanoids are derivatives of arachidonic acid and include the prostaglandins, thromboxanes, and leukotrienes. These substances possess many functions: some eicosanoids cause increased vascular and general smooth muscle tone, whereas others cause vasodilation and decreased smooth muscle tone; some cause platelet aggregation, whereas others inhibit platelet aggregation; some augment immune function and others suppress these functions. Miller-Graziano et al.[49] documented an association between immune suppression and high circulating levels of prostaglandin E_2 (PGE_2) in burn patients with multiple serious infections. They also noted that these patients have a late appearing (more than 12 days) population of T suppressor cells, which stimulate monocyte production of PGE_2, as well as a higher than normal proportion of circulating monocytes with receptors for the Fc portion of the antibody heavy chain. These FcR+ monocytes have been identified as a major source of PGE_2.[47] Interestingly, Kupffer cells in some species have been noted to have a very high percentage of cells with Fc receptors.[50] However, whether or not Kupffer cells have a significant role as PGE_2 producers is not known.

OTHERS

Nitric oxide, also known as endothelial relaxing factor, is released by the enzymatic degradation of L-arginine by endothelial cells and macrophages stimulated in vitro with bradykinin and calcium ionophore. In vivo, nitric oxide is believed to penetrate smooth muscle cells and cause relaxation of vascular tone.[51] It has also been shown to inhibit platelet adhesion and aggregation. Some hypothesize that nitric oxide may affect hepatocellular protein secretion and viability.[52] Superoxide radical has also been mentioned as a possible mediator of hepatocellular injury or death in MOFS. Superoxide is produced by phagocytic cells as part of the respiratory burst used to destroy invading organisms. Although there is great potential for cellular damage by phagocyte-generated oxidants, there is little evidence that oxidant-mediated injury is an important mechanism in the hepatic dysfunction of MOFS.[52]

Kupffer Cells

Kupffer cells make up about 70% of the tissue macrophages in the body and comprise 40 to 80% of nonparenchymal cells isolated from the liver. Kupffer cells are located along the hepatic sinusoids and lie in direct contact with hepatic parenchymal cells. These cells have an immune or phagocytic function and are the primary hepatic source of IL-1, TNF, and eicosanoids. Their numbers increase severalfold in sepsis, a response that can be duplicated by the infusion of lipopolysaccharide or zymosan. Bouwens et al.[53,54] found that about 75% of the Kupffer cell expansion is due to the proliferation of local Kupffer cells, and the additional increase in the Kupffer cell population appears to be due to the recruitment of peripheral macrophage precursors. At least 90% of Kupffer cells proliferate after stimulation with zymosan.[53]

Mazuski et al.[55] found that cultured Kupffer cells release significant quantities of IL-1, TNF, and PGE_2 into the surrounding media when stimulated with endotoxin. Production of IL-1 after lipopolysaccharide stimulation has been shown to be enhanced by the addition of IL-2, suggesting a mechanism for T cell cooperation.[56] IL-2 production is also augmented by incubation of the Kupffer cells with hepatocytes or media in which hepatocytes have been grown.[57] Endotoxin-induced TNF production by Kupffer cells can be further increased by platelet activating factor (PAF), a substance that leads to platelet aggregation and increases platelet adhesion to endothelial surfaces.[58,59]

Activation of Kupffer cell functions by endotoxin is probably mediated by diacylglycerol activation of protein kinase C. Lipopolysaccharide and zymosan also have been shown to activate phospholipase A_2 (PLA_2) in the rat Kupffer cell.[60] Full activity of PLA_2 requires the activity of membrane bound, adenosine triphosphate-dependent, calmodulin enhanced, Ca^{+2} transport.[60] Although rapid intracellular Ca^{+2} fluxes do not induce Kupffer cells to produce mediators, increased Ca^{+2} flux has been shown to be the mechanism by which PAF augments TNF production by macrophages and Kupffer cells.[58,59,61,62] There is also evidence that PGE_2 production depends on changes in intracellular Ca^{+2} [60] as well as an activated $Na^+/H/^+$ exchange.[63]

Hepatocytes

To understand the hepatic dysfunction seen in MOFS on a cellular or molecular basis, one must be able to explain three important histopathologic observations: (1) the histologic presence of centrilobular congestion of hepatocyte necrosis; (2) the decreased ability of the liver to clear substances from the blood, as exemplified by the development of intrahepatic cholestasis and the failure of amino acid clearance; and (3) temporal change in hepatic synthetic function, as manifested by an early increase in acute-phase protein production followed by eventual failure of both acute-phase and nonacute-phase protein synthesis.

The exact pathophysiologic explanation for the hepatocyte damage and death seen in MOFS is not well understood. At present, there are three predominant theories to explain this phenomenon. The first theory is that the combination of decreased hepatic blood flow and increased substrate requirements seen in MOFS leads to cell damage from anoxia or ischemia, or both. This view is supported by evidence that hepatic blood flow is diminished and hepatocyte susceptibility to anoxic damage is increased in MOFS.[20,64] Additionally, transient hepatic ischemia has been shown to cause many of the functional features seen in MOFS.

The second theory is that a bacterial substance, presumably endotoxin, may have a direct toxic effect on the hepatocyte. Direct effects on hepatocellular functions have been shown by incubation of cultured cells with endotoxin; however, little evidence of an hepatotoxic effect has been demonstrated in vitro.[65] The third theory is that some substance produced by the body in response to sepsis has an autotoxic effect. Although superoxide radical had been identified as a likely mediator of hepatocyte damage, further investigation suggests that little superoxide is produced by Kupffer cells. Other possibilities are currently being evaluated.

More information is available concerning the development of intrahepatic cholestasis. Excretion of conjugated bilirubin has been associated with the functioning of Na^+,K^+-ATPase located on the canalicular membrane. This enzyme has been shown to be noncompetitively inhibited by endotoxin.[66,67] IL-1, IL-2 , and γ-interferon appear to have no effect on bile flow.[68] Inhibition of Na^+,K^+-ATPase is not limited to endotoxin; delayed BSP excretion also occurs in rabbits after infusion of a solution containing *S. aureus* or lipoteichoic acid.[28] Cytochrome P450, an enzyme important in degradation of some drugs, has also been shown to be impaired.[69] In fact, Pagani et al.[70] have suggested that the defect in cytochrome P450 activity is due to direct inhibition by endotoxin. However, Ghezzi et al.[71] and Shedlofsky et al.[72] both using endotoxin-sensitive mice, have shown that IL-1 also will decrease cytochrome P450 activity. Therefore endotoxin stimulation of IL-1 production by the Kupffer cells may play a major role in modulating hepatocyte function.

Hepatocyte acute-phase protein synthesis can be induced by several different stimuli, including the products of Kupffer cells. For example, in coculture experiments, when rat hepatocytes and Kupffer cells are incubated together, hepatocyte protein synthesis is increased compared with cultures of hepatocytes alone. Although endotoxin induces a biphasic response in protein synthesis,[71] ultimately both total as well as acute-phase protein synthesis is decreased. This hepatocyte acute-phase protein synthesis response has been further characterized. It is now clear that endotoxin will increase the synthesis of proteins normally expressed by hepatocytes as well as increase the production of new proteins. Among the proteins isolated are antithrombin III and alpha$_1$-proteinase inhibitor.[72,73] The later decrease in total protein synthesis[74] is due in part to suppression of albumin synthesis.[75] These results have been found to be greatly exaggerated when the cocultures are incubated under hypoxic conditions (oxygen tension 18 torr).

When endotoxin is incubated with hepatocytes alone or with hepatocytes cocultured with lymphocytes, there is no evidence of a biphasic protein synthetic response.[74] Endotoxin does induce some hepatic protein synthesis[75,76] and media conditioned by endotoxin-stimulated hepatocytes have been shown to stimulate Kupffer cells to produce IL-1 and TNF as well as prostanoids, such as PGE$_2$.[55] These results have led to the hypothesis that hepatocellular injury is due to a paracrine, amplified cytotoxicity mediated by activated macrophages.

The mechanisms by which hepatocyte-Kupffer cell interactions alter hepatocyte function is an area of intense investigation. IL-1 and TNF have been shown to alter hepatocyte production of serum amyloid-p component, haptoglobin, complement C3, fibrinogen, 1-acid glycoprotein, and albumin.[77–80] Many of these changes seem to be species specific, whereas others have been demonstrated only in transformed cell lines. Therefore these in vitro findings may or may not accurately reflect in vivo hepatocyte function. West et al.,[81] using rat hepatocytes, found that endotoxin-stimulated cocultures produced a wide variety of proteins. The patterns of protein production were not altered by incubation of the hepatocyte cultures or cocultures with additional IL-1 or TNF. This would suggest the existence of an additional as yet unidentified mediator, such as nitric oxide, which is mediating the effect of Kupffer cells on hepatocyte function.

The interaction between Kupffer cells and hepatocytes also appears to be modulated by systemic factors. Billiar et al.[82] showed that germ-free rats had decreased Kupffer cell responses to endotoxin compared with rats fed endotoxin or a solution containing bacteria.[83] In further studies, intestinal overgrowth of bacteria was found to make the Kupffer cells even more responsive than normal.[84]

Treatment

The mainstay of treatment is to prevent or correct the physiologic abnormalities that may lead to hepatic dysfunction. Hemodynamic stabilization is a key factor that must be addressed immediately. This may be best achieved through resuscitation with adequate amounts of intravenous fluids. Dahn et al.[85] observed in humans that resuscitation was not complete until a hyperdynamic splanchnic perfusion could be demonstrated. Thus, pharmacologic manipulation of the cardiac output with dobutamine or nitroprusside to reach a maximal oxygen consumption appears to be clinically indicated to prevent hepatic dysfunction. It must be remembered that hepatic blood flow may be decreased despite a normal- or even hyperdynamic-appearing cardiovascular response. Therefore fluid resuscitation should be initiated early in all patients at risk of developing MOFS and hepatic dysfunction.

Medications that are known to decrease blood flow to the splanchnic circulation should be avoided. Most notable of this group is dopamine, which in the absence of adequate fluid resuscitation or in high doses will decrease splanchnic blood flow. Vasoconstrictors maintain blood pressure by increasing peripheral resistance; thus, they reduce organ blood flow. In some instances, this decrease in circulation affects specific vascular beds to a greater extent than others, as is the case of dopamine's effect on the splanchnic circulation. Adjustment of the cardiac output with fluids and inotropes to provide adequate substrate delivery should be monitored by oxygen consumption and serum lactate to ensure that therapies directed at maintaining cardiovascular homeostasis does not lead to hepatic dysfunction or other complications.

The underlying disease process must also be treated. This entails debridement of injured or necrotic tissue, drainage of abscesses, and treatment of existing infections with appropriate antibiotics.

Nutritional support should be initiated as soon as possible to supplement the body's nutritional requirements. Route of alimentation (enteral versus parenteral) has not yet been shown to be a factor in the incidence of MOFS.[86] Formulas supplemented with additional branched chain amino acids (BCAA) have been recommended, because they may be an important cellular energy source during hypermetabolism and in patients with hepatic dysfunction, they stimulate or support hepatic protein synthesis, and they are associated with a reduced rate of ureagenesis. Wright et al.[87] compared different BCAA formulas in cirrhotic patients and found that formulas containing 35% and 53% BCAA supplementation improved protein synthesis and protein balance compared with other formulas, although none of his patients attained a positive nitrogen balance. These formulas contain little aromatic amino acids, since they have been linked with hepatic encephalopathy. In fact, several studies have suggested improvement in the mental status of patients with hepatic encephalopathy treated with BCAA.[88,89]

The source of fat provided for intravenous nutrition may provide a new direction in treatment. Macrophages from rats fed a diet enriched in ω-3 fats (fish oil) showed a decrease in PGE_2, prostacyclin, and thromboxane A_2 production, as well as a decrease in IL-1 and TNF release in response to endotoxin. After 6 weeks of ω-3 fat therapy, these cells continued to show a decreased production of IL-1 and TNF. Although rats fed a diet enriched in ω-6 fats (safflower oil) showed a decrease in IL-1 and TNF production after 6 weeks of dietary therapy, IL-1 and TNF release was increased after 2 weeks of this diet.[90] These data suggest that dietary manipulation of substrate may be a means of improving survival by altering the response of macrophages to certain stimuli.

Prognosis

The probability of recovery from hepatic dysfunction in the setting of MOFS depends on the degree of hepatic dysfunction as well as the general condition

Table 14–1　Possible Humoral Mediators of MOF

Cytokines
  Interleukin-1
  Interleukin-2
  Interferon-ʃ
  Platelet activating factor
  Tumor necrosis factor
Eicosanoids
  Prostaglandins (PGE$_1$, PGE$_2$, prostacyclin)
  Thromboxanes (TxA$_2$)
  Leukotrienes (LTC$_4$, LTD$_4$)
Mediator amines
  Histamine
  Serotonin
  Epinephrine
  Norepinephrine
  5-hydroxyindoleacetic acid
  Octopamine
  Phenylethanolamine
Opioids and other neurotransmitters
  Enkephalin
  ʝ-endorphin
Hormonal amines and peptides
  Thyroxine
  Growth hormone
  Insulin
  Glucagon
Complement
Kinin
Fibronectin
Growth factors
Enzymes
  Proteases (acid and neutral)
  Other lysosomal enzymes
Steroids
  Corticosteroids
Nitric oxide (derived from L-arginine)
Oxygen-derived intermediates
  Superoxide radical
  Hydroxyl radical
  Hydrogen peroxide

of the patient. Should the patient develop overt hepatic failure, the prognosis is grim. Taking a different perspective, Matuschak et al.[91] studied the prognosis of patients with preexistent liver failure who developed MOFS. In this population of patients awaiting possible liver transplant, the mortality was 100%. With our current state of technology, avoidance of hepatic failure in MOFS is clearly the preferred course.

Table 14–2 Hypermetabolism Versus Starvation

Characteristic	Starvation	Stress
Cardiac output	↓	↑ ↑
Systemic vascular resistance	NC	↓
Oxygen consumption	↓	↑ ↑
Resting energy expenditure	↓	↑ ↑ ↑
Mediator activation	NC	↑ ↑
Regulatory responsiveness	↑ ↑ ↑ ↑	↑
Respiratory quotient	0.75	0.85
Primary fuels	fat	mixed
Proteolysis	↑	↑ ↑ ↑
Protein oxidation	↑	↑ ↑ ↑
Branched-chain oxidation	↑	↑ ↑ ↑
Hepatic protein synthesis	↑	↑ ↑ ↑
Ureagenesis	↑	↑ ↑ ↑
Glycogenolysis	↑	↑ ↑ ↑
Gluconeogenesis	↑	↑ ↑ ↑
Lipolysis	↑ ↑	↑ ↑ ↑
Ketone body production	↑ ↑ ↑ ↑	↑
Rate of development of malnutrition	↑	↑ ↑ ↑ ↑

Table 14–3 Nutritional Requirements for Starvation Versus Hypermetabolism

Setting	Malnutrition	Hypermetabolism or Organ Failure
Basis	Starvation	Metabolic stress
Focus	Emphasis of visceral proteins and lean body mass	Preservation of organ structure and function No substrate limitation facilitation of repair
Fuel utilization		
Glucose	Used if available	Increased (but provides a lesser fraction of total energy needs)
Fat	Increased utilization	Increased utilization
Protein	Spared	Greatly increased utilization
Nonprotein calories per gram nitrogen	≥150/L	≤100/L
Protein g/kg/day	1.0	1.5–2.0
Fat	As tolerated for energy equilibrium in conjunction with glucose	0.5 to 1.0 g/kg/day
Glucose	As tolerated	4–5 gm/kg/day

References

1. Sarfeh IJ, Balint JA. The clinical significance of hyperbilirubinemia following trauma. J Trauma 1978;18:58–62.
2. Nunes G, Blaisdell FW, Margaretten W. Mechanism of hepatic dysfunction following shock and trauma. Arch Surg 1970;100:546–556.
3. Cerra FB. Multiple organ failure syndrome. Perspect Crit Care 1988;1:1–30.
4. Cerra FB, Negro F, Eyer S, Abrams J, Perry J. Multiple organ failure syndrome: Patterns and effect of current therapy. Update in Intensive Care and Emergency Medicine Vol II, 1990; (in press).
5. Gottlieb ME, Stratton HH, Newell JC, Shah DM. Indocyanine green: its use as an early indicator of hepatic dysfunction following injury in man. Arch Surg 1984;119:264–268.
6. Ozawa K, Aoyama H, Yasuda K, Simahara Y, Nakatani T, Tanaka J, Yamamoto Y, Kamiyama Y, Tobe T. Metabolic abnormalities associated with postoperative organ failure. Arch Surg 1983;118:1245–1251.
7. Ruchti C. Pathomorphologische Befunde nach Intensivtherapie. Schweiz Med Wockenschr 1986;116:694–698.
8. Irie H, Mori W. Fatal hepatic necrosis after shock. Acta Pathol Jpn 1986;36:363–374.
9. Mallory TB, Sullivan ER, Burnett CH, Fiorindo AS, Shapiro SL, Beecher HK. The general pathology of traumatic shock. Surgery 1950;27:629–644.
10. Nuytinck JKS, Grois RJA, Weerts JGE, Schillings PHM, Schuurmans Stekhoven JH. Acute generalized microvascular injury by activated compliment and hypoxia: the basis of the adult respiratory distress syndrome and multiple organ failure? Br J Exp Pathol 1986;67:537–548.
11. Cerra FB, Seigel JH, Border JR, Wiles J, McMenamy RR. The hepatic failure of sepsis: cellular versus substrate. Surgery 1979;86:409–422.
12. Gottlieb ME, Sarfeh IJ, Stratton H, Goldman ML, Newell JC, Shah DM. Hepatic perfusion and splanchnic oxygen consumption in patients postinjury. J Trauma 1983;23:836–843.
13. Sarfeh IJ, Balint JA. Hepatic dysfunction following trauma: experimental studies. J Surg Res 1977;22:370–375.
14. Schirmer WJ, Schirmer JM, Townsend MC, Fry DE. Femur fracture with associated soft-tissue injury produces hepatic ischemia. Arch Surg 1988;123:412–415.
15. Schirmer WJ, Schirmer JM, Naff GB, Fry DE. Complement activation in peritonitis. Am Surg 1987;53:683–687.
16. Schirmer WJ, Schirmer JM, Naff GB, Fry DE. Systemic complement activation produces hemodynamic changes characteristic of sepsis. Arch Surg 1988;123:316–321.
17. Fath JJ, St.Cyr JA, Konstantinides FN, Alden P, Ascher NL, Bianco RW, Foker JE, Cerra FB. Alterations in amino acid clearance during ischemia predict hepatocellular ATP changes. Surgery 1985;98:396–404.
18. Becker W, Konstantinides F, Eyer S, Ward H, Fath J, Cerra FB. Plasma amino acid clearance as an indicator of hepatic function and high-energy phosphate in hepatic ischemia. Surgery 1987;102:777–783.
19. Machiedo GW, Hurd T, Rush BF, Dikdan G, McGee J, Lysz T. Temporal relationship of hepatocellular dysfunction and ischemia in sepsis. Arch Surg 1988;123:424–427.
20. Kellar GA, Barke R, Harty JT, Humphrey E, Simmons RL. Decreased hepatic glutathione levels in septic shock. Arch Surg 1985;120:941–945.
21. Seibel R, LaDuca J, Hassett JM, et al. Blunt multiple trauma (ISS 36), femur traction, and the pulmonary failure-septic state. Ann Surg 1985;202:283–295.
22. Amaral JF, Shearer JD, Caldwell MD. Examination of lactate metabolism in the cellular infiltrate of wounded tissue. Surg Forum 1986;37:30–33.
23. Morris AS, Shearer JD, Forster J, Mastrofrancesco B, Henry W, Caldwell MD. The relationship of purine metabolism to the macrophage-mediated increase of high energy phosphates in skeletal muscle. J Surg Res 1986;41:339–346.
24. Wiles JB, Cerra FB, Siegel JH, Border JR. The systemic septic response: does the organism matter? Crit Care Med 1980;8:55–60.
25. Carrico CJ, Meakins JL, Marchall JC, Fry D, Maier RV. Multiple-organ-failure syndrome. Arch Surg 1986;121:196–208.
26. Becker W, Konstantinides F, Cerra F. Interactions between endotoxin, the liver, systemic hemodynamics and amino acid metabolism. Circ Shock 1987;21:301.
27. Hideko A, Ogle CK, Alexander JW, Warden GD. Induction of hypermetabolism in guinea pigs by endotoxin infused through the portal vein. Arch Surg 1988;123:1420–1424.

28. Quale JM, Mandel IJ, Bergasa NV, Straus EW. Clinical significance and pathogenesis of hyperbilirubinemia associated with *Staphylococcus*. Am J Med 1988;85:615–618.
29. Marshall JC, Christou NV, Horn R, Meakins JL. The microbiology of multiple organ failure. Arch Surg 1988;123:309–315.
30. Mochizuki H, Trocki O, Dominioni L, et al. Mechanism of prevention of postburn, hypermetabolism, and catabolism by early enteral feeding. Ann Surg 1984;200:297–310.
31. O'Dwyer ST, Michie HR, Ziegler TR, Revhaug A, Smith RJ, Wilmore DW. A single dose of endotoxin increases intestinal permeability in healthy humans. Arch Surg 1988;123:1459–1464.
32. Bigatello LM, Broitman SA, Fattori L, DiPaoli M, Pontello M, Bevilacqua G, Nespoli A. Endotoxemia, encephalopathy, and mortality in cirrhotic patients. Am J Gastroenterol 1987;82:11–15.
33. Spitzer JA, Nelson KM, Fish RE. Time course of changes in gluconeogenesis from various precursors in chronically endotoxemic rats. Metabolism 1985;34:842–849.
34. Abernathy CO, Bhatena SJ, Recant L, Zimmerman HJ, Utili R. Effects of acute and chronic endotoxin treatment on glucagon and insulin receptors on rat liver plasma membranes. Horm Metabol Res 1982;14:486–471.
35. Pagani R, Protoles MT, Muncio AM. Effect of Escherichia coli lipopolysaccharide on the glucagon and insulin binding to isolated rat hepatocytes. Mol Cell Biochem 1985;65:37–44.
36. Feingold KR, Grunfeld C. Tumor necrosis factor-alpha stimulates hepatic lipogenesis in the rat in vivo. J Clin Invest 1987;80:184–190.
37. Cerra FB, Border JR, McMenamy RH, Siegel JH. Multiple systems organ failure. In Pathophysiology of shock, anoxia, and ischemia. BF Trump, RA Crowly (eds.); Baltimore: Williams and Wilkins, 1982; 254–270.
38. Cerra FB. Metabolic response to injury. In Manual of critical care. FB Cerra (ed). St. Louis: Mosvy, 1987:117–145.
39. Siegel JH, Cerra FB, Coleman B, et al. Physiologic and metabolic correlations in human sepsis. Surgery 1979;86:163–193.
40. Cerra FB, Seigel JH, Coleman B, Border JR, McMenamy RR. Septic autocannibalism. Ann Surg 1980;192:570–580.
41. Harkema JM, Gorman MW, Bieber LL, Chaudry IH. Metabolic interaction between skeletal muscle and liver during bacteremia. Arch Surg 1988;123:1415–1419.
42. Goldberg AL, Baracos V, Rodemann P, Waxman L, Dinarello C. Control of protein degradation in muscle by prostaglandins, Ca^{2+}, and leukocytic pyrogen (interleukin 1). Fed Proc 1984;43:1301–1306.
43. Pittiruti M, Seigel JH, Sganga G, Coleman B, Wiles CE, Belzberg H, Wedel S, Placko R. Increased dependence of leucine in posttraumatic sepsis: leucine/tyrosine clearance ratio as an indicator of hepatic impairment in septic multiple organ failure syndrome. Surgery 1985;98:378–387.
44. Fischer JE, Baldessarini RJ. False neurotransmitters and hepatic failure. Lancet 1971;2:75–79.
45. Durum SK, Schmidt JA, Oppenheim JJ. Interleukin 1: an immunological perspective. Ann Rev Immunol 1985;3:263–287.
46. Robb RJ. Interleukin 2: the molecule and its function. Immunol Today 1984;5:203–209.
47. Smith KA. Interleukin-2: inception, impact, and implications. Science 1988;240:1169–1176.
48. Beutler B, Cerami A. Tumor necrosis, cachexia, shock, and inflammation: a common mediator. Annu Rev Biochem 1988;57:505–518.
49. Miller-Graziano CL, Fink M, Wu JY, Szabo G, Kodys K. Mechanisms of altered myoncyte prostaglandin E2 production in severely injured patients. Arch Surg 1988;123:293–299.
50. Ding A, Nathan C. Analysis of nonfunctional respiratory burst in murine Kupffer cells. J Exp Med 1988;167:1154–1170.
51. Palmer RMJ, Ashton DS, Moncada S. Vascular endothelial cells synthesize nitric oxide from L-arginine. Nature 1988;333:664–666.
52. Billiar TR, Curran RD, West MA, Simmons RL. Toxic L-arginine metabolites produced by endotoxin activated Kupffer cells induce hepatocyte death. Arch Surg 1989; In press.
53. Bouwens L, Baekeland M, Wisse E. Cytokinetic analysis of the expanding Kupffer-cell opulation in rat liver. Cell Tissue Kinet 1986;19:217–226.
54. Bouwens L, Knook DL, Wisse E. Local proliferation and extrahepatic recruitment of liver macrophages (Kupffer cells) in partial-body irradiated rats. J Leukoc Biol 1986;39:687–697.
55. Mazuski JE, Bankey PE, Carlson A, Cerra FB. Hepatocytes release factors which can modulate macrophage IL-1 secretion and proliferation. Surg Forum 1988;39:13–15.
56. Curran RD, Billiar TR, West MA, Bentz BG, Simmons RL. Effect of interleukin-2 on Kupffer cell activation. Interleukin-2 primes and activates Kupffer cells to suppress hepatocyte protein synthesis in vitro. Arch Surg 1988;123:1373–1378.

57. Mazuski JE, West MA, Towle HC, Simmons RL, Cerra FB. Enhanced release of interleukin-1 like activity by hepatocyte:macrophage cocultures. Surg Forum 1987;38:21–23.
58. Bankey P, Carlson A, Singh R, Cerra F. Platelet activating factor signals rapid turnover of phosphatidylinositol in P388D1 Macrophages. Cell Biochem (Abstr.) 1988.
59. Bankey P, Wen YW, Singh R, Carlson A, Cerra FB. Platelet activating factor primes macrophage for lipopolysaccharide signaled tumor necrosis factor release: mechanism by rapid increase in intracellular calcium. (Abstr., Shock Conference).
60. Birmelin M, Marme D, Ferber E, Decker K. Calmodulin content and activity of Ca^{2+}-ATPase and phospholipase A2 in rat Kupffer cells. Eur J Biochem 1984;140:55–61.
61. Bankey PE, Fleigel V, Lee HC, Cerra FB. Kupffer cell activation by lipopolysaccharide is not signaled by rapid intracellular calcium changes. (FASEB Abstr., 1988).
62. Deiter P, Schulze-Specking A, Decker K. Ca^{2+} requirement of prostanoid but not superoxide production by rat Kupffer cells. Eur J Biochem 1988;177:61–67.
63. Deiter P, Schulze-Specking A, Karck U, Decker K. Prostaglandin release but not superoxide production by rat Kupffer cells stimulated in vitro depends of Na^+H^+ exchange. Eur J Biochem 1987;170:201–206.
64. Liu MS, Zhang JN. Glycolytic and tricarboxylic acid cycle intermediates in dog livers during endotoxic shock. Biochem Med 1985;34:335–343.
65. Kellar GA, West MA, Cerra FB, Simmons RL. Multiple system organ failure. Modulation of hepatocyte protein synthesis by endotoxin activated Kupffer cells. Ann Surg 1985;201:87–95.
66. Utili R, Abernathy CO, Zimmerman HJ. Inhibition of Na^+, K^+-adenosinetriphosphatase by endotoxin: a possible mechanism for endotoxin-induced cholestasis. J Infect Dis 1977;136:583–587.
67. Utili R, Abernathy CO, Zimmerman HJ. Studies of nte effects of E. coli endotoxin on canalicular bile formation in the isolated perfused liver. J Lab Clin Med 1977;89:471–482.
68. Rustgi VK, Jones DB, Dinarello CA, Hoofnagle JH. Lymphokines and bile secretion in the rat. Liver 1987;7:149–154.
69. Yoshida M, Egawa K, Kasai N. Effect of endotoxin and its degradation products on hepatic mixed-function oxidase and heme enzyme systems in mice. Toxicol Lett 1982;12:185–190.
70. Pagani R, Portoles MT, Bosch MA, Diaz-Laviada I, Municio AM. Direct and mediated Escherichia coli lipopolysaccharide action in primary hepatocyte cultures. Eur J Cell Biol 1987;43:243–246.
71. Ghezzi P, Saccardo B, Villa P, Rossi V, Bianchi M, Dinarello CA. Role of interleukin-1 in the depression of liver drug metabolism by endotoxin. Infect Immun 1986;54:837–840.
72. Shedlofsky SI, Swim AT, Robinson JM, Gallicchio VS, Cohen DA, McClain CJ: Interleukin-1 (IL-1) depresses cytochrome P450 levels and activities in mice. Life Sci 1987;40:2331–2336.
73. Hoffman M, Fuchs HE, Pizzo SV. The macrophage-mediated regulation of hepatocyte synthesis of antithrombin III and alpha 1-proteinase inhibitor. Thromb Res 1986;41:707–715.
74. West MA, Kellar GA, Hyland BJ, Cerra FB, Simmons RL. Hepatocyte function in sepsis: Kupffer cells mediate a biphasic protein synthesis response in hepatocytes after exposure to endotoxin or killed Escherichia coli. Surgery 1985;98:388–395.
75. Mazuski JE, Ortiz M, Towle HC, Cerra FB. Hepatic protein synthesis can be directly regulated by endotoxin in vitro. The Assoc. for Academic Surgery (Abstr.) 1988.
76. Mazuski JE, Platt JL, West MA, Simmons RL, Towel HC, Cerra FB. Direct effects of endotoxin on hepatocytes: Synthesis of a specific secretory protein. Arch Surg 1988;123:340–344.
77. Baumann H, Onorato V, Gauldie J, Jahreir GP, distinct sets of acute phase plasma proteins are stimulated by separate human hepatocyte-stimulating factors and monokines in rat hepatoma cells. J Biol Chem 1987;262:9756–9768.
78. Mortensen RF, Shapiro J, Lin B, Douches S, Neta R. Interaction of recombinant IL-1 and recombinant tumor necrosis factor in the induction of mouse acute phase proteins. J Immunol 1988;140:2260–2266.
79. Mackiewicz A, Ganapathi M, Schultz D, Kushner I: Monokines regulate glycosylation of acute phase proteins. J Exp Med 1987;166:253–258.
80. Baumann H, Richards C, Gauldie J. Interaction among hepatocyte-stimulating factors, interleukin-1, and glucocorticoids for regulation of acute phase plasma proteins in human hepatoma (HepG2) cells. J Immunol 1987;139:4122–4128.
81. West MA, Billiar TR, Mazuski JE, Curran RJ, Cerra FB, Simmons RL. Endotoxin modulation of hepatocyte secretory and cellular protein synthesis is mediated by Kupffer cells. Arch Surg 1988;123:1400–1405.
82. Billiar TR, West MA, Hyland BJ, Simmons RL. Splenectomy alters Kupffer cell response to endotoxin. Arch Surg 1988;123:327–332.
83. Billiar TR, Maddaus MA, West MA, Dunn DL, Simmons RL. The role of intestinal flora on the

interactions between nonparenchymal cells and hepatocytes in coculture. J Surg Res 1988;44:397–403.

84. Billiar TR, Maddaus MA, West MA, Curran RD, Wells CA, Simmons RL. Intestinal gram-negative bacterial overgrowth in vivo augments the in vitro response of Kupffer cells to endotoxin. Ann Surg 1988;108:532–540.
85. Dahn MS, Lang P, Lobdell K, Hans B, Jacobs LA, Mitchell RA. Splanchnic and total body oxygen consumption differences in septic and injury patients. Surgery 1987;101:69–80.
86. Cerra FB, McPherson J, Konstantinides F, Konstantinides N, Teasley K. Enteral nutrition does not prevent multiple organ failure syndrome from sepsis (MOFS). Arch Surg 1988;104:723–733.
87. Wright PD, Holdsworth JD, Dionigi P, Clague MB, James OFW. Effect of branched chain amino acid infusions on body protein metabolism in cirrhosis of liver. Gut 1988;27(Suppl 1):96–102.
88. Cerra FB, Cheung NK, Fischer JE, et al. Disease-specific amino acid infusion (FO80) in hepatic encephalopathy: a perspective, randomized, double blind controlled trial. JPEN 1985;9:288–295.
89. Fanelli FR, Cangiano C, Capocaccia L, Cascino A, Ceci F, Muscaritoli, Giunchi G. Use of branched chain amino acids for treating hepatic encephalopathy: clinical experiences. Gut 1986;27(Suppl 1):111–115.
90. Billiar TR, Bankey PE, Svingen BA, Curran RD, West MA, Holman RT, Simmons RL, Cerra FB. Fatty acid intake and Kupffer cell function: Fish oil alters eicosanoid and monokine production to endotoxin stimulation. Surgery 1988;104:343–349.
91. Matuschak GM, Martin DJ. Influence of end-stage liver failure on survival during multiple systems organ failure. Transplant Proc 1987;19:40–46.

15

Role of Immediate Surgery in Prevention of Multiple Organ Failure

JOHN R. BORDER, JORGE RODRIGUEZ, LAWRENCE BONE, AND GEORGE BABIKIAN

In patients with blunt multiple trauma, a key observation that has been made is the association between late septic death and a state of pulmonary failure that keeps the patient intubated. In these patients, the onset of pulmonary failure and the need for continued ventilatory support is followed by an increase in the magnitude of the septic state, which ultimately leads to the development of nosocomial infections and multiple organ failure. If this septic state cannot be reversed, the patient ultimately dies a late septic death manifested as terminal cardiorespiratory failure. At autopsy, there is generally no evidence of uncontrolled systemic infection or undrained foci of infection, such as an abdominal abscesses, although many patients do have evidence of bronchopneumonia and/ or urinary tract infections. Thus, today patients dying a late septic death do not die with widespread evidence of bacterial infection, as was the case prior to the development of antibiotics.[1,2]

The advent of modern cardiopulmonary support, intravenous hyperalimentation, and antibiotics has clearly increased the time from the original injury to death. Although these advances have probably also saved a number of lives, this is difficult to prove, since patients dying of multiple organ failure are probably the same patients who used to die of under resuscitated shock (much of the clinical septic shock literature reflects this phenomenon). That is, patients who originally would have died of inadequately treated shock or severe protein-calorie malnutrition, now appear to die of the progressive pulmonary failure septic state. Immediately after the introduction of intravenous hyperalimentation, deaths from calorie malnutrition were largely controlled but nutritional deaths still occurred because of inadequate protein intake. This lack of sufficient protein administration resulted in a syndrome of progressive visceral protein malnutrition. This syndrome occurred in the presence of excess glucose calories and was manifested clinically as hepatic failure and histologically as a fatty liver. Recognition of this protein-calorie mismatch led to the development of nutritional regimens in the late 1970s and early 1980s that were based on meeting protein needs (more than 2g protein/kg/day) while avoiding the excess administration of glucose calories. Under this set of circumstances, we produced patients who, in the absence of preceding cardiopulmonary or hepatic disease, survived for very long periods but remained septic and ventilator dependent. These patients were very fragile and any accidental failure to support oxygen transport vigorously could precipitate oliguric renal failure or death. In contrast, patients with preexisting cardiopulmonary or hepatic disease died much earlier and manifested little or no response to therapy, since they could not mount the high cardiac output and increased hepatic metabolic response required to survive the early postinjury phase.[2] Since all these patients began with some severe crisis of oxygen transport, we attributed this downhill clinical course just described to the original injury. However, this appears not to be the case. Instead, as will be described in the remainder of this chapter, the development of multiple systems organ failure and late septic deaths are not necessarily directly related to the original injury but rather appear to be related to our treatment of that injury.

Immediate Operative Fracture Stabilization Improves Outcome: The Clinical Evidence

In 1975, Ruedi and Wolff[3] published the first article showing that immediate operative fracture stabilization improved patient outcome. The key concept of this approach was that by immediately stabilizing the patient's fractures it was possible to place that patient in an upright position. Thereby, this operative approach, by facilitating early extubation and feeding, greatly reduced the incidence of multiple organ failure and late septic deaths. This extraordinarily important paper is largely unknown, since it was rejected by the English language journals and appeared in German.[3] Its importance rests in the authors' conclusion that the course from injury to multiple systems organ failure and septic death is not necessarily a property of the original injury but rather may be related to the treatment of that injury. This report by Ruedi and Wolff was rapidly confirmed by Riska et al.,[4] who found that the incidence of pulmonary failure after blunt trauma could be reduced from 22 to 4.5% by a policy of early (although not immediate) operative fracture stabilization. They called this syndrome of pulmonary failure developing after skeletal trauma, the "fat emboli syndrome." In a subsequent report, Riska and Nyllynen[5] showed that the incidence of pulmonary problems after skeletal trauma could be reduced from 4.5 to 1.5% by using immediate operative fracture stabilization. Wolff et al.,[6] in a continuation of Ruedi's work, reported in 1978 that only 1 of 117 multiple trauma patients treated with immediate operative fracture stabilization died of progressive respiratory failure. These results were very impressive, since the mortality rate for severely injured multiple trauma patients with nonoperatively treated skeletal fractures ranged from 30 to 50%. However, since none of these series used the Injury Severity Score (ISS) to describe their patients, direct comparisons between patients treated with immediate operative versus conventional fracture management could not be made.

Meek et al.,[7,8] using the ISS, documented that the survival of comparably injured multiple trauma patients was improved by a policy of immediate operative fracture stabilization. In this series, the mortality rate of patients treated with conservative fracture management was 29% (14 of 49 patients), whereas the mortality rate of the patients treated by immediate operative fixation was 5% (1 of 21 patients). The mean ISS of both groups of patients was 37. Since an ISS of 37 was associated with a 30% mortality rate in several large clinical series,[9,10] the mortality rate of 30% in Meek et al.'s conservatively managed patients with fractures was exactly what would have been expected. This study by Meek et al., documenting that immediate operative fracture stabilization improves survival, will probably be the best controlled series we will ever have, even though the study was not prospective or randomized. In this study, both groups of surgeons believed their management was correct, the series was consecutive, and the care in the intensive care unit (ICU) was delivered by an independent group.[7,8]

Despite these early reports, the concept of immediate operative fracture stabilization was slow to gain acceptance. For example, Rockwood et al.,[11] showed in 1978 that aggressive conservation fracture management of patients who quickly achieved the sitting position greatly reduced the frequency of arterial hypoxemia. This article was so contrary to the existing literature that it also was rejected for publication and therefore abandoned.[11] However, eventually the tide began to turn. In 1982, Goris et al.,[12] published a retrospective study comparing conservative versus immediate operative fracture stabilization in blunt trauma patients. In this study, they showed that pulmonary complications could be reduced by the use of prophylactic perioperative ventilatory support. Furthermore, those patients with an ISS of 50 or higher treated with immediate operative fracture stabilization were on the ventilator an average of 4 days and had no late deaths from sepsis, whereas patients treated with conservative fracture management were on the ventilator an average of 16 days and 50% of these patients died a late death from sepsis.[12] Johnson et al.[13] verified the findings of Goris et al. In Johnson et al.'s report on patients with ISS higher than 40, the patients treated with conservative fracture management had a fivefold higher incidence of adult respiratory distress syndrome (ARDS) requiring prolonged ventilatory support than patients treated with early operative fracture stabilization (14 versus 75%).[13] Additionally, none of the 33 patients treated with early fracture surgery died a late death from sepsis, in contrast to the conservative fracture group, in which 4 of 19 patients died a late death from sepsis. These investigators also reported a tight association between delayed (more than 24 hours) operative fracture stabilization and the development of major systemic infection.[13] From these studies, it was becoming clear that by immediate operative fracture stabilization it might be possible to reduce the incidence of both ARDS and late deaths from sepsis.

The concept that pulmonary dysfunction in multiple trauma patients (ISS mean of 36 to 37; minimum, 22) was related primarily to conservative fracture management and not the original injury was further supported by the report of Seibel et al.[14] They found that the conservative treatment of femoral fractures was associated with an immediate increase in the alveolar arterial oxygen tension difference and the need for positive end-expiratory pressure (PEEP). The pulmonary dysfunction associated with femoral traction in these patients was severe enough that these patients could not be extubated as long as they remained in traction. In contrast, patients treated with immediate operative fracture stabilization experienced a rapid decline in alveolar arterial oxygen tension differences that allowed early weaning and extubation, so that the patients were extubated on average 3.4 days postinjury. The differences in pulmonary function between these groups were not due to differences in the magnitude of injury, since the two groups of patients were comparable based on 21 different admission and operating room criteria. In fact, the immediate operative group experienced more chest trauma than the conservatively treated group (12 versus 9 patients). These investigators also reported on a third group of patients who had less severe injuries (mean ISS of 29).[14] These patients were treated with femoral traction and did not receive prophylactic postoperative ventilatory support. All of these patients experienced pulmonary dysfunction, manifested as elevated alveolar arterial oxygen tension differences, and had to be reintubated and placed on ventilatory support with PEEP. Again, their elevated alveolar arterial oxygen tension difference and the need for PEEP precluded extubation until the femoral traction was removed and the patients could sit up.

In this study by Seibel et al.[14] there was no correlation between any measurement of the pulmonary failure or septic state and the initial ISS or the fluid volume required for resuscitation during the first 48 hours postinjury. However, every measurement of pulmonary failure-septic state correlated directly and tightly with days of femoral traction. In addition, the number of positive blood cultures and the number of pulmonary emboli increased in direct proportion to the number of days of femoral traction, whereas neither correlated with the magnitude of the original injury as manifested by the patients' ISS. There were no deaths in this series, probably because of the aggressive protein support supplied. However, two patients who developed advanced multiple systems organ failure and had multiple positive blood cultures almost died. Neither patient was severely injured, but both had been treated with prolonged femoral shaft traction. The septic state cleared and blood cultures became sterile in these two patients only when enteral nutrition was resumed.

Although these studies strongly suggested that immediate operative fracture stabilization was beneficial, none of the studies was prospective or randomized. Thus, there was always the possibility that some aspect of the fracture preselected a more septic group. This last caveat was removed by the results of a prospective randomized study of fracture management by Bone et al.[15] This study was made possible by the development of the locked intramedullary nail, which allowed most femoral fractures to be treated with a single type of closed operative reduction. In most of the preceding studies, operative stabilization was based on open reduction of the femoral fracture. Bone et al. found that the ICU stay of patients (mean ISS 32) treated by femoral traction for just 48 hours was 6 days longer than patients treated with immediate operative fracture reduction. Furthermore, the only late death from sepsis occurred in a patient treated with femoral traction. It must be noted that most delayed fracture surgery previously reported was performed from 7 to 10 days postinjury, so 48 hours of nonoperative therapy is a very short period of time. Bone et al. also showed that, even in patients with isolated femoral fractures, arterial hypoxia was more common in patients treated by femoral traction than immediate operative stabilization.

Thus, the conclusion seems inescapable that the pulmonary failure-septic state that follows severe blunt trauma is not primarily due to the original injury but, instead, is a result of treatment that produces the enforced supine position. This concept is most clearly illustrated in patients with femoral fractures. However, other causes of the enforced supine state, such as lines for intravenous support or monitoring, drainage tubes, or the use of mind-obtunding drugs may also result in a similar pattern of respiratory dysfunction. There are now 11 clinical reports documenting this concept.

Pathophysiology of the Pulmonary Failure Septic State

Role of the Gut Mucosal Barrier

Why is it that femoral shaft traction is tightly associated with an increased incidence and magnitude of pulmonary failure that prevents extubation? We believe that a vicious cycle exists. To maintain the endotracheal tube in place, the patients receive a variety of drugs that obtund consciousness. Although these patients appear relatively stable for the first 2 to 4 days postinjury, they soon begin to become progressively more septic and pulmonary function deteriorates. At this time, because they appear septic, they are frequently receiving drugs to alkalinize their stomach as well as broad-spectrum antibiotics. These measures are associated with an increased ileus (really gastrocolonic stasis) that prevents both food ingestion and defecation. These sedatives, alkalinizing agents, and antibiotics also interfere with the normal antibacterial defense systems of the oropharynx, stomach, airways, and colon. The net result of this sequence of therapeutic maneuvers superimposed on the original injury is gut barrier failure, which then leads to a cascade of physiologic events that enhance the pulmonary failure-septic state.

The gut contains sufficient toxins and bacteria to kill the host millions of times over. These toxins and bacteria are kept out of the body by the barrier function of the gut mucosa. Since the gut mucosa has a high metabolic rate, its nutritional needs must be met on a continuous basis for it to function optimally. Additionally, cellular replication of the mucosa is modulated not only by the available supply of nutrients, but also by a variety of food-responsive hormones and other factors. Mucosal trophic factors include epidermal growth factor, gastrin, the neuroendocrine system, cytokines, and probably the intrinsic nervous system of the gut in addition to orally ingested vitamins, such as vitamin A. The intestine receives its nutrients both from the lumen and the systemic circulation. Nutrients derived from the systemic circulation consist primarily of glutamine and ketone bodies, since the intestine, in contrast to most other tissues, does not use glucose as its main source of energy.[16] In the colon, short chain fatty acids produced by bacterial fermentation of nondigestable fibers are an important lumenal nutrient source.[17] However, the production of short chain fatty acids within the colon is dependent on a normal bacterial flora. Since the septic response largely shuts off ketogenesis and the normal flora may be disrupted in these patients, this leaves glutamine as the primary enterocyte fuel. Glutamine is not provided in standard intravenous amino acid mixtures; therefore, under these circumstances, the primary source of glutamine for the enterocyte is muscle catabolism of valine. The potential importance of this metabolic pathway is highlighted by the findings that one of the indicators of an impending death from sepsis is an increasing plasma valine and a decreasing plasma glutamine.[2,18,19] In fact, the infusion of the enzyme glutaminase into healthy animals results in a decrease in plasma glutamine to undetectable levels, widespread gut mucosal lesions, and death.[20]

The septic response, by virtue of its cytokine/catabolic neuroendocrine response, enhances ambulatory muscle protein breakdown while increasing muscle catabolism of the branched chain amino acids. This process generates energetic substate support for the systemic body in the form of glucose, as well as glutamine for the enterocytes, carnitine for fat oxidation and the production of neurotransmitter precursors. The same process concurrently causes release of a balanced mixture of amino acids from muscle that supports systemic protein synthesis. Thus, the septic response through ambulatory muscle breakdown provides temporary nutritional support to the gut mucosa during the period of ileus. The duration of this temporary metabolic support is limited. Even in a well-muscled man with sepsis, this temporary metabolic support of the gut lasts at most 10 to 20 days in the absence of exogenous nutritional support.[2,21] Thus, prolonged inadequate metabolic support of the gut can result in gut mucosal barrier failure.

Gut mucosal barrier function is also supported by a variety of ancillary but very important processes as described by Deitch in Chapter 4. These factors include a normal gut bacterial flora, secretory immunoglobulin A, bile salts, and gastric acidity. The essential point is that maintenance of the gut mucosal barrier and prevention of disruption of the normal gut bacterial flora and intestinal colonization by pathogenic organisms is highly dependent on oral food ingestion and defecation. Therapeutic maneuvers that induce or prolong the enforced supine position impede oral intake by promoting ileus. In this circumstance, the gut mucosa can be supported for a short time by increased muscle catabolism. This period of gut mucosal support can be extended by high protein (more than 2 g protein/kg/day) intravenous nutritional support regimens, but unless enteral feeding is resumed gut barrier function will ultimately fail. Intravenous nutritional support alone is always inadequate, since none of the processes induced by food ingestion will occur. Thus, the ileus resulting from pulmonary failure results in a lack of food ingestion and defecation, which further contributes to failure of the gut mucosal barrier against bacteria and intralumenal toxins.

Role of Cytokines

Penetration of the gut mucosal barrier by bacteria or endotoxin leads to the activation of the submucosal lymphocyte and monocyte-macrophage populations. These activated cells release cytokines that ultimately reach the liver where they prime the hepatic (Kupffer cell) macrophages. The hepatic macrophage population may be primed or activated in other ways as well in the trauma patient. For example, hepatic macrophages may be activated by cytokines released from the spleen into the portal circulation or during the ingestion of bacteria or endotoxin that have escaped from the gut. These primed or activated hepatic macrophages may in turn release cytokines that act in concert with other circulating soluble or cellular factors to impair distant organ function.

In trauma patients the wound is also a source of biologically active factors, since macrophages, lymphocytes, and neutrophils are activated by devitalized tissue. Once activated, these cells generate oxygen-free radicals, release lysosomal enzymes, and initiate activation of multiple humoral cascades, including the complement and coagulation cascades. Additionally, local macrophages produce and release a host of cytokines, some of which, such as prostaglandin E_2 (PGE_2), serve locally to suppress the immune system. This local immune system suppression at the site of tissue injury may be important in preventing the development of an acute systemic autoimmune response. A variety of characteristics of the wound serve largely to confine these locally produced tissue-destructive, immune-suppressive, products to the wound, with the notable exception of the prostanoids and certain of the cytokines. Mechanical defenses that limit the systemic spread of these products include lymphatic thrombosis and the relatively large diffusion distance from the wound to the patent microvasculature, whereas humoral defenses include the acute-phase proteins.

The usual wound with its minimal retained devitalized tissue had some, but little, systemic consequence, since there is minimal activation of local lymphocyte or macrophage populations and little escape of inflammatory cell-generated, tissue-destructive, immune-suppressive products. The PGE_2 that does escape from the wound is cleared by the normal lung so that it has no systemic consequences. In fact, under normal circumstances, PGE_2 is used in a variety of normal metabolic regulatory systems and its level is regulated on a local generation wash-away basis. Since the lung normally clears the rather large amounts of PGE_2 generated during normal metabolism, it is unlikely that the additional amount of PGE_2 generated in most wounds would be of clinical significance. Nonetheless, it is clear that the wound acts as an endocrine organ via its release of cytokines and prostanoids, especially during the period required to clear the wound of devitalized tissue or bacteria. Many of these same macrophage-monocyte factors induce angiogenesis, collagen synthesis, and tissue remodeling and thus are critical for normal wound healing. However, in the presence of massive amounts of devitalized tissue (30% burn, massive hematoma, dead but partially perfused legs), there is little doubt that these potentially deleterious macrophage products escape from the wound in large amounts. This is especially true if the wound becomes infected.

Retained devitalized tissue had been tightly associated with the development of pulmonary damage and ARDS. One possible mechanism by which devitalized tissue may result in pulmonary injury is through the escape of physiologically excessive amounts of macrophage tissue-destructive products. Potential mediators of lung injury under this circumstance include complement split products, oxygen-free radicals, lysosomal enzymes, prostanoids, and activated leukocytes. There is also evidence that the presence of damaged pulmonary tissue may lead to further tissue injury by directly or indirectly promoting the release of cytotoxic agents by resident pulmonary macrophages. Alternatively, failure of the gut mucosal barrier may result in intestinal and hepatic macrophage activation. Spillover of hepatic macrophage products into the bloodstream is not physiologically difficult to visualize, since the hepatic macrophage lives in a system designed to deliver hepatocyte products directly into the bloodstream.

The basic question therefore arises as to how much the wound macrophage system versus how much the gut-hepatic macrophage system contributes to the pulmonary damage and immune suppression observed in the patient with blunt multiple trauma.

Based on the following clinical observations, we believe that the wound is not the primary source of these injurious factors. It is quite clear that both open and closed internal fixation of femur fractures are equally effective in preventing the pulmonary failure-septic state.[14,15] Although both operative procedures may quickly return the patient to a sitting, largely pain-free, condition, only with open reduction is the large devitalized tissue hematoma removed. Thus, immediate closed reduction is effective in preventing or limiting pulmonary failure, even though devitalized tissue persists. Additionally, since the ISS can be viewed as a reflection of the extent of total devitalized tissue and hematoma, one would expect the ISS value to correlate with the magnitude of pulmonary dysfunction. The lack of statistical correlation between the ISS and any measure of the pulmonary failure-septic state in our or other studies strongly suggests that the wound is not a major source of the factors that induce the pulmonary failure-septic state.[3–8,11–15] We must therefore deduce that the factors produced in the wound are not principally responsible for the development of respiratory failure or the septic state in most patients. This is not to say that large amounts of retained devitalized tissue, especially if infected, cannot result in distant organ injury or induce a systemic inflammatory response. Instead, these clinical observations suggest that in most patients, where devitalized tissue has been debrided, the wound is not sufficient by itself to induce distant organ injury.

In contrast to this deduction regarding the wound macrophage, every known observation strongly suggests that activation of the gut-hepatic macrophage system is tightly associated with the development of the immune suppression, pulmonary failure-septic state. This association was first suggested by the study of Seibel et al.,[14] who found that days of femoral traction correlated not only with the magnitude of pulmonary dysfunction, but also the incidence of positive blood cultures and pulmonary emboli. Others also have documented an association between the incidence of major septic episodes and late deaths from sepsis, and conservative fracture management or delayed internal fixation.[12–15] The beneficial effects of increased enteral protein intake have been documented in two prospective, randomized trials of burn patients.[22,23] In these two studies, Alexander et al.,[22] and Antonacci et al.[23] found that mortality and sepsis could be reduced by increasing the amount of enteral protein administered. These studies are consistent with what is known from metabolic studies predicting outcome during sepsis.[2,24]

Clinical Evaluation of Factors Affecting Outcome in Multiple Trauma Patients

Border et al.,[25] studied this topic in some detail in 66 patients with blunt multiple trauma with a mean ISS of 40. They used a septic severity score to construct a single objective number that characterized the magnitude of the septic state for each ICU day during the patients' course. This septic severity score was based on 16 commonly measured variables. The number generated is dimensionless and is based on standard deviations of change from the mean of normal man. Thus, normal man has a septic severity score of zero, and the 62 surviving patients when discharged from the ICU had a mean score of 34, whereas four patients dying of sepsis had scores in excess of 100. In these patients, the alveolar arterial oxygen tension difference and PEEP correlated tightly with the overall septic severity score. Thus, the score appeared to reflect accurately the physiologic state of the patients.

During the initial 2- to 4-day period postinjury, the septic severity score decreased or remained unchanged. Subsequently, the septic severity score increased and reached its maximal value on about the 14th postinjury day. Despite an increasing septic severity score, all blood cultures obtained prior to day 8 were sterile. After day 8, the incidence of positive blood cultures began to increase and there was a direct correlation between the length of time the patient was on the ventilator and the number of positive blood cultures. The average incidence of positive blood cultures in the patients dying of sepsis (2 of 16) was not different from the surviving patients, who were ventilator dependent for a similar length of time. Thus, the patients who died of sepsis were not in any way bacteriologically different from the patients who survived. In fact, the patients who had the most positive blood cultures were on the ventilator the longest and all survived. Antibiotics had no detectable effect on the magnitude of the septic state or on the clearance of bacteria from the blood. On the contrary, there was a direct relationship between the number of antibiotics used and the magnitude of the septic state. That is, the greater the magnitude of the septic state, the greater the number of antibiotics used. A similar relationship was noted between the amount of intravenous amino acids administered and the magnitude of the septic state. Both of these associations appear to reflect the therapeutic response to an increasing septic state, since as the patients become more septic, additional antibiotics were administered in the expectation that these antibiotics would reduce the magnitude of the septic state. This is clearly not the case. Although an increase in the total number of positive cultures was associated with an increase in the magnitude of the septic state, this association was less significant statistically than the previously mentioned associations.[25] The only factor that was consistently associated with a reduction in the magnitude of the septic state and clearance of bacteremia was increased enteral protein administration. This relationship between enteral feeding and the septic state was present no matter how the data were examined.

As previously shown, internal fixation of femoral fractures was associated with clinical improvement. After internal fixation of fractures, the patients were able to sit, their alveolar arterial oxygen differences decreased, the need for PEEP was reduced, extubation was facilitated, enteral food intake increased, the magnitude of the septic state decreased, and the blood cultures became sterile. Furthermore, early operative fracture stabilization, within the first 24 hours postinjury, was associated with a lesser magnitude of the septic state and more rapid recovery than delayed operative fracture stabilization. In patients, whose operative fracture stabilization was delayed for about 10 days, there was still a distinct relationship between fracture stabilization and recovery. A similar relationship was observed between forced enteral feeding and reduction in the magnitude of the septic state, clearance of blood-borne bacteria, and improvement in pulmonary function. This association between increased enteral feeding and clinical improvement was true for both ventilator-dependent and extubated patients.[25] In contrast, the patients with no enteral food intake became progressively more septic despite receiving twice as much total protein intake as the enterally fed patients. Looked at another way, the patients in femoral traction had low enteral protein intake and became progressively more septic despite receiving intravenous protein at levels equal to that administered to the patients whose fractures were operatively stabilized.

Conclusions and Recommendations

What can we conclude from this study? Femoral shaft traction treatment of a fracture is usually only temporary therapy. Therefore delayed internal fixation of a femur fracture is simply one example of incomplete immediate operative care of a surgical problem. When looked at from this viewpoint, it is tempting to speculate that delayed operations of all kinds may predispose to reduce enteral protein intake and an increased septic state. In our experience, the number of delayed operations is the strongest predictor of the total number of days of ICU care that will be necessary. The second strongest predictor is the day enteral protein intake equaled or exceeded 0.3 g/kg/day. A weaker and probably dependent predictor was the total number of positive cultures.[25]

These data show quite clearly that the lack of enteral food intake produced by being on the ventilator has the strongest association with the pulmonary failure-septic state and that the reason for being on the ventilator is the enforced supine position due to conservative fracture management. There are, of course, a variety of other reasons for the enforced supine position in ICU patients that cannot be quantified as sharply as femoral traction. These include the restraining effects of intravenous fluid and monitoring lines and drainage tubes, as well as the presence of a brain injury or the use of mind-obtunding drugs to prevent accidental extubation. Perhaps the greatest reason is custom. It is highly likely that these other factors, by promoting the enforced supine position, have similar effects as femoral traction on pulmonary function and thereby limit the ability of patients to be extubated. Furthermore, the combination of the supine position and the presence of an endotracheal tube predisposes to pneumonia. The endotracheal tube prevents expulsion of mucus while allowing bacteria to reach the normally sterile lower airways. The enforced supine position produces interstitial pulmonary edema, promotes the retention of secretions, and predisposes to atelectasis, thus providing a fertile soil for bacterial growth.

We began this chapter with the statement that the evidence of infection at postmortem did not seem sufficient to have caused the patients' deaths. It appears that we may now extend that observation, since with modern cardiopulmonary and intravenous nutritional support, there is not sufficient bacteriologic evidence of infection prior to death to explain why many of these patients died.

The Dutch group at Groningen and their intellectual heirs have developed the theory that gut pathogenic bacterial overgrowth leading to nosocomial infections of lungs, blood, bladder, and wounds with gut-origin bacteria adversely affects outcome in major trauma patients. For this reason, they attempted to control gut-origin pathogenic bacterial overgrowth while preserving the normal commensal bacteria by a combination of highly specific systemic and nonabsorbable oral antibiotics (selective antibiotic decontamination). Although this systemic and oral antibiotic regimen clearly reduced the incidence of infection, it did not appear to alter the magnitude or duration of the septic state, nor improve survival.[26–30] Thus, we must conclude as originally suggested by Dr. Baue that infections accompany but do not appear to cause the deaths from sepsis observed in patients with multiple organ failure syndrome.

The most logical deduction to be made from these observations is that the pulmonary failure septic state that leads to multiple organ failure and late deaths from sepsis is due to the failure of the gut mucosal barrier. However, it is the endotoxin and not the bacteria, which cross the mucosal barrier, that leads to the septic state and distant organ failure. In this scheme, intestinal and hepatic macrophages are activated by endotoxin that has penetrated the gut and reached the liver. These activated macrophages subsequently release cytokines and tissue destructive products that directly damage the lung. The magnitude of macrophage-mediated pulmonary damage is enhanced by the enforced supine position. With the patient in this position, pulmonary capillary hydrostasis is increased posteriorly, thereby promoting interstitial pulmonary edema and a larger degree of ventilation perfusion mismatch. In the enforced supine position, not only is the dependent portion of the lung underventilated and therefore relatively hypoxic but, since blood flow to this area is also increased, it is perfused with a greater amount of tissue destructive macrophage products. Other factors, such as atelectasis and the preferential delivery of activated leukocyte and platelet emboli, also disproportionately impair the function of the dependent portions of the lung.[31] The summation of all of these factors contribute to the observed failure of pulmonary oxygen transport and pulmonary damage documented in these patients.

The damaged pulmonary tissue and the embolic products of fat, activated aggregates of leukocytes and platelets, plus the debris from blood transfusions all serve to activate resident pulmonary macrophages. These activated resident macrophages release their own tissue-destructive, immuno-suppressive products directly into the arterial bloodstream. Thus, the lung, instead of clearing these products from the systemic circulation as it normally does, now becomes a source of toxic factors, that are liberated directly into the systemic circulation. Once these factors reach the systemic circulation, they can affect other organs, alter metabolism, and impair systemic immunity. Thus, protein catabolism is increased, which further impairs gut barrier function and the patient becomes further predisposed to systemic infections and the development of the septic state.

Summary

In our proposed scheme, the wound, by inducing the gut mucosa to fail as a barrier, promotes the escape of endotoxin and bacteria from the intestinal lumen. The translocated endotoxin and bacteria then activate intestinal and hepatic macrophages, which release products that increase the magnitude of the pulmonary failure-septic state, while at the same time inducing pulmonary macrophages to liberate products into the systemic circulation. The presence of these macrophage products, directly or indirectly, acts to maintain and frequently worsen the pulmonary failure-septic state. The enforced supine position causes pulmonary failure to occur earlier as well as magnifying the pulmonary failure aspect of the septic state. Nosocomial pneumonias occur as a direct result of the combined effects of intubation, oropharyngeal immune suppression with pathogenic bacterial overgrowth, and the anatomic changes in the lungs resulting from the enforced supine position. The development of a nosocomial pneumonia worsens the degree of pulmonary failure, further activates the pulmonary macrophages, and increases the need for ventilatory support. Embolic factors, such as fat, leukocyte aggregates, or microemboli from blood transfusions also contribute to pulmonary macrophage activation, and yet further increase the magnitude of the pulmonary failure-septic state. The use of broad-spectrum systemic antibiotics and gastric alkalinization contributes to this problem by promoting gastric and intestinal overgrowth with antibiotic-resistant pathogenic bacteria. Lastly, the absence of enteral food intake associated with endotracheal intubation contributes to gut mucosal barrier failure by depriving enterocytes of lumenal-based nutritional support and by stimulation of intestinal food-responsive hormones.

The essential point is that most of these effects are direct consequences of the enforced supine position, which is largely related to the therapy we select and not due to the original injury. If we select therapy that allows and follows a policy that dictates getting these patients immediately mobile and fed, then most of these undesirable consequences can be avoided. Such a policy dictates complete operative care of all treatable injuries or conditions the night of admission.

References

1. Baue AE. Multiple, progressive, or sequential systems failure. A syndrome of the 1970's. Arch Surg 1975;110:779–781.
2. Border J. Trauma and sepsis. In Worth MH (ed): Principles and practice of trauma care. Baltimore: William & Wilkins, 1982:330–388.
3. Ruedi T, Wolff G. Vermeidung posttraumatischer Komplikationen durch fruhe definitive Versorgung von Polytraumatisierten mit Frakturen des Bewegungsapparats. Helv Chir Acta 1975; 42:507–512.
4. Risks EB, von Bonsdorff H, Hakkinen S, Jaroma H, Kiviluoto O, Paavilanen T. Prevention of fat embolism by early internal fixation of fractures in patients with multiple trauma. Injury 1976;6:110–116.
5. Riska E, Nyllynen P. Fat embolism in patients with multiple injuries. J Trauma 1982;22:891–895.
6. Wolff G, Dittmann M, Ruedi T, Buchmann B, Allgower M. Koordination von Chirurgie und Intensivmedizin zur Vermeidung der post traumatischen respiratorischen Insuffizienz. Unfallheilkunde 1978;81:425–442.
7. Meek R, Vivoda E, Crichton H. A comparison of mortality in patients with multiple injuries according to method of fracture treatment. J Bone Joint Surg 1981;63(B):456.
8. Meek RN, Vivoda EE, Pirani S. Comparison of mortality of patients with multiple injuries according to type of fracture treatment—a retrospective age- and injury-matched series. Injury 1986;17:2–4.
9. Baker S, O'Neill B, Haddon W. The injury severity score: a method for describing patients with multiple injuries. J Trauma 1974;14:187–196.
10. Semmlow J, Cone R. Utility of the injury severity score. Health Service Res 1976;11:45–52.
11. Rockwood C, Keever J, Heckman J. Early mobilization of the severely injured patient. Unpublished, 1978.
12. Goris RJA, Gimbrere JSF, Van Niekerk JLM, Schoots FJ, Booy LHD. Early osteosynthesis and prophylactic mechanical ventilation in the multitrauma patient. J Trauma 1982;22:895–903.
13. Johnson K, Cadambi A, Seibert G. Incidence of adult respiratory distress syndrome in patients with multiple musculoskeletal injuries: effect of early operative stabilization of fractures. J Trauma 1985;25:375–384.
14. Seibel R, LaDuca J, Hassett JM, Babikian G, Mills B, Border DO, Border JR. Blunt multiple trauma (ISS 36), femur traction, and the pulmonary failure septic state. Ann Surg 1985;202:283–295.
15. Bone L, Johnson K, Weigelt J, Scheinberg R. Early versus delayed stabilization of femoral fracture stabilization: a prospective randomized study. J Bone Joint Surg, 1989;71:336–340.
16. Souba W, Smith R, Wilmore D. Glutamine metabolism by the intestinal tract. JPEN 1985;9:608–618.
17. Rolandelli R, Koruda M, Settle R, Rombeau J. The effect of enteral feedings supplemented with pectin on the healing of colonic anastomoses in the rat. Surgery 1986;99:703–708.
18. Cerra F, Seigel J, Coleman B, Border J, McMenamy R. Septic autocannibolism: a failure of exogenous nutritional support. Ann Surg 1980;192:570–580.
19. Moyer E, Border J, Cerra F, Chenier R, Oswals F, Watson R, Yu L, McMenamy R. Multiple systems organ failure VI: death predictors in the trauma septic state. J Trauma 1981;21:862–869.
20. Baskerville A, Hambleton P, Benbough J. Pathologic features of glutaminase toxicity. Br J Exp Pathol 1980;61:132–139.
21. McMenamy R, Birkhahn R, Oswald G, Reed R, Rumph C, Vaidyanath N, Yu L, Cerra F, Sorknes R, Border J. Multiple systems organ failure I: the basal state. J Trauma 1981;21:99–114.

22. Alexander J, MacMillan BG, Stinnet JD, Ogle G, Bozian R, Fischer JE, Oakes J, Morris M, Krummnel R. Beneficial effects of aggressive protein feeding in severely burned children. Ann Surg 1980;192:505–518.
23. Antonacci A, Cowles S, Reaves L. The role of nutrition in immunologic function. Infect Surg 1984;3:590–597.
24. Pearl R, Clowes G, Hirsch G, Loda M, Grindlinger G, Wolfort S. Prognosis and survival as determined by visceral amino acid clearance in severe trauma. J Trauma 1985;25:777–783.
25. Border J, Hassett J, LaDuca J, Seibel R, Steinberg S, Mills B, Losi P, Border D. The gut origin septic states in blunt multiple trauma (ISS = 40) in the I.C.U. Ann Surg 1987;206:427–448.
26. Stoutenbeck CP, van Saene HKP, Miranda DR. The prevention of superinfection in multiple trauma patients. J Antimicrob Chemother 1984;14:203–211.
27. Stoutenbeck C, van Saene H, Miranda D. The effect of oropharyngeal decontamination using topical nonabsorbable antibiotics on the incidence of nosocomial respiratory tract infections in multiple trauma patients. J Trauma 1987;27:357–364.
28. Kerver AJH, Rommes JH, Mevissen-Verhage HAE. Prevention of colonization and infection in critically ill patients: a prospective randomized study. Crit Care Med 1988;16:1087–1093.
29. Ulrich C, Haririck-de Wurd ME, Barker NC. Low budget selective gut decontamination: a prospective randomized study. International Congress on Intensive Care Medicine. (Abstr.) Maastricht, 1987.
30. van Dalen R, Andis S. Selective decontamination of the gastrointestinal tract: preliminary results of a prospective randomized study. 15th International Congress on Chemotherapy. (Abstr.) Istanbul, 1987.
31. Border J, Bone L, Rodriguez J. The upright chest and the pulmonary failure septic state. In Cerra F (ed): Perspectives in critical care. St. Louis: Quality Medical Publishers (in press).

16

Pros and Cons of Empiric Laparotomy in Multiple Organ Failure

Nicolas V. Christou

The contribution of intra-abdominal sepsis to the development of multiple organ failure is not fully understood. It is well known that persistent intra-abdominal sepsis may lead to multiple organ failure, but the pathophysiologic events in this process are not known. Recent developments in monokine research, such as the creation of multiple organ failure in rats by the administration of tumor necrosis factor (TNF), have allowed the formulation of new hypotheses to be tested in the laboratory and the clinical setting. One such hypothesis states that a triggering of macrophage activation in the peritoneal cavity by any stimulus, including intra-abdominal sepsis, may create a condition whereby excessive production of monokines, such as TNF, by these activated cells may lead to a cascade of events in which further activation of macrophages and polymorphonuclear neutrophils leads to the release of products of oxidative metabolism that create the tissue damage interpreted as multiple organ failure. If this were so, then eradication of the source of the continuous activation of peritoneal macrophages by any means should improve the established multiple organ failure or reduce the chance of developing this disease. Since a great proportion of patients who die from intra-abdominal sepsis do so with, or as consequence of, multiple organ failure, it makes sense to attempt to clean out the infected or contaminated peritoneal cavity. Also, if this hypothesis is correct, then a patient

Table 16-1   Mortality Rates from Peritonitis

Clinical Condition Causing Peritonitis	Mortality Rate (%)
Ruptured appendix[27]	0–10
Perforated peptic ulcer[28]	10–18
Rupture of obstructed viscous[29]	24–35
Bile peritonitis[30]	25–35
Postoperative anastomotic disruption[31]	50–75

with multiple organ failure should have an empiric laparotomy to ensure that the peritoneal cavity does not contain "occult sepsis," which propagates the driving mechanisms of multiple organ failure syndrome. The issues discussed in this chapter are: (1) should a patient with multiple organ failure have an empiric laparotomy to eradicate the presumed intra-abdominal sepsis? and (2) should radical methods such as the "open abdomen" approach be used in patients with peritonitis in order to prevent the persistence of intra-abdominal sepsis and thus reduce or eliminate the development of multiple organ failure.

Mortality of Peritonitis and Occult Intra-Abdominal Sepsis

The mortality of peritonitis varies between 0 and 80% depending on the study and the period that the results were collected (Table 16–1). Even in present-day surgical practice with the availability of broad-spectrum antibiotics, these results have not changed dramatically when conventional surgical therapy is used. This conventional approach to diffuse peritonitis includes the correction of the inciting problem, irrigation of the abdomen with or without antibiotic-containing fluids, and closing the abdomen and observing the patient in the postoperative period. If the patient deteriorates clinically and demonstrates new or persistent signs of sepsis or multiple organ failure, he usually gets reoperated on. This is based on the belief that multiple organ failure is a sign of occult intra-abdominal injection. It is also believed that the primary cause of this increased mortality is the persistence of intra-abdominal infection. Dellinger et al.[1] carried out a multicenter review of 187 patients with a variety of intra-abdominal infections. The overall mortality was 24%. Twenty-seven of the 44 patients who died had persistent abdominal infection.[1] When a patient presents with sepsis and no clear cause, the abdomen can hide a focus of infection and must be considered in the course of the evaluation. There are certain groups of patients who do not exhibit the usual signs and symptoms of intra-abdominal infection and therefore constitute the population at risk for occult abdominal sepsis. These patients, for one reason or another, have an unreliable history or physical examination. If a thorough evaluation of the abdomen reveals a possible source of infection, a measured medical and surgical approach can be undertaken, depending on the etiology. If no source is found, the question of a diagnostic laparotomy arises in certain cases. Without a previous history of abdominal surgery or pathologic condition, and with no other clinical evidence of intra-abdominal infection, a nondirected laparotomy can be safely performed when organ failure is not present but usually will not reveal a treatable lesion. Multiple organ failure may indicate the presence of a hidden abdominal source of infection; however, the window for successful surgical intervention is not always clear. Multiple organ failure does not mandate laparotomy when there is no clinical or radiographic basis for suspecting an abdominal source of infection. This is especially true if an alternative source of sepsis has been defined.

Should a Patient with Multiple Organ Failure Have an Empiric Laparotomy?

Patients with peritonitis by definition have an inflammation of the peritoneal cavity and the surgeon can elicit signs of peritoneal irritation, unless the patient has severe central nervous depression. Thus, the diagnosis of "de novo" secondary peritonitis can be made with some certainty. The microbiology of this form of peritonitis can usually be predicted to contain gram-negative enteric bacteria, gram-positive bacteria, and one or several anaerobes of the bacteroides group. The patient with intra-abdominal infection in the form of one or multiple abscesses is more difficult to diagnose. Intra-abdominal abscess, resulting either from primary intraperitoneal disease or as a complication of surgery, remains a serious problem with high patient mortality if not treated early and adequately. The initial attempt at diagnosis rests on strong clinical evidence supported by nonspecific laboratory findings. The most helpful advance over conventional radiographic studies has been the advent of noninvasive imaging techniques, such as ultrasonography or computed tomography (CT). Radioisotopic scanning with gallium or indium makes possible a generalized survey of the peritoneal cavity, but only after a delay from the time of injection. Ultrasonography is very operator dependent and somewhat limited in utility in the left subphrenic space. CT scanning when available remains the technique with the highest resolution. These noninvasive imaging techniques also have the potential for directed percutaneous catheter drainage. Diagnosis of an intraperitoneal or retroperitoneal abscess can be made in more than 50% of the cases by accurate interpretation of abdominal plain films. If combined with ultrasonography, diagnosis is possible in almost 90% of the cases. CT also may show the exact localization and extension of the lesion and is very useful in planning further treatment.[2] The use of radiolabeled leukocytes for detecting intra-abdominal abscesses is only useful in conjunction with other imaging methods. In every region of the body, a variety of lesions other than foci of bacterial infection can produce a positive uptake of the labeled leukocytes.[3] Thus, most radiologists agree that imaging with labeled leukocytes is valuable for demonstrating sites of infection in conjunction with other diagnostic methods, usually with an accuracy of about 85%. Overall, CT, because it is less operator dependent than ultrasound, probably does provide the most accurate means to detect an intra-abdominal abscess.[4] Three points are clear from the plethora of literature concerning this subject: the need to individualize the clinical and imaging approach to each patient suspected of having an abnormal fluid collection or abscess, the need to individualize the imaging procedure based on what is done best at that institution, and the need for percutaneous aspiration of all fluid collections for diagnosis. No single imaging test is totally sensitive or specific for the detection of an infected fluid collection.

There is a form of "tertiary" peritonitis that is seen in patients with prolonged stays in the surgical intensive care unit following an initial laparotomy for intra-abdominal sepsis. These patients do not form well-localized abscesses and have a higher mortality because of the associated failure in other organ systems.[5] Not only are these patients unable to clear their infections but the microbiology is different from that of secondary peritonitis. In place of the usual *Escherichia coli* and *Bacteroides fragilis*, one finds *Staphylococcus epidermidis*, Candida, and Pseudomonas as the most commonly isolated organisms. The source of these organisms is not clear but may be coming from the gut. Marshall et al.[6] cultured the proximal gastrointestinal tract of such patients and found that the same three organisms found in tertiary peritonitis were found in the stomach and duodenum. Furthermore, there was a high association between multiple organ failure and identification of these organisms. Mortality was enhanced in those patients with systemic invasion by any of these three organisms. These patients usually had high multiple organ failure scores.

These observations may explain the findings that nondirected laparotomy performed for the presence of multiple organ failure is a futile procedure, as exemplified by the data of Bunt[7] who reviewed 2657 primary laparotomies performed over a 50-month period. Of these, 192 patients underwent urgent relaparotomy within 21 days of the original operation for complications of the primary laparotomy. Most had correction of a dehisced abdomen or drainage of a well-defined intra-abdominal abscess with a 12.8% mortality. There were 46 relaparotomies in patients with nonlocalized or systemic infection or multiple organ failure. In these 46 patients, 31 relaparotomies were "directed" either by positive peritoneal signs or CT, ultrasound, or radionuclide imaging examinations. Ninety-four percent (29 of 31) yielded positive findings and mortality was acceptable (about 50%) for this high-risk patient group. Fifteen were nondirected, that is, no examination pointed to an intra-abdominal focus of infection, but the surgery was done in an effort to uncover an occult source of continuing sepsis in patients with multiple organ failure. This yielded only a 13% (2 of 15) positive findings rate, but a 93% (14 of 15) mortality. This retrospective study showed that relaparotomy for sepsis directed by positive radiologic or clinical findings can be reliably expected to demonstrate a surgical focus whose correction may improve patient survival. In contrast, a nondirected relaparotomy seldom demonstrates a focus of infection and does not contribute to survival.

Hinsdale and Jaffe[8] reviewed 87 abdominal reexplorations (1.6% of total laparotomies over a 2-year period between 1981 and 1983) performed on 77 patients for sepsis. Fifty-one patients were reexplored solely on clinical grounds (localized tenderness, fever, and absent bowel sounds), 21 on clinical plus radiographic criteria, four solely on radiographic grounds, and 11 for multiple organ failure. The overall mortality rate was 43%. In the 11 patients explored solely for multiple organ failure, six patients had drainable pus despite no clinical signs and negative radiographic studies. Two of these patients survived. The other five patients had negative laparotomies and all died. The combined mortality of 88% is similar to that of Bunt.[7] The fact that all patients who were explored with negative findings died reiterates the futility of nondirected laparotomies for occult sepsis in multiple organ failure. These investigators believe, however, that the small chance of finding drainable pus in the abdomen in patients with multiple organ failure and the possibility of some survivors justifies the nondirected second-look procedure.

There was no attempt made at stratification of the cases as to severity of illness in either of the previously mentioned studies. This makes interpretation of the outcome data difficult, since there is no reference to the degree of "illness" of each patient. A scoring system such as the Acute Physiologic and Chronic Health Evaluation II (APACHE II) proposed by Knaus et al.[9] is essential in these studies. Knaus et al. have reanalyzed their data using multiple logistic regression where APACHE II was used as one of the independent variables that influence the dependent variable, which is mortality. Multiple logistic regression assigns the relative weights of each independent variable by a statistical technique known as maximum likelihood and expresses the result as a probability. The logistic regression equation takes the form:

$$\text{P}|\text{death}| = 1/\{1 + e^{(3.157 - 0.146^*(\text{APACHE II score}) - 0.603(\text{postemergency} = \text{yes}) - (\text{diagnostic category weight})}\}$$

The diagnostic category weight is the one precipitating the admission to the intensive care unit (ICU) and is chosen from a separate list. It is imperative that any study involving therapeutic interventions in patients with multiple organ failure, such as empiric laparotomy, should use a stratification scheme in order to make the outcome data more meaningful and comparative among various centers. This is imperative, since studies addressing the question of empiric laparotomy in multiple organ failure will require a multicenter approach.

Should Radical Methods Such as the "Open Abdomen" Approach be Used in Patients with Peritonitis to Prevent the Development of Multiple Organ Failure?

In the last 10 to 15 years some alternate, aggressive means have been proposed to treat patients with persistent peritonitis. All these methods aim to reduce the high mortality of this condition by preventing multiple organ failure. They are based on the hypothesis that eradication of the peritoneal infection or the necrotic material therein removes the "activation" signal for peritoneal macrophages and the cascade of events leading to multiple organ failure. There are three methods to consider, radical peritoneal debridement, continuous peritoneal lavage, and the packed open abdomen.

Radical peritoneal debridement was first proposed by Hudspeth.[10] He proposed that all fibrinous exudates and abscess walls be meticulously and completely removed. In his nonrandomized trial, which included a high proportion of patients with perforated appendicitis and gynecologic infections, the mortality was extremely low. Indeed, there were no deaths in 95 cases, no abscess formation, and no wound infections. A well-done randomized study, which followed his report,[11] did not demonstrate any advantage over conventional therapy. Most surgeons find that only very early cases of peritonitis are amenable to adequate debridement and that in advanced cases the resulting hemorrhage is significant. Also, infection that has invaded the peritoneal wall is difficult to debride. This approach does not offer any benefit, and the tedious dissection required to "debride" all of the abdominal cavity may actually do harm.

The second option is continuous postoperative peritoneal lavage (CPPL). In this technique, the problem inciting diffuse peritonitis is corrected at surgery, the abdomen is washed with saline and drains are placed in the paracolic gutters and other accessible areas for infusion of peritoneal dialysis solution with provisions that the solution is drained through strategically placed drains with the aid of gentle suction. The aim is to "wash out," the peritoneal products of sepsis, including the bacteria, and prevent the further development of intra-abdominal collections. The best study using this technique was reported by Stephen and Lowenthal[12] who reviewed their experience with 29 patients. Criteria for using this technique included a blood pressure below 100 mmHg, multiple organ failure with multiple abscesses, fecal peritonitis and anastomotic breakdown causing peritonitis. They used CPPL with dialysis fluid and antibiotics for 72 hours postsurgery. Mortality was reduced to 22 from 48% based on historical controls. Half the studies reported in the literature support this technique, the other half refute it.[13] None are prospective and randomized, and none use any form of illness stratification as discussed earlier. Thus, the efficacy of this approach remains to be proved.

The third technique involves variations of the open abdomen approach to treat peritonitis. The earlier studies just packed the abdomen open with gauze, mousse, or polyurethane. The first such report was by Steinberg[14] in 1979, who left the abdomen open and packed with 4 inch gauze for 72 hours. The abdomen was closed with previously placed wire sutures. Thirteen of 14 patients survived.[14] Some achieved very good results, but in others there was a high rate of intestinal fistula formation, which, coupled with massive fluid imbalances, made matters worse for both the patient and the surgeon. An additional problem of just packing the abdomen open is the requirement for prolonged ventilatory support. This was shown clearly in the study of Duff and Moffat[15] who treated 18 patients with severe peritonitis (eight with necrotizing wound infections) by leaving the peritoneal cavity open following exploration for intra-abdominal infection. No stay sutures were used. Petrolatum-impregnated gauze soaked in antibiotics was used as dressing. Thirteen of the 18 patients had prolonged ventilatory failure requiring intubation for an average of 44 days. The observed mortality rate was 39% compared with the expected 50 to 80% derived from historical controls. Similar methods were used by Maetani and Tobe[16] with 13 patients with an 8% mortality. The curious observation made by these investigators was that four abscesses formed regardless of leaving the abdomen open.[16] Hollender et al.[17] carried out a critical evaluation of 22 cases with serious diffuse purulent or fecal peritonitis treated by open abdomen following surgical intervention. Seven (32%) patients died, three because of continuing sepsis and one because of acute hemorrhagic necrotizing pancreatitis. Three others died of general complications, one due to hepatic coma and two due to massive embolisms; at autopsy their abdominal cavities were entirely free of infection. Mughal et al.[18] used the name "laparostomy" for this treatment. Following laparotomy for severe intra-abdominal sepsis, the abdominal cavity was left open to heal by granulation in 17 patients. In 14 patients, operation was required because of recurrent gastrointestinal perforation or anastomotic dehiscence. In three patients, the indication for this procedure was recurrent pancreatic abscess. Of the 17 patients in this study, 13 had previously undergone multiple operations that had failed to control sepsis. Laparostomy was performed as a primary procedure in only one case, a patient with fulminating pancreatitis requiring pancreatic debridement. The overall mortality was 28%. No patient eviscerated and only 9 (50%) required mechanical ventilation for a median duration of 5 days. The median time for wound healing was 10 weeks and six patients have subsequently undergone definitive surgery with satisfactory results. In contrast, Anderson's data does not support open peritoneal drainage.[19] They treated 20 patients by packing the abdominal cavity with gauze (including the paracolic gutters) and replacing these packs every 48 hours until the patient was well or died. Their mortality was 60% compared with 33% for historical controls. One can see another example of the difficulty of interpretation of such data due to lack of proper study design. There is no objective stratification of patient illness, nor appropriate controls. Witness the variability in mortality of historical controls in these studies. Because of the potential complications of leaving the peritoneal cavity open, various surgeons have used Marlex mesh,[20] or placation of the bowel with rubber tubing[21] and use of gravity drainage by means of a circular bed. Thus, leaving the abdomen open may reduce the mortality rate in patients with severe diffuse peritonitis. By reducing the bacterial contamination and the suspected macrophage activation, it may reduce multiple organ failure. No studies addressing this question have been published. Complications of the open abdomen technique include severe fluid and protein loss through the wound, intestinal fistulas, evisceration, prolonged respiratory insufficiency, and abdominal wall hernias.

More recently, most of these problems have been minimized by the use of a mesh support sutured to the abdominal wall fascia followed by cutting a hole in the mesh and suturing a zipper in it so that the abdominal cavity could be "explored," sometimes up to three times per day, and all intra-abdominal infection dealt with and drained. Hay et al.[20] were the first to use this Marlex mesh technique with repeated exploration of the abdominal cavity at the bedside using analgesia. Mortality was reduced from 66% (historic controls) to 35%. Etappenlavage, which has been in use in Europe since 1979, is a new concept of scheduled multiple laparotomies with abdominal lavage for diffuse peritonitis.[23] The purpose of etappenlavage is to ensure exclusion of the infected source, promote maximal elimination of toxic necrotic material, and allow prompt recognition of complications to effect immediate repair. Patients with diffuse peritonitis at high risk of developing multiple system organ failure (as assessed by high scores in the Peritonitis Index Altona and Acute Physiology and Chronic Health Evaluation classifications) were routinely reexplored on a daily basis until evidence of improvement or healing was noted. From 1980 to 1984, 61 patients with intra-abdominal sepsis were treated. Thirty-four cases were due to spontaneous perforation of an intestinal viscus, and 27 cases were secondary to postoperative infections. In 51 cases, the primary process was present for more than 48 hours. A total of 235 etappenlavages were performed (mean, 3.9 per patient). In ten cases, additional bowel lacerations were noted and repaired at the second laparotomy. In the last 31 patients, closure with a zipper has facilitated reoperation. No drains were used. After definitive closure, primary wound healing was seen in 79% of cases. The overall mortality in this high-risk group was 22.9%. Similar results have been presented by Walsh et al.[24] They used a zipper technique that allowed effective continuing drainage of the septic abdomen, permitted early diagnosis of organ damage, minimized ventilator dependency and gastrointestinal complications, was well tolerated by the patients, and produced a modest 65% survival rate in the first 34 critically ill patients in whom it was used. The investigators caution that this "is a technique that must not be undertaken lightly but that appears to have life-saving potential." The report by Garcia-Sabrido et al.[25] was the first to attempt patient stratification by use of the APACHE II system. This study was based on the concept that by reducing intra-abdominal macrophage activation through the removal of necrotic tissue or septic foci, the continued "activation" of host processes that in turn may lead to multiple organ failure and death can be abrogated. They hypothesized that by providing wide-open drainage of the abdominal cavity and not allowing intra-abdominal collections to form, they should be able to reduce mortality in these patients. Since 1982, they treated 49 patients with necrotic pancreatitis and related infections and 15 patients with severe intra-abdominal sepsis from intestinal perforations. The surgical treatment was based on the provision for daily laparotomies in the intensive care unit with the patient under epidural anesthesia by using an "open-abdomen" technique (zipper alone or a zipper-mesh combination). The APACHE II score was used to derive expected mortalities. The patients with intra-abdominal sepsis had a mean APACHE II score of 25 and an expected mortality of 45% versus the 26.5% mortality that was observed. The lowest mortality in the necrotic pancreatitis group was associated with noninfected pancreatic necrosis (6%) and single abscess (9%) versus 22% mortality rate in the patients with infected pancreatic necrosis. The mean expected mortality in this group was 47% versus the observed 22%. They attributed this result to the daily abdominal explorations that achieved a complete excision of infected or necrotic tissue. Again, most of the studies that report improvements in the mortality of patients with diffuse peritonitis and multiple organ failure use historical controls. None are prospective and randomized and most lack adequate patient stratification.[26]

Summary

The question of empiric laparotomy in multiple organ failure has not been answered in this review. There is no clear answer by reviewing what is written on the subject. My personal interpretation is that the concept of restoring the peritoneal cavity to "normal" as quickly as possible after peritonitis or trauma is valid. This should eliminate the signal or signals that trigger activation of peritoneal host defenses. Such triggering and propagation of events in the presence of an insult that the body can handle without the need for an ICU is probably beneficial. If the system of peritoneal host defense "overshoots," then this can have detrimental effects. Without a surgical ICU (SICU) this is of no consequence as one would die. With the help of the SICU, the body is kept alive for the detrimental effects of this "overactive" host defense system to become evident. The most obvious is the development of multiple organ failure. Some patients in whom this process can be stopped will survive. Techniques such as empiric laparotomy or packed open abdomens present the dilemma that the cure may be worse then the disease. The patient with a packed open abdomen may be no better off then one in whom the abdomen is closed and contains no or minimal bacterial infection. The difficulty arises in matching the patient to the appropriate treatment. Pack open a patient with little intra-abdominal infection and you may continue the "unnatural" state of his abdominal cavity, which may worsen multiple organ failure. On the other hand, leave massive infection in the abdominal cavity and the end result is the same. The question of empiric laparotomy, packed open abdomen, or open abdomen with daily or on demand laparotomies for the reduction or elimination of multiple organ failure and the accompanying high mortality remains to be answered by appropriately designed prospective randomized multicenter trials. We still do not know how to match the patient to the cure, and we do not know how to prevent the peritoneal host defenses from "overshooting."

References

1. Dellinger EP, Wertz MJ, Meakins JL, Solomkin J, Allo M. Surgical stratification for intra-abdominal infection. Arch Surg 1985;120:21–29.
2. Krestin GP, Beyer D, Steinbrich W. Radiologic diagnosis of intra-abdominal abscesses by stepwise use of imaging procedures. Roentgenblatter 1984;37:295–304.
3. McAfee JG, Samin A. In-111 labeled leukocytes: a review of problems in image interpretation. Radiology 1985;155:221–229.
4. Baker ME, Blinder RA, Rice RP. Diagnostic imaging of abdominal fluid collections and abscesses. CRC Crit Rev Diagn Imaging 1986;25:233–278.
5. Rotstein OD, Pruett TL, Simmons RL. Microbiologic features and treatment of persistent peritonitis in patients in the intensive care unit. Can J Surg 1986;29:247–250.
6. Marshall JC, Christou NV, Horn R, Meakins JL: The microbiology of multiple organ failure. The proximal gastrointestinal tract as an occult reservoir of pathogens. Arch Surg 1988;123:309–315.
7. Bunt TJ: Non-directed relaparotomy for intra-abdominal sepsis. A futile procedure. Am Surg 1986;52:294–298.
8. Hinsdale JG, Jaffe BM. Re-operation for intra-abdominal sepsis; indications and results in modern critical care setting. Ann Surg 1984;199:31–36.
9. Knaus WA, Draper EA, Wagner DP, Zimmerman JE. APACHE II: a severity of disease classification system. Crit Care Med 1985;13:818–829.
10. Hudspeth AS. Radical surgical debridement in the treatment of advanced generalized bacterial peritonitis. Arch Surg 1975;110:1233–1236.
11. Polk HC Jr, Fry DE. Radical peritoneal debridement for established peritonitis: the results of a prospective randomized controlled trial. Ann Surg 1980;192:350–355.
12. Stephen M, Lowenthal J. Generalized infective peritonitis. Surg Gynecol Obstet 1978;147:231–234.
13. Kinney EV, Polk HC Jr. Open treatment of peritonitis: an argument against. Adv Surg 1987;21:19–28.

14. Steinberg D. On leaving the peritoneal cavity open in acute generalized peritonitis. Am J Surg. 1979;137:216–220.
15. Duff JH, Moffat J. Abdominal sepsis managed by leaving the wound open. Surgery 1981;90:774–778.
16. Maetani S, Tobe T. Open peritoneal drainage as effective treatment of advanced peritonitis. Surgery 1981;90:804–809.
17. Hollender LF, Bur F, Schwenck D, Pigache P. The "left-open abdomen": technic, indication and results. Chirurg 1983;54:316–319.
18. Mughal MM, Bancewicz J, Irving MH. "Laparostomy": a technique for the management of intractable intra-abdominal sepsis. Br J Surg 1986;73:253–259.
19. Anderson ED, Mandelbaum DM, Ellison EC, et al. Open packing of the peritoneal cavity in generalized bacterial peritonitis. Am J Surg 1983;145:131–135.
20. Wouters DB, Krom RAF, Sloof MJH, et al. The use of Marlex mesh in patients with generalized peritonitis and multiple system organ failure. Surg Gynecol Obstet 1983;156:609–614.
21. Vasquez MT, Speare OR. Gravity drainage in the treatment of patients with near fatal recurrent intra-abdominal sepsis. Milit Med 1981;148:597–599.
22. Hay JM, Duchatelle P, Elman A, et al. The abdomen left open. Chirurgie 1979;105:508–510.
23. Teichmann W, Wittmann DH, Andreone PA. Scheduled reoperations (etappenlavage) for diffuse peritonitis. Arch Surg 1986;121:147–152.
24. Walsh GL, Chiasson P, Hedderich G, Wexler MJ, Meakins JL. The open abdomen. The Marlex mesh zipper technique: a method of managing intraperitoneal infection. Surg Clin North Am 1988;68:25–40.
25. Garcia-Sabrido JL, Tallado JM, Christou NV, Polo JR, Valdecantos E. Treatment of severe intra-abdominal sepsis and/or necrotic foci by an "open-abdomen" approach. Zipper and zipper-mesh techniques. Arch Surg 1988;123:152–156.
26. Maddaus MA, Simmons RL. Leave the abdomen open for peritonitis: yes, no, maybe? Adv Surg 1987;21:1–12.
27. Kazarian KK, Roeder WJ, Mershamer WL. Decreasing mortality and increasing morbidity for acute peritonitis. Am J Surg 1970;119:681–685.
28. Kozoll DD, Meyer KA. Effects of surgery on mortality and morbidity in acute gastrointestinal perforations. Am J Surg 1962;103:577–588.
29. Colletti L, Edmunds R, Togut AJ, et al. Mechanical small bowel obstruction, Am J Surg 1962;104:370–375.
30. Voigt J, Hantschmann N. Bile peritonitis after perforation of the gallbladder. Dtsch Med Wochenschr 1974;99:133–137.
31. Prandi D, Rueff B, Roche-Sicot J et al. Early diffuse septic peritonitis. Ann Chir 1976;29:835–840.

17

Multiple Organ Failure: Summary and Overview

Edwin A. Deitch

As described by Dr Baue in Chapter 1, our recognition of the multiple organ failure syndrome (MOFS) as a distinct clinical entity is a relatively recent event dating from the mid-1970s. Since that time, multiple organ failure (MOF) has emerged as a common final pathway leading to death in a wide variety of patients. Organ failure in this syndrome is unique, since in MOF the organs that fail are not limited to or even necessarily involved in the original injury or infection. Instead, MOFS appears to be a stereotyped response to a major physiologic insult, in which the sequence of organ failure follows a largely predictable course. In the typical patient, pulmonary failure occurs first, followed by hepatic (metabolic), intestinal, and finally renal failure. However, as pointed out by Fry (Chapter 2), individual patients may not follow this classic pattern of MOF. This departure from the typical sequence of organ failure is especially common in persons with preexistent organ disease. Thus, hepatic failure usually occurs earlier in the patient with cirrhosis, whereas renal failure occurs earlier in patients with chronic renal failure. These clinical exceptions illustrate an important biologic principle. That is, although the systemic responses are similar in patients developing MOFS, the sequence of organ failure can be significantly modulated by the patient's physiologic reserve. Common factors influencing the patient's response include age, nutritional status, the presence of preexistent diseases, immunologic reserve, and the exact nature of the physiologic insult that precipitated the sequence of organ failure.

In Chapter 2, Fry reviews the epidemiology, diagnosis, and prognosis of MOF.

285

This chapter presents evidence documenting that in most series there is a tight clinical association between shock, infection, severe tissue injury, or trauma and the development of MOF. Furthermore, in most series, prognosis is related more to the number of organs that have failed than to the underlying process that initiated the MOFS. For example, in Fry's clinical series, as the number of organs that failed increased from one to four, the mortality progressively increased from 30 to 100%. This concept has been recently verified and expanded in a prospective multi-institutional study on the prognosis of acute organ failure.[1] In this study of 5677 medical and surgical intensive care unit (ICU) patients with acute organ failure, a direct relationship was found between the number of organs that failed and mortality. In addition, a direct relationship also was found between the length of time the patient was in organ failure and mortality. Thus, prognosis appears to be related directly to both the number of organs that fail and the length of time the patient is in organ failure.

Despite these prognostic and epidemiologic studies, problems still exist in identifying the high-risk patient and in comparing the results of studies from different institutions. As stated by Baker in Chapter 3, one major clinical challenge has been to identify and stratify accurately patients at increased risk of developing MOF prior to the onset of organ failure. A second challenge has been to develop a system for stratifying the severity of MOF in this heterogeneous group of patients. Until these two challenges are met, it will remain difficult, if not impossible, to evaluate critically the potential efficacy of therapeutic and prophylactic treatment regimens carried out at different institutions, as well as to identify the patient for whom further therapy is not warranted. For these reasons, many investigators are attempting to develop clinically accurate scoring systems that can be used to identify or stratify patients with MOF. Although no scoring system presently exists that is accurate enough to be used for the individual patient, over the next several years it is reasonable to hope that such a system will become available. Thus, the current lack of an objective, reproducible system for identifying and stratifying patients for inclusion in potential clinical trials is a major factor limiting the evaluation of prophylactic and therapeutic regimens in these high-risk patients.

Mechanisms and Pathophysiologic Aspects of Multiple Organ Failure

MOFS has been the focus of extensive clinical and laboratory studies over the past decade. These studies have led to the generation of several distinct hypotheses to explain the mechanisms responsible for the development and perpetuation of acute organ failure. However, the exact mechanisms remain controversial. In evaluating any of these current hypotheses, several clinical facts must be considered. First, in most patients who develop MOFS, the organs that fail are not necessarily directly injured or involved in the primary disease process. Second, there is a lag period of days to weeks between the initial or subsequent physiologic insults and the development of distant organ failure. These two clinical observations strongly indicate that MOFS is a systemic process mediated

Table 17–1   Clinical Paradoxes in MOF

1. Organs that fail frequently are not directly injured in the initial insult
2. There is a lag period of days to weeks between the initial insult and the development of organ clinical failure
3. Not all patients with clinical sepsis with MOF have microbiologic evidence of infection (Septic state)
4. No septic focus can be identified clinically or at autopsy in more than 30% of bacteremic patients dying of clinical sepsis and MOF
5. Identification and treatment of suppurative infections in patients with MOF may not improve survival

by endogenous or exogenous circulating factor or factors, whose effects are not apparent immediately after the initiating event. Since these patients appear to be clinically septic and several groups have documented an association between an untreated septic focus and the development of MOFS, it was proposed in the late 1970s that MOF was the external expression of an occult septic focus.[2,3] Although it is clear that an untreated focus of infection can induce MOF, it is equally clear that not all patients dying with MOFS have untreated infections.[4] This appears true in bacteremic as well as nonbacteremic patients. Furthermore, identification and treatment of an occult septic focus in the patient with established MOF has not been consistently associated with survival.[5,6] These clinical paradoxes are summarized in Table 17–1.

One point deserving special emphasis is the physiologic similarities between systemic infection (sepsis), MOF, and a septic state in which there is no evidence of infection. The concept that patients displaying systemic signs of infection may not have underlying infections has led many investigators and clinicians to adopt the terms "septic state" or "sepsis syndrome" to describe this phenomenon. In fact, all too frequently it is impossible to differentiate clinically the patient with systemic infection from the patient who appears septic (septic state) but does not have evidence of systemic infection. All three states appear to share certain physiologic similarities, such as altered intermediary metabolism, a hyperdynamic state, and signs of systemic inflammation. Thus, it appears likely that the mediators responsible for the external expression and pathogenesis of these three clinical syndromes are similar. For this reason, some investigators have begun to use the term "mediator disease" to describe these syndromes. The concepts underlying the use of the terms "septic state" and "mediator disease" are likely to result in a better understanding of the pathophysiologic factors responsible for the development and perpetuation of MOF.

Although we do not know the exact cause of MOF, certain associations appear to be clear. The development of MOF is most commonly associated with one or more of the following clinical conditions: infection (endotoxemia), trauma with retained necrotic tissue, or shock. All three of these clinical conditions are associated with distant organ injury. It appears that these clinical conditions can initiate distant organ failure in a number of ways. They can impair gut barrier function resulting in systemic endotoxemia or bacteremia (Chapter 4), generate or induce the release of endogenous mediators (Chapter 5), promote reticu-

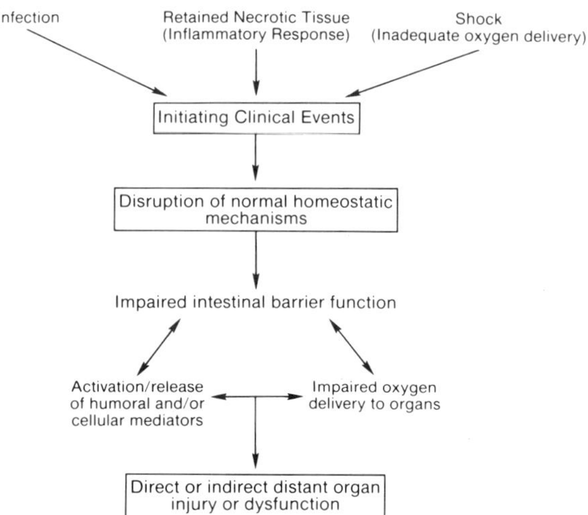

Figure 17–1.   Schematic diagram of potential relationship of various clinic events to the development of distant organ injury.

loendothelial system dysfunction (Chapter 6), or disrupt oxygen delivery to the tissues (Chapter 7). Although my own bias is that gut barrier failure plays a key role in promoting or potentiating the development of MOF, it is likely that these mechanisms interact to produce organ failure. Figure 17–1 schematically outlines a simplified version of how this might occur.

First, there is an initiating clinical event that disrupts multiple normal homeostatic mechanisms. These altered homeostatic mechanisms then interact to amplify or modulate each other. For example, during shock, oxygen delivery to the gut is impaired, resulting in increased intestinal permeability. Increased permeability of the gut subsequently results in luminal bacteria and endotoxin reaching the portal and systemic circulations, where they activate resident macrophages and circulating neutrophils, as well as activate multiple humoral plasma protein cascades. Products of these activated leukocytes and plasma protein cascades in turn may further impair oxygen deliver by their effects on the microcirculation, as well as potentiate the continued translocation of products from the gut by increasing the degree of intestinal permeability. A similar scenario may occur during infectious or inflammatory states where activation of endogenous inflammatory mediators leads to changes in tissue oxygen delivery as well as impairment of intestinal barrier function. Therefore it appears that under the right conditions, the cumulative disruption of multiple interacting systems may ultimately result in distant organ injury.

Currently, it is not known with certainty why some organs fail before others, or whether on a cellular level different organs exhibit different abilities to resist the specific putative mediators of cellular injury, such as oxidants, proteases, or cytokines. A necessary corollary of this multifactorial hypothesis of MOF is that the prevention and treatment of MOF must be multimodal. Therefore, based on our current limited understanding of MOF, it is unlikely that any single

Table 17–2   Prevention of MOF

1. Early definitive treatment of all treatable injuries
2. Mature clinical judgment
3. Rapid cardiovascular resuscitation
4. Maximized oxygen delivery
5. Nutritional support
6. Early diagnosis and treatment of infectious complications

therapeutic maneuver will be fully effective in the prevention or treatment of MOF.

Therapeutic Options

General Concepts

Clearly, the best treatment for MOF and its potential sequelae would be prevention (Table 17–2). As early as 1977, Eiseman et al.[7] stressed that intraoperative and postoperative errors in technique or judgment were contributing factors in more than 50% of patients who develop MOF. Their report highlights the fact that there is no substitute for mature clinical judgment and good operative technique in the prevention of MOF. By debriding necrotic tissue, controlling bacterial contamination, and preventing the development of postoperative seromas and hematoma, not only is the milieu in which bacteria multiply removed, but the delivery of host antibacterial defense factors to sites of injury and infection is improved. Early definitive primary or reoperative surgery leading to the removal of necrotic tissue, the drainage of abscesses, and the control of peritoneal soilage may bolster host defenses by reducing circulating levels of inflammatory mediators as well as by limiting the period of stress. Border, in Chapter 15, expands on this concept and presents evidence that immediate definitive treatment of all injuries, especially long bone fractures, is effective in preventing the development of MOF in the multiple trauma patient.

In addition to good clinical judgment and immediate operative treatment of injuries, other factors may be important in preventing or limiting distant organ failure. These include maximizing oxygen delivery (Chapter 7), aggressive nutritional support (Chapters 8 and 9), and the early diagnosis and treatment of infections (Chapter 10).

In Chapter 7, Harkema and Chaudry present evidence that inadequate oxygen delivery may play a role in the development or perpetuation of organ injury or dysfunction. Under normal circumstances, tissue oxygen consumption is not limited by the rate of oxygen delivery, since if oxygen delivery decreases the amount of oxygen extracted from the delivered blood will increase. Likewise, during periods of hypermetabolism, when tissue oxygen demands increase, the amount of oxygen extracted will increase concomitantly to match the higher

Table 17–3   Daily Nutritional Needs

	Normal	*MOF*
Calories (BMR)*	1700–2000	150–200% of BMR
Protein	1 g/kg	1.5–2.5 g/kg
Non-protein calorie: nitrogen ratio	150:1	125:1 to 100:1

*BMR: basal metabolic rate is based on Harris-Benedict equation.

level of metabolic demand. Thus, under most conditions, oxygen consumption is not supply dependent. In contrast, there is evidence that this physiologic situation changes at some point in patients who develop adult respiratory distress syndrome (ARDS) or MOF. In these patients, oxygen consumption is directly related to oxygen delivery and oxygen consumption is therefore supply dependent. In this situation, the delivery of supranormal amounts of oxygen improves survival.[8,9] Although the exact mechanisms explaining how increasing oxygen delivery improves organ function and survival are not known, it appears prudent to optimize oxygen delivery in all high-risk patients. Methods of improving oxygen delivery will be discussed later in this chapter.

As stressed by many of the authors, adequate nutritional support is critical in these patients. In Chapter 8, Kispert and Caldwell outline the metabolic alterations that occur as patients pass through the different metabolic states leading from uncomplicated trauma through sepsis to MOF. Although they stress that these changes form a continuum, the end result of this process is a hyperglycemic, catabolic, immunocompromised patient with marked muscle wasting and organ failure. In this chapter, they discuss the metabolic pathways involved in substrate utilization and cycling under normal conditions and how these metabolic pathways are altered during periods of stress, sepsis, and organ failure. Knowledge of the differing metabolic responses to stress, trauma, and infection have allowed investigators to develop various nutritional protocols to meet the specific nutritional needs of these hypermetabolic patients.

Bessey, in Chapter 9, described the principles underlying nutritional support. In order to provide optimal nutritional support, it is necessary to calculate the patient's estimated nutritional needs, to document the amount of nutritional support that is being administered, and to verify that the level of calculated nutritional support is meeting the patient's actual requirements. Although controversy still exists over the optimal nutrient mix for the individual patient, it is clear that patients with or at risk of developing MOF require higher levels of energetic substrates (calories) as well as protein (Table 17–3). Although both the amount of calories and protein required to meet the metabolic demands of these patients are increased, relatively more protein than calories are required. Thus, the optimal nonprotein calorie:nitrogen ratio is lower in the critically ill patient (100:1) than in healthy persons (150:1). The route of nutrient delivery also is important, since enteral alimentation appears to be physiologically superior to parenteral alimentation. Although it is frequently impossible to administer all the required nutrients enterally, the gut should be used to deliver at least a portion of the patient's needs whenever possible. On a practical level, this means

Table 17–4   Therapeutic Approach to Infection

Established concepts
  1. Drainage or mechanical control of focus of infection when possible
  2. Antibiotics based initially on Gram-stain results and clinical status of patient
     Antibiotic regimen is modified based on patient's clinical response and results of cultures
  3. General supportive therapy, including intravenous fluids and nutrition
  4. Steroids should not be used
Unestablished adjuvant therapy
  1. Opioid antagonists such as naloxone
  2. Cryoprecipitate (fibronectin)
  3. Monoclonal or polyclonal antibodies directed against endotoxin

that most patients will be receiving nutrients by both enteral and parenteral routes.

Infection appears to be a major predisposing factor in approximately two thirds of the patients who develop ARDS or MOF. In Chapter 10, Dunn outlines the role of infection and the use of antimicrobial agents during MOF. The first step in the patient suspected of being infected is a thorough search for the focus of infection. In many of these patients, surgery or drainage will be required, in addition to antibiotics, to control the infectious process adequately. Examples of patients requiring mechanical treatment of their infections range from the intubated patient with suppurative sinusitis to the patient with a perforated viscus or leaking anastomosis. When a site of infection is found, the initial empiric antibiotic regimen chosen is based on the results of a Gram's stain. In instances in which no infectious focus is identified, empiric antibiotic therapy is based primarily on the patient's clinical status, specific disease processes, and the suspected pathogens. Based on the patient's clinical response and the results of cultures, the empirically chosen antibiotic regimen may be left unchanged or modified. The role of steroids in the treatment of severe infections is no longer controversial. Two recent prospective randomized trials have clearly established that corticosteroid administration during septic shock will not improve survival and in some patient subgroups may even increase mortality.[10,11] In addition to antibiotics, mechanical drainage, and general physiologic support, other treatment modalities are being investigated in the infected patient with MOF (Table 17–4). However, these adjuvant therapies have either not been adequately tested clinically or the results of clinical studies have been controversial (see Chapter 10 for details).

A question that continues to plague clinicians is the role of empiric laparotomy in the patient with MOF, a topic covered in Chapter 16. The concept that MOF is the external expression of an occult septic focus led to a general belief that the presence of MOF in the absence of an identifiable focus of infection is an indication for an empiric laparotomy. However, as more patients with MOF without clinical or radiographic evidence of intra-abdominal sepsis were explored, it became obvious that the vast majority of these patients do not have intra-abdominal infectious processes. Thus, MOF does not mandate laparotomy when there is no clinical or radiographic evidence suggesting intra-abdominal disease. This is especially true when an alternative focus of infection has been identified, such as pneumonia. Thus, my current approach to this difficult clinical problem is to perform serial clinical and radiographic (computed tomography scanning preferred) abdominal examinations in these patients. In the absence of evidence of an intra-abdominal focus of infection, laparotomy is not performed. If a fluid collection is found, needle-directed aspiration under ultrasound guidance is performed when feasible to verify whether or not this fluid collection is an abscess. If needle aspiration documents the presence of an abscess and the abscess can be successfully drained percutaneously, this is performed. If the abscess cannot be adequately drained percutaneously or the fluid collection cannot be sampled for any reason, a laparotomy is performed.

Organ-Specific Therapeutic Options

One of the complexities in treating patients with MOF is that failure or dysfunction of one organ frequently contributes to the failure of other organ systems. Although the pathophysiologic assessment and therapy of specific organ systems are discussed individually in Chapters 11 through 14, in reality none of the organ systems function in isolation. Since injury to one organ may result in injury or dysfunction of other organs, it is critical to support each organ system to prevent dysfunction of that organ system contributing to the failure of other organ systems. In the remaining portion of this section, a distillate of clinical recommendations for the support and therapy for each of the major organ systems will be presented.

Cardiovascular

Less attention has been focused on the heart than other organs, since, generally, cardiac output is increased in sepsis, after major trauma, and in patients with established MOF. The transition from a hyperdynamic to a hypodynamic state in these patients is a late event and occurs preterminally. Only recently has it become well appreciated that the presence of normal or even increased cardiac output does not mean that cardiac function is adequate to deliver sufficient oxygen to meet all the body's metabolic needs. This finding appears to be related to the fact that in patients with MOF oxygen consumption becomes directly related to oxygen delivery. Therefore, maintenance of oxygen delivery at sufficient levels to optimize oxygen consumption at the tissue level is critical.

The three major factors that influence oxygen delivery are cardiac output, arterial oxygen saturation, and the level of hemoglobin (Table 17–5). Therefore each of these variables should be optimized in high-risk patients as well as in patients with established MOF. Table 17–5 outlines specific therapeutic maneuvers that can be used to improve oxygen delivery (see Chapter 11 for details).

In these patients, sufficient fluids should be administered to maintain a clinically optimal preload and hence cardiac output. Only when cardiac output

Table 17–5   Clinical Approach Toward Improving or Maintaining Oxygen Delivery

Oxygen delivery = (cardiac output) (oxygen saturation) (hemoglobin)

Cardiac output
  Fluids to maintain preload
  Inotropic agents; dobutamine or norepinephrine (with or without dopamine) if
  required to maintain cardiac index 4.5 L/min/M^2 or more

Oxygen saturation
  Maintain PaO_2 saturation more than 90% (PaO_2 = 60 torr)
  Supplemental oxygen via mask or ventilator
  CPAP or PEEP to decrease ventilation:perfusion (V:Q) mismatches

Oxygen-carrying capacity
  Maintain hemoglobin at 10 to 12 g/100 ml

cannot be maintained at sufficient levels by fluid therapy are cardiotonic agents required. Initially, dobutamine is used. When dobutamine is not effective norepinephrine may be tried. However, norepinephrine or dobutamine at high doses may impair mesenteric and renal blood flow because of their peripheral vascular effects. Therefore low-dose dopamine should be administered concomitantly with these vasoactive agents to maintain renal and mesenteric perfusion. Arterial hypoxemia should be avoided and arterial oxygen tension (PaO_2) saturation kept at greater than 90% (PaO_2 greater than 60 torr). To accomplish this, supplemental oxygen may be administered by mask in the patient with adequate respiratory dynamics or by mechanical ventilation in the patient with incipient respiratory failure. Since a major cause of hypoxia in patients with MOF and ARDS is increased shunting of blood across the pulmonary circulation due to ventilation and perfusion mismatches, continuous positive airway pressure (CPAP) or positive end-expiratory pressure (PEEP) should be added to recruit collapsed alveoli to increase functional residual capacity of the lungs and reduce the shunt fraction. Additionally, since oxygen-carrying capacity is directly related to the hemoglobin level, the hemoglobin level should be kept greater than 10 to 12 g/dl. It is important to remember that once oxygen consumption becomes supply dependent, a decrease in any one of these three determinants must be compensated for by an increase in the other two factors. For example, a decrease of 30% in the level of hemoglobin below normal requires a compensatory increase of the cardiac output by 30%.

Application of these general approaches toward improving oxygen delivery in the individual patient is based on a thorough study of the patient's cardiovascular state. This topic is covered in detail by Conrad and coauthors in Chapter 11. Lastly, it is important to mention the fact that meeting the body's oxygen needs can be improved by decreasing oxygen demand as well as by increasing oxygen delivery. For example, by decreasing the work of breathing, controlling fever, and preventing overfeeding, one can decrease oxygen demands and thereby improve the relationship between oxygen delivery and oxygen consumption.

Table 17–6 Prophylactic and Therapeutic Options in Patients with or at Risk of Developing ARDS

General	*Organ Directed*
Prophylactic options	
Definitive therapy of injuries	Assisted ventilation with PEEP
Nutritional support	Pulmonary toilet
Optimize oxygen delivery	
Therapeutic options	
Treatment of underlying infections	Ventilatory support
	(Reverse inspiratory to expiratory)
	(Jet ventilation)
Empiric antibiotic therapy	Antibiotics for pneumonia
	Bronchodilators for bronchospasm
	Extracorporeal membrane oxygenation
	Vasoactive mediators (PGE_1)

Pulmonary

Increased microvascular permeability resulting in hypoxia, atelectasis, and increased pulmonary shunting are the basic pathophysiologic changes seen in patients with ARDS. Since the exact mediators responsible for lung injury and the development of ARDS are not known, therapy is directed at preventing or limiting pulmonary injury in the patient at increased risk of developing ARDS. Once ARDS had occurred, therapy is primarily supportive. For example, in the multiple trauma patient, prophylactic therapy includes early definitive therapy of all injuries, including operative stabilization of unstable bony injuries, assisted mechanical ventilation with PEEP prior to respiratory failure, and early optimal nutritional support. As discussed in Chapter 15, early definitive fracture stabilization appears to reduce the incidence of pulmonary failure and ARDS by limiting the changes in microvascular permeability. Mechanical ventilation and PEEP prevent atelectasis and improve oxygenation by limiting ventilation-perfusion mismatches (Table 17–6).

Once signs of ARDS are present, the therapeutic options are limited. These options include continuance of prophylactic maneuvers plus directed therapy to treat underlying pulmonary or nonpulmonary factors (Table 17–5). For example, if the patient cannot be adequately oxygenated or ventilated using standard ventilator settings plus PEEP, the use of high-frequency jet ventilation[12] or reverse inspiratory to expiratory ratio may be helpful. Extracorporeal membrane oxygenation has been used in patients dying of ARDS who are refractory to supportive therapy. Although initial studies suggested that this modality may improve survival,[13] subsequent studies have not verified its clinical utility.[14] Thus, at the present time, extracorporeal membrane oxygenation is not recommended in these patients.

A number of vasoactive agents have been examined for their ability to improve pulmonary function in experimental models of lung injury as well as in patients with ARDS. Currently, the most promising of these agents is prostaglandin E_1

(PGE$_1$), which has been tested in two randomized prospective studies.[15,16] In these studies, pulmonary function of patients receiving PGE$_1$ was superior to those patients receiving placebo. The beneficial effect of PGE$_1$ appears to relate primarily to its ability to vasodilate the vasoconstricted pulmonary circulation and thereby improve arterial oxygenation and cardiac output, the net result of which is improved oxygen delivery. However, a recent multi-institutional study has called into question the clinical efficacy of PGE$_1$ in patients with established ARDS.[17]

The role of empiric antibiotics in these patients is not clear. However, if pneumonia is suspected clinically, it seems prudent to initiate empiric antibiotic therapy early. Of special importance is a thorough search for nonpulmonary foci of infection, such as an intra-abdominal abscess. In the absence of a focus of infection, a trial of empiric antibiotics is clearly warranted if infection is suspected.

Renal

The mortality rate of acute renal failure (ARF) has not changed significantly over the last decade and remains at about 50%. ARF may occur before or after other organs have failed. When ARF occurs prior to the failure of other organs, it is generally a consequence of inadequate volume resuscitation or severe hemorrhage. In contrast, renal failure developing after other organs have failed may be due to ischemia, microemboli, nephrotoxic drugs, such as the aminoglycosides, or be a manifestation of uncontrolled infection or endotoxemia. Although the pathophysiologic pattern of ARF at the cellular level is not known, it is clear that a decrease in effective renal blood flow is a common cause of renal injury. In this circumstance, as renal vascular resistance increases renal blood flow decreases and blood is shunted from the renal cortex to the juxtamedullary and medullary regions in an attempt to maintain an adequate glomerular filtration rate (GFR). However, at some point renal vascular resistance increases to the point that renal perfusion falls below a level sufficient to maintain an adequate GFR. This decrease in GFR is generally manifested as oliguria and an increasing serum creatinine.

Since the kidneys receive 20 to 30% of the cardiac output under normal circumstances, decreasing renal blood flow increases the proportion of the cardiac output available to perfuse more oxygen-dependent organs, such as the heart and brain. Although decreased renal blood flow may be beneficial in the short term, ARF will occur unless effective renal blood flow can be restored. Therefore a major goal of therapy is the prevention of ARF by restoring or maintaining effective renal blood flow. Unfortunately, it is not always possible to prevent ARF. Thus, a second major goal of therapy is to convert oliguric to nonoliguric renal failure, since the mortality rate of oliguric renal failure (50%) is about twice that of nonoliguric or high output renal failure (25%). Table 17–7 outlines various therapeutic options available to prevent ARF as well as the major therapeutic modalities that have been used in an attempt to convert oliguric to nonoliguric renal failure.

Table 17–7   Principles of Prevention and Treatment of Renal Failure

Prevention of renal failure
    Maintenance of effective renal perfusion
        Volume administration
        Cardiovascular support
        Low-dose dopamine
    Maintenance of oxygen delivery
    Avoidance of nephrotoxic injury

Converting oliguric to polyuric renal failure
    Volume administration to pulmonary arterial wedge pressure of 15 to 18
    High-dose mannitol (2.5 g)
    Loop diuretics (furosemide 100–300 mg)
    Low-dose dopamine

Therapy of renal failure
    Dialysis
    Continue nutritional support
    Modification of drug dosing
    Control of sepsis

Avoidance of renal ischemia and maintenance of effective renal perfusion and oxygen delivery are key factors in the prevention of ARF. Therefore therapy is directed toward maintaining an adequate circulating blood volume by ensuring adequate fluid resuscitation and cardiovascular function as well as by avoiding hypoxia (Table 17–7). In some patients, this requires the use of a Swan-Ganz catheter to ensure that cardiovascular hemodynamics are optimal. As mentioned under the section on cardiovascular function, it may be necessary to administer low-dose dopamine to maintain renal perfusion when other vasoactive drugs are used. It is also important to avoid nephrotoxic renal injury by monitoring serum levels of aminoglycosides and ensuring that endogenously produced nephrotoxic substances, such as myoglobin, are effectively cleared. Since the mortality rate of nonoliguric renal failure is about half that of oliguric renal failure, it is important to attempt to convert oliguric to nonoliguric renal failure. Thus, if oliguria develops that is not responsive to volume administration, a trial of furosemide and mannitol is warranted. As mentioned in Chapter 13, in several uncontrolled clinical series,[18,19] the combination of mannitol and furosemide successfully converted oliguric to nonoliguric renal failure in about two thirds of the patients. Although not fully proven, there is also some clinical evidence that low-dose dopamine (2 to 5 μg/kg/min) also may be beneficial in converting oliguric to nonoliguric renal failure.[20]

Once renal failure is established, dialysis may be required to maintain fluid and electrolyte balance as well as to limit the extent of uremia. Nutritional support should not be reduced in these patients, even if daily dialysis therapy is required to maintain homeostasis, since these patients are catabolic and have an increased susceptibility to infectious complications. Since sepsis is commonly associated with the development of renal failure, septic foci should be treated when found.

Table 17–8   Concepts in Therapy Directed at Improving Intestinal and Hepatic Function

1. Maintenance of effective splanchnic and hepatic blood flow
   Optimize oxygen delivery and organ perfusion
2. Treatment of underlying disease processes
   Early definitive surgery
   Debridement of necrotic or injured tissue
   Drainage of abscesses and antibiotic treatment of existing infection
3. Nutritional support
4. Prevention of stress-induced upper gastrointestinal bleeding
   Sucralfate, antacids, H_2 blockers
5. Prevention of nosocomial pneumonias in intubated patients
   Sucralfate superior to antacids or H_2 blockers
6. Maintenance of intestinal barrier function

Gastrointestinal and Liver

The mainstay of treatment is to prevent or correct the physiologic abnormalities that may induce intestinal or hepatic dysfunction. Hemodynamic stabilization is a key factor in preventing injury to these organs. Thus, fluid therapy and, when necessary, pharmacologic manipulation of the cardiac output should be instituted to allow oxygen delivery to reach levels sufficient to meet oxygen requirements (Table 17–8). Since splanchnic or hepatic blood flow may be decreased despite a normal or even hyperdynamic-appearing cardiovascular response, fluid resuscitation should be initiated in all patients at risk of developing MOF, intestinal, or hepatic dysfunction. As mentioned previously in this chapter, underlying disease processes must be treated and adequate nutritional support must be initiated promptly. Once liver dysfunction has occurred or intestinal barrier function has been lost, there are no specific therapeutic agents available that will selectively restore these functions. Thus, prophylaxis is critical to prevent or limit hepatic and intestinal dysfunction or injury, since the transition from clinical hypermetabolism to frank MOF is accompanied by the failure of hepatic metabolic function.

Gastrointestinal bleeding and ileus are well-recognized complications in critically ill patients and traditionally therapeutic goals have centered on prevention of stress-induced bleeding. However, the gastrointestinal tract is now recognized to have important endocrine, immunologic, metabolic, and barrier functions, as well as its traditional role in nutrient absorption. Therefore, gastrointestinal-directed therapy must include more than prophylaxis of stress bleeding and nasogastric decompression during the period of ileus. This concept is supported by the recent finding that despite the ability of antacids or H_2 blockers to reduce the incidence of stress bleeding, these agents have not improved survival.[21,22] In a recent study of 200 patients on ventilators, the mortality rate of those patients treated prophylactically with cimetidine was significantly higher than those not receiving cimetidine.[23] The explanation for why antacids and H_2 blockers are not effective in improving survival in intubated patients appears to be related to the fact that these agents promote the development of nosocomial pneumonias. It has been postulated that by alkalinizing the stomach, these drugs promote bacterial colonization of the stomach and thereby the subsequent development of pneumonia. If this concept is valid, then the use of a prophylactic agent against stress bleeding that preserves the gastric acid barrier against bacterial overgrowth (sucralfate) should be clinically superior to antacid or H_2 blockers. This concept was verified in a prospective randomized trial documenting that sucralfate is as effective as antacids or H_2 blockers in preventing stress-induced bleeding while minimizing the risk of pneumonia.[24]

Although there are potential relationships between loss of intestinal barrier function, bacterial translocation, and endotoxemia in the development of organ dysfunction and MOF, few therapeutic clinical studies have been completed in this area. The studies that have been carried out have been directed at controlling the intestinal microflora and not at improving the intestinal barrier (see Chapter 4 for details). Although the use of orally administered and topically applied nonabsorbable antibiotics to decontaminate the gut selectively reduces the incidence of systemic infections in several groups of patients, its effect on improving survival has been disappointing. What this means clinically is that control of the gut microflora is unlikely to be fully effective in preventing bacteremia or endotoxemia in patients with a damaged intestinal mucosa. Although currently there is no established therapy to maintain or augment barrier function, future options include the development of therapeutic approaches to prevent, limit, or speed the repair of the intestinal mucosal injury that may occur after shock, sepsis, or trauma. Future therapeutic possibilities include the enteral delivery of nutrients, the administration of growth factors, and the use of agents to prevent oxidant-mediated intestinal injury.

Conclusion

The goal of this chapter has been to summarize and put into perspective the material presented in the previous chapters of this book. Although many facets of MOFS remain shrouded in mystery, confusion, or controversy, progress is being made. Testable hypotheses on the cause and pathophysiologic features of organ failure have been generated and a consensus has been reached on multiple aspects of the care of these patients. Since good clinical practice and health care policy follow from good science, the results of future laboratory and clinical studies should improve our ability to treat patients with this complex syndrome.

References

1. Knaus WA, Draper EA, Wagner DP, Zimmerman JE. Prognosis in acute organ-system failure. Ann Surg 1985;202:685–693.
2. Fry DE, Pearlstein L, Fulton RL, et al. Multiple system organ failure: the role of uncontrolled infection. Arch Surg 1980;115:136–140.
3. Baue AE. Multiple, progressive, or sequential systems failure: a syndrome of the 1970s. Arch Surg 1975;110:779–781.

4. Goris RJ, Beokhorst PA, Nuytinck KS, et al. Multiple organ failure: generalized autodestructive inflammation. Arch Surg 1985;120:1109–1115.
5. Norton LW. Does drainage of intra-abdominal pus reverse multiple organ failure? Am J Surg 1985;149:347–351.
6. Bunt TJ. Non-direct relaparotomy for intraabdominal sepsis: a futile procedure. Am Surg 1986;52:294–298.
7. Eiseman B, Beart R, Norton L. Multiple organ failure. Surg Gynecol Obstet 1977;144:323–326.
8. Shoemaker W, Appel P, and Kram, et al. Clinical trial of an algorithm for outcome prediction in acute circulatory failure. Crit Care Med 1982;10:390–395.
9. Shoemaker W. Relation of oxygen transport patterns to pathophysiology and therapy of shock states. Intensive Care Med 1987;13:230–243.
10. Bone RC, Fisher CJ Jr, Clemmer TP, Slotman GJ, Metz CA, Balk RA, the Methylprednisolone Severe Sepsis Study Group. A controlled clinical trial of high-dose methylprednisolone in the treatment of severe sepsis and septic shock. N Engl J Med 1987;317:653–658.
11. The Veterans Administration Systemic Sepsis Cooperative Study Group. Effect of high-dose glucocorticoid therapy on mortality in patients with clinical signs of systemic sepsis. N Engl J Med 1987;317:659–665.
12. Hurst JM, Dehaven CB. Adult respiratory distress syndrome: Improved oxygenation during high-frequency jet ventilation/continuous positive airway pressure. Surgery 1984;96:764–769.
13. Gattinoni L, Pesenti A, Masheroni D, et al. Low-frequency positive-pressure ventilation with extracorporeal CO_2 removal in severe acute respiratory failure. JAMA 1986;256:881–886.
14. Hickling KG. Extracorporeal CO_2 removal in severe adult respiratory distress syndrome. Anaesth Intensive Care 1986;14:46–53.
15. Holcroft JW, Vassar MJ, Weber CJ. Prostaglandin E_1 and survival in patients with adult respiratory distress syndrome. Ann Surg 1986;203:371–378.
16. Shoemaker WC, Appel PL. Effects of prostaglandin E_1 in adult respiratory distress syndrome. Surgery 1986;99:275–280.
17. Bone RC, Slotman G, Maunder A, et al. Randomized double-blind multicenter study of prostaglandin E_1 in patients with the adult respiratory distress syndrome. Chest 1989;96:114–119.
18. Eliahou HE. Mannitol therapy in oliguria of acute onset. Br Med J 1964;1:807.
19. Luke RG, Briggs JD, Allison MEM, et al. Factors determining the response to mannitol in acute renal failure. Am J Med Sci 1970;259:168.
20. Graziani G, Cantaluppi A, et al. Dopamine and furosemide in oliguric renal failure. Nephron 1984;37:39.
21. Groll A, Simon JB, Wigle RD, et al. Cimetidine prophylaxis for gastrointestinal bleeding in an intensive care unit. Gut 1986;27:135–140.
22. Pinilla JC, Oleniuk FH, Reed D, et al. Does antacid prophylaxis prevent upper gastrointestinal bleeding in critically ill patients? Crit Care Med 1985;13:646–650.
23. Craven DE, Kunches LM, Kilinsky V, et al. Risk factors for pneumonia and fatality in patients receiving continuous mechanical ventilation. Am Rev Respir Dis 1986;133:792–796.
24. Tryba M. Risk of acute stress bleeding and nosocomial pneumonia in ventilated intensive care patients: sucralfate versus antacids. Am J Med 1987;83 (Suppl 3B):117–124.

Index